CANCER
Etiology,
Diagnosis,
and Treatment

D1127744

CANCER
Etiology,
Diagnosis,
and Treatment

Walter J. Burdette, A.B., A.M., Ph.D., M.D.

McGraw-Hill
HEALTH PROFESSIONS DIVISION

New York   St. Louis   San Francisco   Auckland
Bogotá   Caracas   Lisbon   London   Madrid
Mexico City   Milan   Montreal   New Delhi   San Juan
Singapore   Sydney   Tokyo   Toronto

McGraw-Hill

A Division of The McGraw·Hill Companies

CANCER: Etiology, Diagnosis, and Treatment

Copyright © 1998 by The McGraw-Hill Companies, Inc. All rights reserved. Printed in the United States of America. Except as permitted under the United States Copyright Act of 1976, no part of this publication may be reproduced or distributed in any form or by any means, or stored in a data base or retrieval system, without the prior written permission of the publisher.

1 2 3 4 5 6 7 8 9 0 DOCDOC 9 8 7

ISBN 0-07-008992-2

This book was set in Times Roman by The PRD Group.
The editors were James Morgan and Peter McCurdy;
the production supervisor was Richard Ruzycka;
the cover designer was Robert Freese.
The index was prepared by B. Littlewood.
R.R. Donnelley & Sons was printer and binder.

This book is printed on acid-free paper.

Library of Congress Cataloging-in-Publication Data

Burdette, Walter J.
    Cancer: etiology, treatment, and diagnosis/Walter J. Burdette.
      p. cm.
    Includes index.
    ISBN 0-07-008992-2
    1. Cancer. I. title.
    [DNLM: 1. Neoplasms. QZ 200 B951c 1998]
    RC261.B88 1998
    616.99′4—dc21
    DNLM/DLC
    for Library of Congress   97-25674
                               CIP

CONTENTS

PREFACE

The management of cases of cancer usually requires the expert application of more medical disciplines than is the case for any other disease. The gravity of the diagnosis is grasped immediately by all involved, and the urgency of obtaining solutions needs no additional emphasis. Because of the complexity implied, this volume has been written to provide a comprehensive but succinct account of the professional resources available and, when possible, how they may be combined appropriately. It is hoped that it will be useful for those who share the responsibilities of diagnosis and treatment and their patients. Gratitude is expressed to all who helped with the preparation of the manuscript and illustrations, especially Dr. Susan Burdette Radoux. Others are Drs. Samuel Bean, Dennis Beck, Byron Bohnn, Arthur Faris, Nelson Fernandez, Barbara Gibbs, Alfred Hernandez, John Jones, Howard Moench, John Pagani, Marvin Romsdahl, and the editor, James Morgan.

INTRODUCTION

There is no specialty in medicine in which doctors are trained to give all the types of treatment required and available for the care of most cases of cancer. The specialties most likely to be involved are surgical oncology (general surgery and the applicable surgical specialties), medical oncology (chemotherapy), and radiation oncology (radiotherapy). With the recent advent of more treatment given as outpatient therapy, family practice physicians have taken a larger role in treatment. It is most important to have the management given by physicians in each specialty correlated with that given by the other participants. In order to review all possible treatments, many hospitals and clinics have tumor seminars, boards, or clinics affording the opportunity to review all the information about a given case by a group of practitioners experienced in the management of neoplastic diseases with the objective of selecting the best plan of treatment for the case reviewed. These panels are frequently available to all doctors and their patients in a community. Care by more than one doctor is most easily obtained in a hospital, but outpatient therapy is often possible and more desirable if the patient's condition permits and the treatment can be given in that fashion. Irradiation usually entails fractionation of the dosage in multiple treatments and often is given as an outpatient procedure. The same is true for multiple courses of oral and/or intravenous chemotherapy after the treatment has been initiated. Some biopsies and minor surgical excisions also can be done as outpatient procedures. Those most responsible and affected by medical decisions are the physician(s), the patient, and the patient's immediate family. This should be kept in mind when evaluating suggestions by others about management.

TREATMENT TRIAD

Surgical procedures available vary widely from biopsies and vascular access for hydration and chemotherapy to complicated procedures such as hepatic lobectomy and transplantation. They differ depending on the type of cancer being treated and are discussed most profitably in that context. Not only has the use of an increasing variety of drugs advanced the treatment and improved palliation and provided some cures, but also hormonal therapy and biological agents such as interferons, interleukins, and monoclonal antibodies have been used increasingly, alone or in combination with other therapy. Also, it is now possible to transport tumor supressor genes utilizing viral and other vectors to transfect human tumors, making gene therapy for cancer more than a remote possibility. Again, discussion of this medical therapy is most profitable in the section devoted to a specific type of cancer. However, an initial general discussion of methods and the physical basis for radiotherapy is appropriate.

Radiotherapy may be used alone to treat neoplastic disease or as a supplement to operation or chemotherapy or both. Although the machines used to generate irradiation are imposing, fortunately the treatments are not at all painful. Several types of irradiation constitute the armamentarium of the radiotherapist. The source may be a radioactive element such as radium or cobalt or an apparatus such as an x-ray machine. Irradiation is a very powerful and effective therapeutic tool; the beam is capable of killing cells that are malignant. Unfortunately, it will damage normal cells as well, and the radiation oncologist must administer the therapy in such a manner that a maximum effect on the malignant cells will be obtained with minimal damage to normal cells, permitting their recovery. At his command is a panoply of types of irradiation and methods for administering each. From a practical standpoint he must determine the position and size of the neoplasm and direct the beam of irradiation to that location with as little inclusion of normal tissue surrounding the tumor as possible. Of course the field of irradiation must be sufficiently large to include the peripheral extent of the neoplasm as well. The dosage of irradiation will depend on the intensity of irradiation, the distance of the tumor from the origin of the beam, and the number of ports used for cross-firing the target. By cross-firing through multiple ports on the surface, the dosage of irradiation at the tumor target is additive, whereas the dosage on the skin and deeper normal tissues is not. Obviously, it is important to maintain exactly the same pattern of ports if multiple treatments over a period of days are indicated, which usually is the case. The ports are outlined on the skin with an indelible marker, and it is imperative for the patient to retain them until the course of therapy is completed. Also, rigid restraints may be used occasionally to maintain the same position of the target each time it is irradiated. Depending on the circumstance and the type of treatment, irradiation may be associated with side effects locally and systemically. These occur at variable times after the initiation of therapy and may continue for several weeks afterward. Medication may alleviate the symptoms. Except in the case of lymphomas and leukemias, irradiation is directed toward a localized neoplastic target, the location of which is known with precision. The results of treatment extend over a longer period than the course of therapy, and the final result cannot be determined immediately at the conclusion of treatment.

Irradiation therapy may be administered with the source near the targeted tumor (brachytherapy) or at a distance (teletherapy). The former is more likely to originate from a radioisotope or a superficial x-ray therapy machine or an arrangement permitting intraoperative therapy. The use of radioisotopes in the treatment of cancer began shortly after the discovery of radium-226 by Pierre and Marie Curie in 1898. Many other useful isotopes have been used for treating neoplasms since that time, but their use has declined with the development of other means for producing irradiation. Some sources such as radium are shielded inside metal containers or needles and are implanted temporarily at a suitable location. All sources are constantly decaying, the rate of decay expressed as the *half-life*. The half-life of radium 226 is 1600 years; that of radon 222, the heaviest of the noble gases, is 3.82 days. Therefore, the latter contained in tiny seeds can be left in place in the tissue permanently. Radon is an emanation from radium and was used more frequently in the past than at the present time. Examples of radioisotopes that are available for therapeutic use are cesium 137, cobalt 60, gold 198, iodine 125, iodine 131, iridium 192, phosphorus 32, radium 226, and radon 222. Individual isotopes have characteristic energy and decay products. When properly shielded, cobalt 60 can be used effectively for teletherapy.

Machines that produce radiation are devices that increase the energy of nuclear particles, such as electrons. By using a gradient of voltage to direct electrons at an anode, an x-ray machine is set up to utilize the electromagnetic wave of energy (x-rays) that results from the collisions. This beam of energy is then used for superficial therapy in the range of 60 to 140 kilovolts and for teletherapy in the case of orthovoltage machines in the range of 250 to 500 kilovolts. Betatrons and linear accelerators are machines utilizing higher voltages, ranging up to 18 Mev. Cyclotrons are used only in a research setting.

The dosage of irradiation is measured in small chambers as the number of ion pairs produced in the field of irradiation measured by the current between the plates of the chamber. The unit of radiation exposure is the *roentgen* and is denoted by the symbol R. It is defined as the exposure dose of X or gamma irradiation liberating electrons and positrons producing ions carrying positive and negative charges of 2.58×10^{-4} coulombs* per kilogram of air. More important to the radiotherapist is the amount of energy absorbed by the tissues. This unit is the *Gray* and is the equivalent of 100 rads[†]; the centiGray (cGy) is the equivalent of 1 rad. X-ray machines are calibrated

---

*A coulomb is the amount of electricity conveyed in one second by the current produced by an electromotive force of one volt acting in a circuit having a resistance of one ohm.

†A rad is the unit of absorbed dose equal to 100 ergs per gram.

periodically, but supervoltage machines may be calibrated throughout each treatment using more complex dosimeters than the simple ionization chamber for measurement of dosage in air. When a patient with cancer undergoes irradiation therapy, the dosage may be expressed in centiGrays. Also the number, size, and position of ports, the length of each treatment, the number

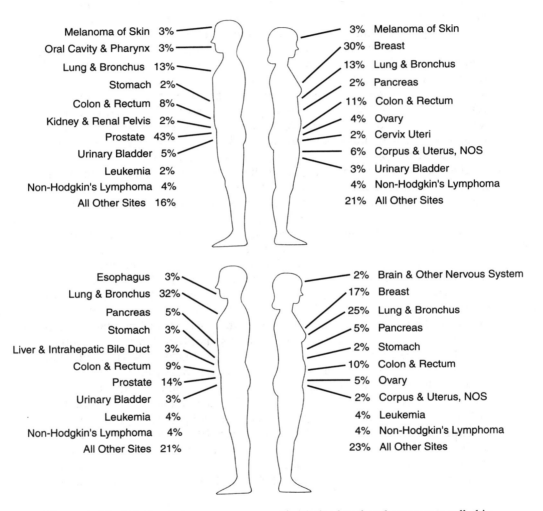

Figure 1 (*Top*) Estimated new cancer cases (excludes basal and squamous cell skin cancer and carcinoma in situ except bladder). The ten leading sites by sex, United States, 1997. (*Bottom*) Estimated cancer deaths (excludes basal and squamous cell skin cancer and carcinoma in situ except bladder). The ten leading sites by sex, United States, 1997. (Used with permission of *Ca—A Cancer Journal for Clinicians*.)

of treatments, and the expected tumor dose at the end of treatment must be included in the description of the treatment.

It is necessary not only to treat through identical ports from one treatment period to the next, but it is also necessary to maintain the position of the patient or the part of the body being treated in relation to the table or chair holding the patient and the source of irradiation. In order to insure that the location of the patient and ports is maintained throughout the course of treatment, an extremity may be held in place with appropriate restraints applied each time or a mold or cast of a portion or the entire body may be made and utilized each time one of a series of treatments is given. The advent of computed tomography and nuclear magnetic resonance imaging has increased the accuracy of treatment with irradiation by defining the image of neoplasm and surrounding tissues in great detail as well as making available the inhomogeneity of tissues at the target. Laser beams properly aligned with the treatment machine and table are used for appropriate alignment of the subject to be irradiated. The comfort of the patient is always kept in mind in the use of any means to maintain his position in relation to the external beam of irradiation. Diagnostic x-ray studies of the area of each port and an additional study of this area plus the surrounding area of the body for orientation may be taken before treatment starts and during the course of treatment as well. The contour of the port desired may be irregular and may not conform to the limits of the beam of irradiation to be used. In that case, shielding may be devised of appropriate shape to exclude the undesirable portion.

For brachytherapy, tubes containing radioactive isotopes such as cesium 137, cobalt 60, and radium 226 may be used. Isotopes may be used as needles, seeds, fluids, or intracavitary implants. The apparatus to contain the isotope may be placed at the appropriate site, its position checked radiologically, and the isotope loaded after the patient returns to his room. The apparatus is designed at times to displace adjacent structures susceptible to irradiation but not involved with the neoplastic growth. The isotope is then removed when the desired length of time to give the dosage required has elapsed, except in the case of seeds containing an isotope with short half-life.

UNIFORM CLASSIFICATION AND STAGING OF CANCER

Any neoplasm has a natural history of growth and spread. In order to label each stage in the course of the disease, agreement has been reached internationally by the medical profession to use the TNM scheme of staging, in order to have a classification of the characteristics of cancer under different environmental and genetic conditions. This allows assessment of the results of treatment objectively. Originally the idea of staging arose from the observation that cancer diagnosed and treated in the early stage when it is localized is associated with higher rates of survival than when first detected later when the malignancy has spread beyond the site of origin. Progression usually consists of growth locally, spread to regional lymph nodes, and metastatic foci consisting of malignant cells carried through the lymphatic and circulatory systems beyond the site of origin. This progression must be determined by objective clinical and laboratory findings. The TNM system is a simple system of classifying the extent of the disease. T catalogs the size of the primary neoplasm, N records the absence or presence and extent of malignant cells in the regional lymph nodes, and M the absence or presence of distant metastases in the following general classification.

Primary Tumor (T)

TX	Cannot be assessed
T0	No evidence of primary tumor
Tis	Cancer in situ
T1 etc.	Size and extension

Regional Lymph Nodes (N)

NX	Cannot be assessed
N0	No nodal metastases
N1 etc.	Evidence of nodal metastases

Distant Metastases

MX	Cannot be assessed
M0	No distant metastases
M1	Distant metastases

The general heading of stages of cancer are:

Stage 0	Carcinoma in situ
Stage I	Localized cancer
Stage II	Limited local extension and/or limited spread to regional lymph nodes
Stage III	More extensive spread locally or to regional lymph nodes
Stage IV	Spread to distant sites

Clinical classification (cTcNcM) is that resulting from all studies, physical examination, biopsies, etc., prior to the first definitive treatment of the disease. Pathologic classification (pTpNpM) is based on examination of the tumor tissue removed. Microscopic examination of metastatic lesions results in classification of metastatic disease (pM). Retreatment classification (rTNM) ensues when additional treatment is planned after recurrence following an interval without symptoms or signs of the disease. For each anatomic site of origin, T, N, and M headings are grouped into stages, depending on the advancement of the neoplasm at the time of classification. The details of staging each specific type of cancer are indicated initially when the management is delineated.

Although it may seem at first to be rather an academic exercise without practical purpose, TNM classification and staging has proved to be very valuable for comparing the results of different treatments, as an indication of the likely future course of the disease, for planning treatment, and for evaluating the results of medical management. In addition, standardized performance scales which have been adopted for objective comparison of the physical condition and exercise tolerance of patients also have been found useful. An outline of the performance scales of Karnofsky and the Eastern Cooperative Oncology Group appears below.

Karnofsky Performance Scale

No Care Needed
100%:	No symptoms of disease; active
90%:	Minor signs of disease; active
80%:	Minor signs of disease; active with effort

Cannot Work; Able to Live at Home
70%:	Can care for self
60%:	Needs assistance at times
50%:	Much assistance & frequent medical care required

Requires Institutional Care or Equivalent
40%:	Disabled
30%:	Severely disabled
20%:	Hospital care required
10%:	Moribund

Eastern Cooperative Oncology Groups Performance Scale

Grade 0:	Active
Grade 1:	Strenuous activity restricted
Grade 2:	Cannot work
Grade 3:	Requires assistance for a portion of care
Grade 4:	Disabled; confined to chair or bed

CLINICAL TRIALS

After preliminary laboratory and clinical studies have been completed a new method of treatment may seem promising. In order to determine whether the new treatment is truly effective, a clinical trial may be instituted to compare it to current methods of management. This requires a protocol demanding certain characteristics of the patients to be tested and the various modes of treatment to be studied. Often, groups of patients are entered in such studies from widely scattered locations geographically. A physician taking care of an individual may inquire whether the patient wishes to be enrolled and will agree to continue with the trial plan of treatment for its expected duration. The new treatment may be given to some patients and others are used as a control, with only supportive treatment or with treatment known to be effective. In any event, the patient should understand exactly how the trial is to be conducted. All clinical trials are evaluated by an ethics committee to be certain that patients are properly informed about the potential risks and benefits involved in participation in the trial. In a double blind study neither the doctor nor the patient may know whether they are a part of the control group given a placebo or the group being given the new treatment until after the trial is concluded. By discussing the proposed trial with the treating physician, the patient can make an informed decision as to whether to enter the study and accept the regimen prescribed. Many advances in the treatment of cancer have evolved from clinical trials, and they are likely to continue to be a feature of the decisions confronting the patient with neoplastic disease. Participation may not only benefit the patient entering the trial but also the many patients having the same type of malignancy, if the trial confirms the management as a successful improvement. Results are stated in terms of survival advantage, palliation, length of symptom-free period, and complications.

At the present time, the governmental examination of new therapeutic substances for use in cancer therapy has required much less time before release for clinical use than formerly. Examples are Camptosar (irinotecan) for possible use in cases of metastatic colorectal carcinoma salvage, Doxil (liposomal doxorubicin) for refractory Kaposi's sarcoma, Gemzar (gemcitabine) for pancreatic carcinoma, Hycamptin (topotecan) for metastatic ovarian cancer, Navelbine (vinorelbine) for non-small cell carcinoma of the lung, and Taxotere (docetaxel) for metastatic carcinoma of the breast. As usual, the final judgment about usefulness will require additional experience. Unfortunately, the cost of many of the new compounds continues to be exceedingly high.

CANCER
Etiology,
Diagnosis,
and Treatment

ONE

NEOPLASMS OF THE SKIN

With as many as one million cases reported annually, cancer of the skin is the type of neoplasm found most frequently by far in the United States. The three predominant types, squamous cell and basal cell carcinomas and malignant melanomas, arise from epidermal keratinocytes, basal cells, and melanocytes, respectively. (The origin of basal cell cancer remains somewhat controversial. Possibly, it may arise from a pluripotential cell in the pilosebaceous epithelium.) Although mortality from malignant melanomas is much higher than that from other skin cancers, malignant melanomas occur less often, with an incidence of not more than 40,000 cases a year. Malignant melanomas are discussed in a separate chapter.

The finding of scrotal skin cancer in chimney sweeps was reported by Percivall Pott in 1775. Since that time, evidence has accumulated demonstrating that skin carcinoma can arise from exposure to ionizing radiation, chronic ulceration and infection, exposure of mucous membranes of the mouth to tobacco, papilloma viral infection, prolonged exposure to arsenic, xeroderma pigmentosum, the presence of immunosuppression from any cause including transplantation, and the presence of the autosomal dominant causing nevoid basal cell carcinoma (Gorlin's syndrome). The predominant cause of these cancers is exposure to ultraviolet B radiation ranging from 190 to 350 nm. This has been attributed to mutation at up to nine foci within the *p53* tumor suppressor gene resulting in mutations with reversal of cancer suppression. The damage occurs in the region of DNA where pyrimidine bases are juxtaposed, and susceptibility to cancer is promoted by the vitiation of the *p53*

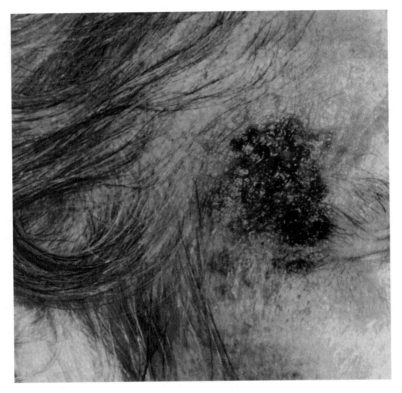

Figure 2 Mixed squamous and basal cell carcinoma of the face.

influence to prolong repair and to promote excision of damaged genes and apoptosis of affected cells. The hereditary Gorlin's syndrome resulting in multiple basal cell carcinomas is the result of mutation occurring at a site other than that for the *p53* tumor suppressor gene. Among other hereditary syndromes with cutaneous manifestations are those of Gardner, Ferguson-Smith, Torre, Peutz-Jeghers, and Carne. Sarcomas occurring in the skin include fibrous histiocytomas, dermatofibrosarcomas, and fibroxanthomas.

BASAL CELL CARCINOMAS

Basal cell carcinoma is the most common carcinoma of the skin. It occurs most frequently in whites and rarely in those with pigmented skin. These neoplasms spread insidiously, do not respond to 5-fluorouracil very well, and have a tendency to spread along tissue planes. They appear chiefly on the head and neck and can be very difficult to treat with desired cosmetic results

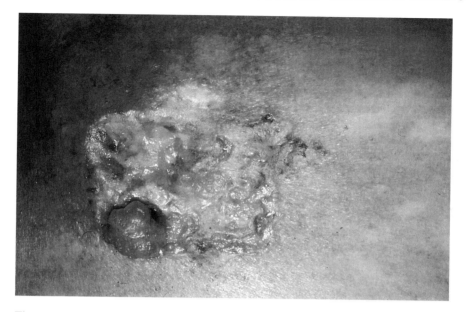

Figure 3 Basal cell carcinoma of the skin following irradiation.

when they are located on the alar groove and tip of the nose, cartilage of the ears, and inner canthus of the eye. They rarely metastasize to regional nodes, with only a few hundred cases reported in the global literature. They have a tendency to recur and should be treated aggressively, with careful microscopic study of the margins resected. Dermal fibrosis always accompanies the basal cells and possibly may be the reason for infrequent metastatic behavior. The three types of basal cell carcinomas in descending order of frequency are nodular, superficial, and sclerosing. Superficial basal cell carcinomas can spread very widely and are usually treated by cryosurgery or other means to remove the superficial neoplastic cells with a wide margin. Recurrences must be managed with frozen section control either surgically or with the Mohs' technique. They occur more frequently on the trunk and extremities than the head and neck where other types of basal cell cancers are more likely to be found. Nodular basal cell cancer expands radially from the original site without commensurate increase in thickness. The usual method of management is resection for the larger lesions; very small lesions can be treated successfully with electro- and cryosurgery. Neoplasms located on the nose, ears, and infra-orbital area are more prone to recur and must be followed carefully. Sclerosing basal cell carcinomas and basosquamous neoplasms are the most aggressive of the basal cell tumors with characteristic infiltration and a tendency to recur. They must be removed surgically with adequate margins relying on the evidence from frozen sections at the time of operation.

KERATOSES AND SQUAMOUS CELL CARCINOMAS

Solar (actinic) keratoses are superficial anaplastic benign precursors of squamous carcinomas. They appear wherever the skin is exposed to the sun. They usually respond to topical 5-fluorouracil. If not, cryosurgery or curettage can be effective for management. Keratoacanthomas are interesting tumors that may grow at an alarming rate, but they usually regress spontaneously within 12 months. Plastic repair or irradiation is used in some cases because scarring may result after spontaneous remission of large tumors. Carcinoma in situ in skin exposed to the sun and Bowen's disease in skin with no history or minimal exposure respond to electrodissection, cryosurgery, curettage, and topical 5-fluorouracil. Larger tumors, recurrences, and primary squamous cell carcinomas require resection with frozen sections to establish margins free of cancer cells. Carcinomas of the lip should be excised widely; they metastasize to regional nodes which then must be resected. These neoplasms occur more frequently on the lower lip and often require plastic restoration.

METASTATIC CANCER OF THE SKIN

Up to 10 percent of malignant tumors metastasize to the skin. Cutaneous metastases seen most frequently are those from cancer of the breast in females and cancer of the lung in males. Other cancers that spread to the skin are gastrointestinal and renal in origin along with hypernephromas, T-cell lymphomas and leukemias, acute myelogenous leukemias, ovarian neoplasms, melanomas, and Kaposi's sarcoma (in patients with AIDS). Those cancers spreading by hematogenous routes tend to be found in the skin. Occasionally cutaneous metastases are identified before the primary site is discovered.

The diagnosis of both primary and metastatic carcinoma of the skin must be established by biopsy and microscopic study of the specimen. These neoplasms should be excised completely with margins checked by microscopic study of frozen sections when indicated. This is especially important in the case of basal cell carcinomas, which may be resistant to treatment with 5-fluorouracil and must be excised with sufficiently wide margins to reduce the likelihood of any malignant cells remaining. Also they should be followed carefully for recurrence. When dermal metastases are the first manifestation of primary tumors elsewhere, a search for the primary neoplasm should be initiated immediately in each case.

CHAPTER TWO

MELANOMA

Melanomas are usually pigmented neoplasms that appear chiefly in the skin with peak incidence from ages 20 to 45. They are increasing in incidence in the United States more rapidly than any other neoplasm. They appear more frequently in whites than in others, and exposure to ultraviolet light is undoubtedly a major cause of the disease, possibly as a result of the shift to an outdoor lifestyle in recent years resulting in the remarkable increase in incidence. The risk for developing a melanoma is greatest in those with a fair complexion, in the presence of one or more hereditary dysplastic nevi, with a familial history of melanoma, and in the presence of a previous melanoma. They appear more frequently on the extremities in women and on the trunk in men. Although more uncommon, other sites for melanomas are the eye, mucous membranes, anus, and genitalia.

Based on their pattern of growth, melanomas have been classified into four groups. The type appearing most frequently is the superficial spreading melanoma, which may evolve over several years before being diagnosed. Occurring later, often in middle age in about half as many patients, are the small, deeply pigmented nodular melanomas. Their growth may be rapid and behavior alarming. Lentigo maligna melanomas occur with still less frequency, are usually somewhat larger lesions, and are less likely to metastasize. They usually occur in older patients and appear chiefly on the face or neck. The acral lentiginous or palmar-plantar-mucosal melanomas are not encountered as often as the others and appear in darker as well as lighter skin. They are most often found on the soles of the feet but also originate in the nail bed (most frequently of thumb or great toe) and palms. With the passage of time, melanomas grow to larger size and usually with irregular margins; they often

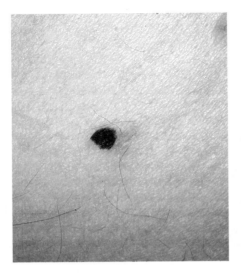

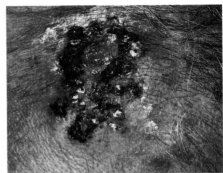

A   B

Figure 4 Melanoma of the skin. A. small melanoma in fair skin. B. large melanoma in dark skin.

become ulcerated and are pigmented in various shades of red and blue with areas of white and black. The neoplasms may itch and bleed. Amelanotic melanomas frequently exhibit more aggressive behavior than those that are pigmented. The antecedent cell which becomes malignant in a melanoma is the melanocyte. These cells originate during embryonic development in the neural crest and subsequently migrate to the skin, mucous membranes, and eye where they are responsible for the pigmented appearance. This inherent ability to migrate is believed by some investigators to be the reason for the potential of melanomas to metastasize.

Fortunately the outlook for cure of small melanomas detected early is excellent after surgical excision. Unfortunately approximately one-third of melanomas have spread beyond the primary site at the time diagnosis is first made. About half of these metastases are to regional nodes. Early in the course of the disease the adjacent skin and subcutaneous tissues are invaded. Later the lymph nodes then the lungs and liver, bone, gastrointestinal tract, and brain can become involved. Eventually almost half of the patients have metastases in the tissues of the central nervous system with most of the attendant symptoms related to hematomas originating from the invasion.

One system of staging frequently used for melanomas consists of four stages based on thickness of the primary lesion found on pathologic examination of the biopsy specimen and the presence and extent of metastases.

Stage IA	Localized 0.75 mm or less
Stage IB	Localized 0.76–1.5 mm
Stage IIA	Localized 1.50–4.0 mm
Stage IIB	Localized >4.0 mm
Stage III	Nodal metastases limited to fewer than five in transit or one solitary nodal area
Stage IV	Advanced regional metastases

The risk involved is divided more evenly among the four categories than in other schemes for staging. The outlook for various presentations of the disease has been delineated extensively in numerous studies. The prognosis is less favorable in thicker lesions, in those with greater tumor volume and mitotic rate, in those with more extensive metastases, in men than women, in lesions of the scalp and face than the extremities, in older rather than younger patients, and in lesions found to be ulcerated, tender, and/or bleeding.

The diagnosis of melanoma requires biopsy or complete excision of the malignancy wherever found with microscopic study of sections of the specimen(s). Careful examination for nodal involvement must be included with the supplementation of lymphangiography and lymphatic mapping when indicated. Radiographic studies, computerized tomograms, and nucleomagnetic resonance studies are necessary when metastases are suspected. Staging based on the dimensions, size, and location of each lesion is mandatory for determining the most effective plan of treatment.

The surgical management of melanomas has been the traditional treatment and continues to be the primary basis of curative treatment. Therapy has been expanded and supplemented with irradiation, chemotherapy (both general and regional), and various types of biotherapy, which are in initial stages of trial. Many questions about the selection of various single and multiple forms of treatment remain unanswered, but definitive studies are in progress. The initial operative treatment can be curative and consists either of excisional or diagnostic biopsy. The additional risk of biopsy with subsequent excision seems to be minimal when compared with that of initial excisional biopsy.

In the past very wide margins were thought desirable when excising all lesions, but since prognosis has been found to be related to the thickness of the lesion, more superficial melanomas can be excised safely with narrower margins. Micrometastases are present in less than 5 percent of cases with lesions less than 1.5 mm thick to two-thirds of the cases with tumors greater than 4 mm thick. The rate of survival for 5 years is approximately 95 percent for lesions less than 0.76 mm thick, 90 percent for those less than 1.5 mm thick, 70 percent for those less than 4 mm thick, and 50 percent for those more than 4 mm thick. Although the width of margins ultimately depends on the judgment of the operating surgeon, those usually used are approximately

1 cm for lesions less than 1.5 mm thick, 1.5 cm for lesions less than 1.5 mm thick, and no more than 3 cm for those greater than 1.5 mm thick.

It may not be possible to obtain greater than a 1.0-cm margin when excising head and neck and facial lesions such as those about the eye and ear, and the resulting defect may offer a considerable challenge to provide a satisfactory plastic repair. Melanomas beneath the nail or skin of a finger frequently require amputation. As much length as possible is saved, particularly that of the thumb, as long as the objective of complete removal is achieved. Leaving some surface on the sole of the foot to bear weight when possible also is an important consideration when the melanoma is located there.

The problem of how to detect and manage involved regional lymph nodes is difficult to solve with certainty. Choices range from regional node dissection at the time the diagnosis is made to waiting until later—up to the time when invasion is apparent from physical examination. Lymphangiography may be helpful, and recently lymphatic mapping using injection of radioactive colloid an hour before operation and blue dye (Lymphazurin, Isosulfan) at the time of operation around the primary site before it is excised has been useful to determine whether the most proximal or sentinal node contains micrometastases. In the case of lesions of the trunk, lymphoscintography may be advisable before the day of operation because lymphatic drainage may be into more than one basin. At the time of operation, the most radioactive site is detected with a scinti-scanner probe covered with a sterile protective sheath. The incision is made at the site; in addition to excision of the neoplasm, the node stained most intensively is removed and frozen sections are obtained. If micrometastases are discovered, then the regional nodes are removed. If negative, then serial sections and immunohistologic methods are used in careful assessment; removal of the nodes beyond the sentinal node then proceeds in a subsequent operation only if micrometastases are found. False negatives occur in less than 5 percent of cases, and deferring resection of regional nodes and beyond on the basis of negative results is justified as long as the patient is followed carefully. When nodal metastases are found, extending a femoral to an iliac node resection depends on involvement of sentinal node and thickness of the primary neoplasm. Resection of regional nodes with metastatic disease from the lower extremity requires covering the defect with the sartorius muscle and using diuretics, antibiotic coverage, and compression hose to avoid subsequent edema. When there is axillary nodal involvement, axillary dissection should be thorough and complete with preservation of the pectoralis minor muscle, suction drainage of the wound, and antibiotic coverage. The management of metastatic disease from primary disease located on the trunk may be much more complex.

Intraocular melanoma, the most common neoplasm in this location in the white population, arises from uveal melanocytes. They were formerly managed by enucleation, but more recently in many cases a more conservative approach has been used. It is unfortunate that there has been insufficient experience to reach a consensus on all the problems involved in treatment. The doubling time of a growing tumor varies from months to 2 years. The absence of lymphatics in the eye removes the problem of lymphatic spread, although hematogenous extension to distant sites such as the liver may occur as the malignancy grows. There appears to be little controversy with the view that large choroidal melanomas and melanomas of the ciliary body should be treated with enucleation. In those of intermediate size, more variation in management is currently encountered. Radiation is an option when vision is adequate and the affected eye is the only one functional. The 5-year survival is not appreciably different when results in large groups of patients treated conservatively are compared with those in patients treated with enucleation. In small melanomas, numerous approaches to treatment are advocated by various therapists, including observation, local resection, radiation, photocoagulation, ultrasonic hyperthermia, and enucleation. Melanoma of the iris is usually treated very conservatively with local resection considered before enucleation, since spread of the malignancy is much less aggressive than at other sites in the eye. Episcleral extension of ocular melanomas is associated with great risk, but the value of exenteration in these cases remains controversial.

The recurrence of a localized melanoma, if small, can be treated by excising it again. When the size is larger, then regional perfusion or irradiation along with hyperthermia should be considered. The presence of metastases in transit indicates consideration of perfusion or infusion of isolated limb with hyperthermia. Radical neck dissection is done for cervical metastases and includes parotid nodes when they are involved. Modified neck dissection has the advantage of saving the spinal accessory nerve and sternocleidomastoid muscle. Complications of node resections vary from edema of extremities to chylous leak from the thoracic duct after cervical operations, and preventive precautions must characterize the technique used during the operative procedure to avoid problems in the postoperative period. Adjuvant treatment with irradiation has yielded some help in inhibiting recurrence following operation. The appearance of a melanoma on an extremity is often treated by a combination of operation to remove the neoplasm and regional nodes and regional perfusion with arteriovenous isolation. The procedure is done most frequently for regional involvement of lower extremities using a choice of nitrogen mustard, melphalan, carmustine, and dacarbazine as a perfusate. Regional therapy can also be carried out as a less complicated procedure consisting of infusion with a tourniquet to isolate the region to be treated.

Melanomas spread to distal sites in skin, lymph nodes, lung, liver, bowel, brain, adrenals, kidneys, and bones in descending order of occurrence. Careful clinical and laboratory follow-up must continue after the diagnosis of melanoma is made initially. When computerized tomograms, nucleomagnetic resonance imaging, clinical examination, and other information identify distant metastases, the therapist must consider both the specific site(s) involved and the patient's expected length of survival to advise wise management with operation, irradiation, or systemic therapy. At times no treatment is the best course to follow, especially when the metastatic tumors are progressing slowly and are asymptomatic and when the condition of the patient does not permit the management otherwise indicated. In patients who represent reasonable risks for the procedure, excision of lesions of brain, lung, those that are superficial, and visceral metastases with symptoms is justified at times. As would be anticipated, solitary lesions yield the best results. Craniotomy to remove a hematoma associated with cerebral metastatic disease is indicated in some cases. Even multiple metastatic pulmonary lesions can be removed successfully at times. Irradiation of superficial lesions and those in brain and bone may be helpful as well. Metastases to the alimentary tract are frequently multiple and are usually found in the jejunum or ileum with symptoms of bleeding and anemia, abdominal tenderness, and at times intussusception. Resection of these lesions may be necessary.

Some radiologists favor using high fractional doses for metastatic disease. Using fractions as high as 800 cGy to the whole brain at times yields responses for an extended period. The addition of hyperthermia can be advantageous when metastases in soft tissues are irradiated. Chemotherapy is usually reserved for those with spread to skin and subcutaneous tissue, lymph nodes, and lungs. Usually more than one distal site is invaded during the later stages of this malignancy.

The most favorable circumstances for obtaining responses to chemotherapy are found in patients younger than 65 years of age with good performance status, normal hepatic and renal function and hemogram, no history of previous chemotherapy, lesions involving soft tissue with spread to few or no visceral sites, and no known metastases to the central nervous system. Pulmonary metastases may be very sensitive in these patients as well. Chemotherapy is not used customarily as standard therapy or for stage IV disease by many medical oncologists, since there is no effect on survival.

The most useful compound when used as a single agent is dacarbazine (DTIC). Approximately one-fifth of patients receiving it show some response. It is administered intravenously in an interrupted schedule. Response occurs in involved skin and subcutaneous tissue, lymph nodes, lung, and at times liver, bone, and brain. Side effects that must be alleviated are nausea and vomiting, local pain at the site of injection, symptoms similar to influenza, diarrhea, thrombocytopenia, leukopenia, hepatic failure, and photosensitivity. The nitrosoureas also have elicited some, but fewer, responses. They are soluble in lipids, and for that reason at first it was hoped that they would be especially effective for treating metastatic cerebral foci, but anticipated results have not materialized. As a group, cumulative toxicity is a disadvantage. Among those found useful are carmustine (BCNU), formustine, lomustine (CCNU), semustine (Methyl-CCNU), and tauromustine (TCNU). Other agents with somewhat limited action are alkylating agents, cisplatin (Platinol), carboplatin, dactinomycin (Actinomycin D), detorubicin, dibromodulcitol (Mitolactol), ifosfamide, pirirexin, procarbazine, the vinca alkaloids (vinblastine and vindesine), and Taxol. High dosages with rescue by autologous transplantation of bone marrow as a means for trying to extend the response to these agents carries great risk and should be understood by the patient when attempted. Peritoneal and pleural effusions at times respond to instillations of bleomycin, dacarbazine, radioactive colloidal gold (^{198}Au), radioactive chromic phosphate (^{32}P), or thiotepa.

Various combinations of chemotherapeutic agents have and are being tested in clinical trials either as combinations of drugs known to be active against melanomas or as combinations of active drugs and others without known activity. Experience so far suggests activity when DTIC and melphalan or ifosfamide are combined and when combinations with BCNU, such as melphalan and cyclophosphamide or cisplatin, are used. Other combinations are cisplatin, DTIC, and vinblastine; BCNU, cisplatin, DTIC, and tamoxifen; and CCNU, procarbazine, and vincristine. Some combinations have resulted in greater activity against melanomas than single agents. It is unfortunate that this may be at the expense of greater toxicity. The choice of chemotherapy in managing this neoplasm is difficult not only because of the refractory behavior of the malignancy itself and the limited choice of effective agents but also because the most advantageous method of administering agents on hand is not yet clear from trials still in process.

Also being developed is a panoply of biologic treatments, which are being tested against melanomas. They have as primary objective the use of immune mechanisms to combat these malignancies and include monoclonal antibodies, the cytokines (interleukins and interferons), and methods for inducing active immunity. Monoclonal antibodies alone and as conjugates with toxins and radioisotopes have yielded promising results in laboratory experiments. The response rate has been as high as 20 percent in clinical trials. Clinical trials using interleukin-2 and activated lymphocytes with cyclophosphamide have been initiated backed by encouraging laboratory results showing responses in animals in similar trials. Interleukin-2 can exhibit severe toxicity, and treatment requires hospitalization in special centers. Responses have been in the range of 15 to 20 percent. Recombinant interferon-α has exhibited activity against melanomas, but no significant advantage so far in randomized clinical trials. Whether interferon-β offers any advantage when compared with interferon-alfa has not been determined. Both interferon-alfa and the interleukin tested have side effects that increase with dosage. Results so far are suggestive that they may be useful and should be studied more extensively. Interlesional therapy with bacillus Calmette-Guérin (BCG) has initiated some local response in melanomas and more rarely at other sites. Interferon alfa-2b is accepted as adjuvant therapy for patients at high risk of relapse after resection of positive nodes.

After definitive treatment patients should be followed with periodic physical examinations and radiographic studies of the chest along with frequent self-examination for a period of at least 2 years for primary lesions less than 0.75 mm thick and for 5 years for those greater than this thickness.

American Joint Cancer Commission/Union Internationale contre le Cancer classification and staging of melanoma

Primary tumor

Tx	Cannot be assessed
T0	No evidence of primary neoplasm
Tis	Melanoma in situ
T1	Tumor ≤ 0.75 mm thick, invading dermis
T2	Tumor >0.75 to 1.5 mm thick and/or invading dermis
T3	Tumor >1.5 to 4 mm thick and/or invading dermis
T3a	Tumor >1.5 to 3 mm thick
T3b	Tumor >3 to 4 mm thick
T4	Tumor >4 mm thick and/or invades subcutaneous tissue and/or satellite(s) within 2 cm of primary
T4a	Tumor >4 mm thick and/or invades subcutaneous tissue
T4b	Satellite(s) within 2 cm of primary

Lymph nodes

Nx	Regional nodes cannot be assessed
N0	No nodal metastases
N1	Nodal metastasis ≤ 3 cm
N2	Nodal metastasis >3 cm and/or in transit
N2a	Nodal metastasis >3 cm
N2b	Metastasis in transit
N2c	Both metastasis >3 cm and in transit

Distant metastasis

Mx	Cannot be assessed
M0	No distant metastasis
M1	Distant metastasis
M1a	Metastasis beyond regional nodes in skin, subcutaneous tissue, or lymph nodes
M1b	Visceral metastasis

Stage

I	T1	N0	M0
II	T2	N0	M0
III	T3	N0	M0
	Any T	N1	M0
	Any T	N2	M0
IV	Any T	Any N	M1

Grade

Gx	Cannot be assessed
G1	Well differentiated
G2	Moderately well differentiated
G3	Poorly differentiated
G4	Undifferentiated

THREE

CARCINOMA OF THE BREAST

Carcinoma of the breast is the type of cancer second most frequently encountered by women in the United States, only exceeded very recently by bronchogenic carcinoma. It is probably the neoplasm most dreaded by women because of its prevalence, the familial occurrence of the disease, and the fear of disfigurement and undesirable side effects of therapy. Approximately one out of eight women will be afflicted with this disease. Much progress has been made in recent years in the search for the genetic cause of mammary cancer. Two mutant genes, *BRCA1* and *BRCA2,* have been discovered, localized on chromosome 17, and found to be associated with cancer of the breast. A DNA screening test is available for identifying carriers with these genes. It is unfortunate that the test is quite expensive at the present time, and the problem is further complicated because those affected may be denied insurance when the results are known. Approximately one-tenth of Ashkenazim with German semitic inheritance are estimated to carry the *BRCA1* gene, but in the population at large its prevalence is no more than 1 in 500. The distribution of the *BRCA2* gene is less certain. Changes in susceptibility of immigrants have been attributed to change in diet, but the components responsible are unknown. Exposure to intensive or prolonged irradiation is known to cause the disease, but no virus similar to that causing murine mammary cancer has been identified in the human disease. Current information about the inheritance of cancer of the breast offers new means to explore the possibility of gene therapy in the future.

The detection of neoplasms of the breast is most effective when it occurs early in the course of the disease when the tumor is small and remains localized. Cooperation between the patient and the doctor she has chosen is necessary to use the few means available for making an early diagnosis. Examination of the breasts by the patient at regular intervals of not greater than 1 month and by the physician when any change in contour or density is discovered and at intervals not longer than 6 months is essential. In addition, mammograms should be a part of the planned regimen. When there is a question of whether a palpable lesion or one seen on radiographic study is cystic, ultrasonography is useful in making the determination. There is some controversy about how often and at what age mammography should be done based on the positive results obtained in large series of cases studied objectively. Individuals often are reluctant to defer using this means of diagnosis despite the statistics indicating a low percentage of positive mammograms in younger patients, fearing that their case may be an exception to the rule. It should be understood always that a cancer can be present and not be palpable and can be present with a negative mammogram. The only way to be certain is to have a biopsy of the breast with immediate microscopic study by a pathologist when a palpable mass, a positive mammogram, or both are found.

Cancer of the breast is classified by the appearance of sections of the neoplasm when examined under the microscope. These malignancies may be localized and referred to as cancer in situ, or they can be infiltrating and invasive. The localized lesions have not spread beyond the base of the epithelium. Three quarters or more of all carcinomas of the breast are labeled infiltrating ductal carcinomas. They have the poorest prognosis of those appearing most frequently with approximately 60 percent survival at 5 years and 40 percent at 15 years. Another type of carcinoma prone to occur at multiple sites, including the opposite breast, is infiltrating lobular cancer, constituting approximately one-tenth of all neoplasms of the breast. Other types of mammary cancer are classified as colloid or mucinous, comedo, medullary, and papillary. The rates of survival in ascending order are ductal, lobular, medullary, colloid, comedo, and papillary. Two additional types of malignant tumors are called Paget's disease of the breast and inflammatory carcinoma of the breast. Paget's disease consists of eczematoid changes in the appearance of the nipple with crusting and bleeding at times. The majority of these lesions are associated with an underlying mass. Usually the most malignant of all carcinomas of the breast are inflammatory cancers. They have the appearance of an inflammatory process, but few inflammatory cells are present, and the dermal lymphatics are invaded with malignant cells. Usually there is no associated palpable mass. A diagnosis of the histologic type of tumor is made from a study of the tissue removed at the time of biopsy and/or resection. A complete expectant plan of treatment awaits this information.

Biopsy of the breast may be carried out with a needle, or the lesion can be excised with the scalpel. Many surgeons are skeptical about the wisdom of relying on the former, since negative needle biopsies cannot be used to rule out the presence of a neoplasm. Ideally, biopsies should be carried out under circumstances permitting immediate definitive operation for treating the cancer. When the needle is used, a negative biopsy yields only a small fragment of tissue, and the chance that a neoplasm has been missed is always

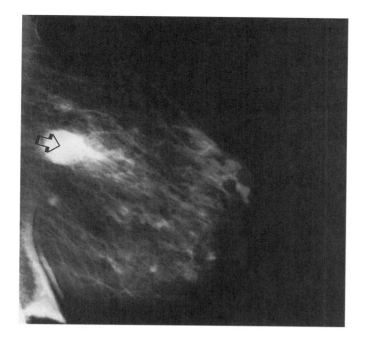

A

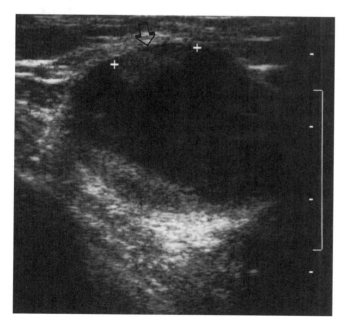

B

Figure 5 Papillary cystic adenocarcinoma of the breast. A. Mammogram showing the tumor. B. Ultrasound study showing mural tumor (*arrow*), cyst, and fluid.

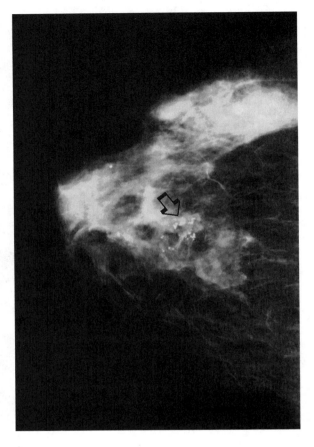

A

Figure 6 Positive mammogram without palpable mass. A. Mammogram of the breast.

present. If positive, an operation is indicated anyway. By using a circumareolar incision the surgeon can biopsy a tumor in any part of the breast with very good cosmetic result if the lesion is benign. The radiologist can localize a lesion visible radiographically at the point of a localizing needle to be left in place to help the surgeon identify the exact locus at the operating table. Experienced surgeons find this help necessary only in the occasional case. When a possible cystic lesion is seen by the radiologist doing the sonogram, needle aspiration of the fluid is usually done and the fluid examined for malignant cells immediately. In those patients with cystic disease of the breast, tumors may appear at intervals and biopsies indicated whenever this occurs. In unusual cases with a history of multiple operations, subcutaneous mastectomy with preservation of the nipple and cosmetic augmentation may consti-

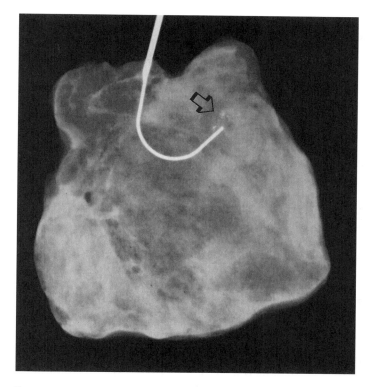

B

Figure 6 *(Continued)* B. Roentgen study of biopsy specimen with calcium localized by needle inserted preoperatively.

tute the best solution. The surgeon always keeps in mind the possibility of malignancy at more than one location in doing both diagnostic examinations and other studies and at the time of operation.

Some characteristics of cancers of the breast are useful to help forecast the patients' progress in the future. Estrogen and progesterone receptors should always be determined as part of the examination of the excised malignant tissue. If present, especially with a high titer, management of the disease is more successful. Other characteristics suggesting a more favorable prognosis are the absence of a positive test for carcinoembryonic antigen (CEA), small size of the primary neoplasm, and absence of detectable metastases. On the other hand, an increase in the number of cells in the S phase of DNA synthesis in the cell cycle, the greater departure from the normal diploid number of chromosomes, the amplification of cancer genes (oncogenes), the presence of metastases in lymph nodes or elsewhere, larger size of the tumor, and the histologic type of the tumor such as inflammatory carcinoma, infiltrating ductal carcinoma, and carcinoma detected during pregnancy are suggestive of a less favorable outcome of treatment when compared with the management of patients with cancers having different characteristics.

Malignancies of the breast require operation after a definitive tissue diagnosis is made from microscopic studies. The type of operation recommended has changed with the passage of time since the radical operation recommended by Halsted and Meyer in 1895 was first performed. Controversy has arisen about the best procedure to use; in this discussion a noncontroversial approach is used throughout. Radical mastectomy, which includes removal of the pectoralis major muscle, is no longer performed today. The choice is between a modified radical mastectomy and one popularly known by a rather inelegant and misleading term, *lumpectomy*. The mastectomy done for cancer of the breast preserves the large pectoralis major muscle of the chest wall and is no longer associated with swelling of the arm and other complications encountered in the past. It also includes removal of the axillary lymph nodes through the primary transverse incision. The breast, including the overlying skin and nipple, the entire tumor, and the axillary nodes are removed with sufficient skin remaining to close the wound without tension. In the case of the usual tumor, the operative incisions are made beyond the margins of the neoplasm, the site of the previous biopsy having been closed. The other operation consists usually of an incision over the site of the tumor with removal of the tumor and multiple biopsies at its periphery until microscopic study of the specimens removed fail to reveal any malignant cells. This wound is then closed, and a second incision is made in the axilla through which the axillary nodes are removed. Without exception, the remaining portion of the breast is irradiated. It is obvious that this procedure is more than a simple lumpectomy.

After a modified radical mastectomy described above, irradiation may not be required if the lymph nodes do not contain any metastastic foci. The results of the two types of procedures are comparable. A simplistic viewpoint is whether the patient wishes the entire breast to be removed, including any malignant cells contained in it, or whether reliance is placed in irradiation to kill residual cancer that could have been missed in the portion of the breast preserved. After modified radical mastectomy, a cosmetic operation to restore the contour of the breast and reconstruct the nipple can be performed.

The patient and surgeon jointly should choose the type of surgery after the patient thoroughly understands the options. Other factors such as the presence of extremely large breasts may alter the recommendation of the therapeutic radiologist. Central lesions may indicate removal of the nipple along with the malignancy. Multicentric lesions may suggest that a mastectomy is a wiser choice. The surgeon should explain carefully all factors to the patient. Most surgeons are quite capable of performing either operation. Although some of the original data used to determine the value of lumpectomy were

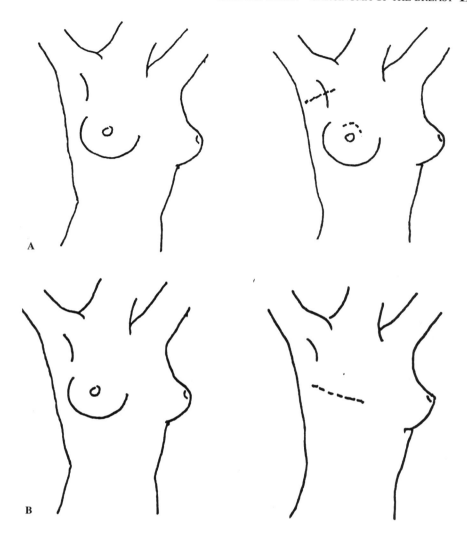

Figure 7 Operations for carcinoma of the breast. A. "Lumpectomy" including axillary node dissection and radiation and/or chemotherapy. B. Modified radical mastectomy requiring a single transverse or oblique incision with postoperative chemotherapy and/ or radiotherapy only in selected cases. (Prosthetic or muscular augmentation can be done for plastic restoration.)

found to be spurious and were discarded, those remaining have substantiated the original conclusions that modified radical mastectomy and lumpectomy yield equivalent clinical results.

Paget's disease of the breast requires wide removal of the malignancy, including the nipple and surrounding skin, as a minimal approach. Inflammatory cancer must be treated on an individual basis depending on the characteristics of the tumor. The prognosis is discouraging in any case. Carcinoma of the breast occurring during pregnancy has been treated more successfully in recent years, but it remains a challenge. The tendency of infiltrating lobular cancer to occur in multiple sites, including the opposite breast, has led to bilateral mastectomy in the past, but this approach is used less frequently now. In advanced cancer of the breast, mastectomy and radical removal of much of the tumor may be indicated to reduce the bulk of the neoplasm to facilitate radiotherapy and/or chemotherapy. Carcinoma of the breast occurs rarely in men, but even bilateral cancer of the breast has been reported in males. They are usually treated by a modified radical mastectomy.

The aim of chemotherapy in early disease is to destroy micrometastases, and the results and side effects must be evaluated both for the short and long term. In more advanced disease the goal is somewhat more circumscribed to increasing the patient's comfort, diminishing pain, reducing the size of the population of tumor cells, and promoting the functional capacity for work and enjoyment. There are a number of agents that are differentially cytotoxic for tumor cells. The optimum dosage of chemotherapeutic agents that is most effective does not always correspond to the maximum safe dosage. The results of many clinical trials indicate that the combination of drugs in a program of chemotherapy frequently increases the effectiveness of treatment when compared with results of treatment with a single agent. As many patients can corroborate, these compounds are toxic for normal cells, and side effects occur. The therapist wishes to obtain the maximum tumoricidal effect which can be obtained with dosage that causes acceptable side effects. Factors that alter the program are those of risk characteristic of the specific cancer being treated, the titer of hormone receptors in the neoplasm, the age and physical condition of the patient, whether the patient is pre- or postmenopausal, and the stage of the disease.

In premenopausal patients without detectable nodal metastases, classified as low risk with estrogen receptors negative, and tumors less than 1 cm in diameter, no chemotherapy may be acceptable. However, in patients with larger tumors and/or at higher risk a regimen of chemotherapy and tamoxifen is appropriate. In those with negative receptors, usually the tamoxifen is omitted. Premenopausal women with positive lymph nodes are treated similarly. All postmenopausal women are given tamoxifen; those younger than 70 years are given chemotherapy in addition, if the estrogen receptors are negative. Tamoxifen therapy is known to be associated with increased risk for uterine cancer. Therefore great care to follow a regimen designed to detect early cancer of this organ must be followed when tamoxifen is prescribed.

Agents known to be effective in altering the progression of breast cancer are cyclophosphamide, doxorubicin (Adriamycin), epirubicin, 5-fluorouracil, methotrexate, vinblastine, thiotepa, fluoxymesterone (Halotestin), mitomycin, and mitoxantrone. They are used in various combinations and may be combined with hormonal and/or biologic agents. Other agents known to yield responses are paclitaxel, docetaxel, vinorelbine, and 5-fluorouracil. The regimens most commonly used are AC (Adriamycin, cyclophosphamide four cycles), CAF (cyclophosphamide, Adriamycin, and 5-fluorouracil), CMF (cyclophosphamide, methotrexate, 5-fluorouracil six cycles), and FEC (5-fluorouracil, epirubicin, cyclophosphamide six cycles). Toxic side effects may necessitate altering the dosage and timing of the regimen chosen. Neural, renal, hepatic, cardiac, cystic, gastrointestinal, dermal, and hemic toxicities are always carefully monitored by the oncologist responsible for therapy so as to be able to alter the plan of management when undesirable response to treatment indicates that a change is necessary. Patients are always encouraged by the fact that the rate of survival is increased by chemotherapy in premenopausal women with positive nodes following operation and in postmenopausal women with positive nodes and treated with tamoxifen. Often combinations of agents are more effective than single agents.

Since cancer cells in the breast may retain sensitivity to endocrines in varying degrees, the determination of titer of estrogen and progesterone receptors in the cancer tissue allows the oncologist to prognosticate the response of a given neoplasm to this type of treatment. In the premenopausal patient estrogen antagonists such as tamoxifen are quite useful, and a great amount of information has been accumulated over the years about the usefulness of surgical and radiologic oophorectomy. Also, antiestrogen therapy is used in the management of cancer of the breast in postmenopausal women as well, since it is known to stimulate inhibitory factors and inhibit growth factors. Endocrine therapy is less likely to be effective when the titers of estrogen and progesterone receptors are low. The use of endocrine therapy frequently is accompanied by other modes of treatment, and management of an individual case requires careful assessment of the most promising sequence and combination with operation, irradiation, and chemotherapy. Ablation of ovaries, adrenal glands, and pituitary along with manipulative therapy with androgens, estrogens, antiestrogens, and progestins are all available for possible inclusion in the treatment of patients with carcinoma of the breast.

Therapy for metastatic disease can include radiotherapy and hormonal therapy as well as chemotherapy. Among useful agents are Taxol, Taxoline, Venovelbin, 5-fluorouracil, and leucovorin. Those patients who are at higher risk of relapse and those with metastatic disease and who have appropriate performance status and are able to tolerate intensive chemotherapy can be offered autologous bone transplantation.

Classification and staging of carcinoma of the breast (American Joint Committee on Cancer)

Classification

Primary tumor

Tx	Cannot be assessed
T0	No evidence of primary neoplasm
Tis	Carcinoma in situ
T1	≤2 cm

      T1a ≤0.5 cm

      T1b >0.5 cm, not >1 cm

      T1c >1.0 cm, not >2 cm

T2	>2 cm, not >5 cm
T3	>5 cm
T4	Any size with extension to chest wall or skin
T5	T4a Extension to chest wall
	T4b Edema, ulceration, satellite nodules same breast
	T4c T4a + T4b
	T4d Inflammatory carcinoma

Regional lymph nodes

NX	Cannot be assessed
N0	No nodal metastases
N1	Movable ipsilateral axillary nodes
N2	Fixed metastases ipsilateral nodes
N3	Metastases ipsilateral internal mammary nodes

Distant metastases

MX	Cannot be assessed
M0	No distant metastases
M1	Distant metastases

Stage grouping

Stage 0	Tis	N0	M0
Stage I	T1	N0	M0
Stage IIA	T0	N1	MQ
	T1	N1	M0
	T2	N0	M0
Stage IIB	T2	N1	M0
	T2	N0	M0
Stage IIIA	T0	N2	M0
	T1	N2	M0
	T2	N2	M0
	T3	N1, N2	M0
Stage IIIB	T4	Any N	M0
	Any T	N3	M0
Stage IV	Any T	Any N	M1

FOUR

CANCER OF THE HEAD AND NECK

Cancer of the head and neck appears in all divisions of this portion of the body, and there is a surgical specialty devoted to these areas alone, since surgical treatment requires special training and experience to meet the unique problems each region presents for therapy to be successful. This specialty and the classification of cancers in the region do not include neoplasms of the brain. The TNM classification for a specific tumor allows comparisons between the case being studied and the results of therapy and the natural history of similar neoplasms. The accompanying table gives a summary of this classification for these cancers along with the staging criteria.

The regions bearing benign and malignant neoplasms in the head and neck are salivary glands, nasal cavity and paranasal sinuses, lips and oral cavity, buccal mucosa, alveolar ridge and floor of the mouth, tongue, oropharynx, hard palate, tonsils and tonsillar pillars, soft palate, pharyngeal wall, nasopharynx, hypopharynx, and larynx. The diagnosis of neoplasms arising in this region consists of obtaining a careful history and physical examination and biopsy with microscopic study of sections of the specimen. From the pharynx downward this requires endoscopic visualization for observation and biopsy. The determination of invasion of lymph nodes, bone, and distant sites is also essential and requires radiographic examination when suspected.

Surgical resection and radiation therapy have been used and refined over many years of experience. Chemotherapy currently plays a lesser role in treatment, and for many sites experience is somewhat rudimentary. In general, the most useful chemotherapy is cisplatin plus 5-fluorouracil; methotrexate; and isotretinoin. It is hoped that additional clinical trials and relevant basic research will provide greater success and additional effective drugs and biologic agents.

TNM classification and staging of tumors of the head and neck

Tumor

T0	No tumor
T1	≤2 cm
T2	>2 to 4 cm
T3	>4 to 6 cm
T4	>6 cm

Lymph nodes

NX	Cannot be determined
N0	None
N1	1 ipsilateral node ≤3 cm
N2A	1 ipsilateral node >3 to 6 cm
2B	Multiple ipsilateral nodes ≤6 cm
2C	Multiple bilateral nodes ≤6 cm
N3	1 or more nodes >6 cm

Distant metastases

MX	Cannot be determined
M0	None
M	Any number

Staging

Stage I

T1	N0	M0

Stage II

T2	N0	M0

Stage III

T1	N1	M0
T2	N1	M0
T3	N0	M0
T3	N1	M0

Stage IV

T4	N0	M0
T4	N1	M0
Any T	N2	M0
Any T	N3	M0
Any T	Any N	M

Surgical biopsy provides the tissue diagnosis essential for initiating treatment. A positive biopsy provided by aspiration with a fine needle or removal of a small cylinder of tissue can be as useful. The resection of the neoplasm requires consideration of the removal of metastatic cancer as well. In the head and neck the adjacent lymph nodes are frequently invaded, and surgical treatment has and continues to include the resection of lymph nodes in addi-

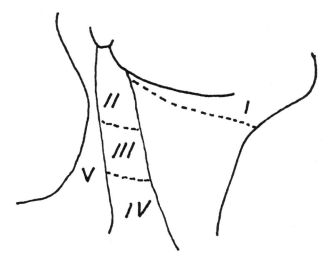

Figure 8 Regions in the neck with designations useful in planning resections of cervical lymph nodes.

tion. Removing them as a prophylactic measure may be justified when the natural history and size and extent of the primary cancer is taken into consideration. In the past a radical neck dissection was included in the treatment of many cancers of the head and neck, including removal of the sternocleidomastoid muscle, the jugular veins, the regional lymph nodes in the neck, and the spinal accessory nerve. This radical procedure is seldom done at the present time, since more conservative operations have given comparable results. The sternocleidomastoid muscle and spinal accessory nerve are usually preserved, and variations of modified neck dissections are the approaches followed. The regions of the neck have been designated I through V as a convenient indication of the lymph nodes removed. This anatomic division is illustrated in the accompanying table.

Radiation therapy may be given as photon irradiation, neutron irradiation, electron beam therapy, or brachytherapy with radioisotopes carried in interstitial containers left in place permanently or temporarily. Teletherapy is delivered to areas outlined on the surface in multiple doses. These ports are scattered about the surface with the irradiation target converging on the tumor, thus reducing the dosage to uninvolved tissue and concentrating additive dosages on the tumor. Radiologists have become skilled in using three-dimensional models for planning how the ports and cross-firing angles are arranged to increase the tumor dose and diminish the dosage received by normal tissue. Radiation dermatitis and mucositis and loss of hair are side effects localized

Location of cervical lymph nodes

Margins	Superior	Anterior	Inferior	Posterior
Level I	Mandible	Midline	Hyoid bone	Digastric muscle
Level II	Jugular foramen	Digastric muscle	Carotid bifurcation	Posterior border sternocleido-mastoid muscle
Level III	Carotid bifurcation	Digastric muscle	Omohyoid muscle	Posterior border sternocleido-mastoid muscle
Level IV	Omohyoid muscle	Midline	Clavicle	Posterior border sternocleido-mastoid muscle
Level V	Posterior border sternocleido-mastoid muscle	Posterior border sternocleido-mastoid muscle	Omohyoid muscle	Trapezius muscle

in the portal areas and, if the beam is sufficiently penetrating, at the site of exit. Loss of taste and dry mouth and dry eyes resulting from irradiation of salivary and lachrymal glands, respectively, are acute effects. These are delayed in appearance but then subside with the cessation of treatment. Residual problems depend on the extent of the dosage and the kind of irradiation. Inclusion of the mandible in the field of irradiation may result in the loss of teeth, and extraction beforehand may be advisable. Most often irradiation is given postoperatively, but preoperative therapy is given at times.

The value of chemotherapy with single agents and combinations of two or more has been tested for cancer of the head and neck in many clinical trials. Chemotherapy with compounds such as methotrexate and cisplatin can be used for palliation following recurrence after resection and for metastatic disease. Other agents that have been used are bleomycin, carboplatin, 5-fluorouracil, ifosfamide, and leucovorin. Combination therapy has generally been more successful than therapy with single agents. Also chemotherapy can be used to enhance the effect of radiotherapy. Improved approaches to utilizing chemotherapy await additional clinical trials and agents. The number of courses, best combinations, value of induction therapy, adjuvant therapy, and chemoradiation, and how chemotherapy should be combined with resection and irradiation deserve additional study. It is hoped that contributions will be in the rate of cures as well as in the sphere of improving the quality of life.

SALIVARY GLANDS

Minor salivary glands are scattered throughout the upper digestive and respiratory tract and are most numerous in the palate and elsewhere in the oral cavity, including the nasal passages and sinuses. The remaining three glands are paired. The largest is the parotid gland located anterior to the ear and extending around and beneath the mandible. It is traversed by the five major external branches of the facial nerve. There are no true lobes of the gland, but that portion external to the facial nerve and its branches is often referred to as the superficial lobe and the portion beneath the nerve and its branches the deep lobe. Tumors of the deep portion of the gland can be confused with tumors originating in the oropharynx and parapharyngeal space. Computerized tomograms or nuclear magnetic imaging may be required for differentiating them. It is fortunate that many more benign and malignant tumors originate in the superficial portion of the gland. Lymphatic drainage is into intraparatoid lymph nodes, which in turn drain into the deep upper and middle cervical chain of nodes. The periparotid preauricular nodes drain into the superficial cervical nodes and seldom are involved in the spread of parotid malignancies. The submandibular salivary glands are located beneath and medial to the anterior portion of the mandible. They drain into submental lymph nodes, which drain into the upper deep jugular nodes. The sublingual glands are situated beneath the mucosa of the anterior floor of the mouth and have lymphatic drainage similar to that of the submandibular glands.

Tumors of the salivary glands present themselves as masses within the major glands and submucosal tumors of the minor salivary glands. Those of sublinguinal and submandibular glands are revealed best by bimanual examination. The work-up can be extended profitably by computerized tomography and/or nuclear magnetic imaging, but sialograms outlining the ducts of the major glands are not used as frequently as in the past. Fine needle biopsy is useful as a diagnostic tool as long as it is realized that a negative biopsy does not necessarily rule out the presence of a neoplasm. The tumors may grow slowly and later become tender and painful. More rapid growth, firm consistency, and symptoms of nerve damage such as numbness of the buccal mucosa and tongue and weakness of facial muscles characteristic of lesions of the branches of the motor facial nerve are suggestive that a tumor is malignant.

Benign tumors of the salivary glands consist of the following types: mixed (pleomorphic adenoma), lymphoepithelioma, monomorphic adenoma, oncocytoma, and papillary cystadenoma lymphomatosum. Malignant neoplasms found in these glands are classified as acinic cell carcinoma, adenocarcinoma, adenoid cystic carcinoma, mixed tumor (malignant), mucoepidermoid carcinoma, and squamous (epidermoid) carcinoma. Separation of benign from malignant tumors on the basis of microscopic study is sometimes difficult, but fortunately most of the tumors are benign. The malignant neoplasms can exhibit perivascular, perineural, and lymphatic invasion not seen in the benign tumors. Mucoepidermoid carcinomas are the kind encountered most frequently in the parotid gland. The aggressiveness of the neoplasm varies widely from characteristics of slow growth and benign appearance to more rapid spread and invasion. Adenoid cystic carcinomas occur more frequently in minor than in major salivary glands. Although their growth may be exceptionally slow, they can metastasize to distant sites with fatal outcome. Mixed tumors present special problems because the benign variety (pleomorphic adenoma) is difficult to distinguish from the malignant. Also a malignant mixed tumor may arise at the site of a pleomorphic adenoma which has been growing slowly. Many pathologists believe that the malignant mixed tumors are always malignancies arising de novo at a given location and do not represent a transformation of benign to malignant mixed tumor.

The treatment of tumors of the major salivary glands is primarily surgical. Resection of malignancies of the parotid is complicated by the presence of branches of the facial nerve coursing through the center of the gland. Every effort is made to preserve the branches of the nerve while taking care to remove all vestige of the neoplasm. In most cases the nerve can be preserved and irradiation added when indicated. When resection of a portion of the nerve is unavoidable for complete removal of the neoplasm, nerve grafts have been transplanted successfully. Every effort is made to remove the entire malignancy during the initial operation. Access to the deep lobe of the parotid gland containing a malignancy can be facilitated by techniques of removal that include partial resection of the mandible. Recurrence, particularly within the parotid gland, presents much more difficult problems when resection is necessary again than those encountered during the initial procedure. Even when the parotid gland contains a large malignant tumor, the cosmetic result of the operation is quite acceptable when the incision is placed appropriately. Irradiation is added when margins contain evidence of residual malignant cells, the neoplasm is high-grade or advanced, tumor cells are spread during the operation, regional lymph nodes contain malignant cells, the deep lobe of the parotid lymph nodes contain malignant cells, the deep lobe of the parotid contains malignant cells, the malignancy is an adenoid cystic carcinoma, or the neoplasm is recurrent. The presence of metastatic nodal disease initially or discovered at the time of operation by nodal resection warrants the extension of the field irradiated with a total tumor dose as much as 7500 cGy. Neoplasms of the minor salivary glands warrant extended radiation fields up to the base of the skull when perineural spread is present. In general, external beam photon ports can be used alone or with electron beam radiation. Also brachyradiation therapy has been a helpful addition to combined treatment especially in treating cancers of the oral cavity. Neutron therapy is advocated by some radiologists for advanced malignancies. The method of local removal is not the usual one applicable to treating cancer of the salivary glands. The surgeon is meticulous and careful to remove the entire neoplasm from the gland when possible, even though a radical approach with wide resection of all tissue is not used, as in former years. Enucleation is never advisable for these tumors even when it becomes necessary to remove a benign lesion.

Chemotherapy for neoplasms of the salivary glands has been given utilizing single agents including cisplatin, cyclophosphamide, doxorubicin, 5-fluorouracil (5-FU), and methotrexate. Although there have been some responses, the experience has not been great because of the relative scarcity of patients with these neoplasms suitable for testing. Combined therapy has also been tried with combinations such as cisplatin, cyclophosphamide, and doxorubicin with and without 5-FU. Neoadjuvant and adjuvant therapy may be a worthwhile addition to treatment, but much more information from clinical trials is needed for final assessment. Currently, combination therapy with multiple agents is a reasonable approach to extension of therapy for high-grade, extensive, and metastatic cancer of the salivary glands. In preliminary studies, undifferentiated and mucoepidermoid carcinomas seem to respond to different combinations of agents when compared with responses of the remainder of the cancers of the salivary glands.

NASAL CAVITY AND PARANASAL SINUSES

Neoplasms originating in the nasal cavity and paranasal sinuses are usually grouped together because of their proximity and the likelihood that a single cancer will affect both. The paranasal sinuses consist of the maxillary, frontal, ethmoid, and sphenoid sinuses located in a lateral, anterior, medial, and posterior relationship. The nasal cavity consists of a pyramidal inferior entrance lined with skin containing hair follicles and sebaceous glands designated the vestibule and the superior and posterior antrum lined with mucosa and containing the superior, middle, and inferior turbinates extending from the lateral wall medially. The nasal septum divides the nasal cavity into two symmetric chambers. Most of the neoplasms located in these anatomic sites are squamous carcinomas, but a variety of other malignancies occur in these locations as well. The type and results of treatment depend on the type of tumor being treated. Some of these cancers are found much more frequently in the Orient and elsewhere than in the United States. The occurrence of some of them is attributable to industrial carcinogens. The prognosis and method of treatment follows the extent of the tumor at the time of discovery. It is unfortunate that this is discovered later than desirable in almost all cases. Symptoms and signs consist of nasal obstruction, intermittent bleeding, pain, and swelling. When the neoplasm has extended into the orbit, mouth, and mandible the patient may complain of diplopia, loose dentures, and trismus. More rarely the tumors can extend upward into the cranial cavity. In addition to careful physical examination, computerized tomograms are quite useful in determining the margins of the tumor.

Surgeons have developed great skill in removing these tumors and have had considerable success in curing the less advanced cancers. It is usually not customary to include a dissection of regional lymph nodes in the procedure adopted unless there is good evidence that the nodes have been invaded, since this is a late event in the usual progress of the disease. The chief problem is local recurrence. For that reason combined management with operation and irradiation is not infrequently used either as the primary treatment or when recurrence ensues. The occurrence of cancer of the maxillary antrum usually is managed by maxillectomy followed by irradiation. The primary tumor designation for the TNM staging of tumors of the maxillary antrum appears below (The remainder is the same as for other locations in the head and neck.)

TX	Primary not accessible
T0	No evidence of primary
Tis	Carcinoma in situ
T1	Tumor antral mucosa
T2	Tumor with erosion of hard palate
T3	Tumor invading skin, orbit, ethmoid, or maxillary sinus
T4	Invading widely including base of skull and nasopharynx

Irradiation alone is used in early lesions and often effects a cure when the cancer is small and more localized. When the situation is suitable, chemotherapy has been used with irradiation, and the result, when successful, may be more satisfactory cosmetically than when an operation is performed. Intraarterial chemotherapy can be used instead of the intravenous route, since some investigators believe that higher doses can be delivered to a specific localized field without diffusion into a wider area. Bleomycin, cisplatin, and 5-fluorouracil have been used alone and in combination. When the cancer has invaded the orbit, enucleation may or may not be necessary. Various surgical techniques have been used for support when the defect is repaired before closure when exenteration is not done. Diplopia and other complications can ensue, and the surgeon must be very skilled to make a wise choice about the procedure adopted.

ORAL CAVITY

Cancer of the oral cavity includes those of the lip, floor of the mouth, alveolar ridge, tongue, and oropharynx. The tumor staging common to all these sites appears below. The remainder is identical with other divisions of the head and neck.

TX	Primary not accessible
T0	No evidence of primary
Tis	Carcinoma in situ
T1	Tumor <2 cm
T2	Tumor >2 to 4 cm
T3	Tumor >4 cm
T4	Tumor invading soft tissues and/or bone

LIP

Cancer of the lip is most frequently epidermoid carcinoma and grows slowly. Among tumors of the head and neck, it occurs with a frequency only second to cancer of the skin and occurs in men more often than in women. It is usually attributed to the use of tobacco or exposure to the sun. The lower lip is the location where the tumors are found most frequently. Almost all the neoplasms encountered are squamous carcinomas along with some basal cell cancers. In addition, salivary gland malignancies occur infrequently. The lesions develop as an ulcerated or exophytic lesion with firm edges. Lymphatic drainage is to submental or submaxillary nodes. Spread to these locations is relatively late, and initial treatment of T1 and T2 lesions usually does not require resection or irradiation of regional nodes. The neoplasms may be somewhat painful and bleed, but many patients do not seek medical advice until this type of cancer is far advanced. In the case of T1 and T2 lesions, irradiation gives results that compare with those from resection. It is especially useful for lesions occupying a position at the commissures. A most useful and frequent approach to treatment is resection, however. Hyperkeratoses and carcinomas in situ require only superficial excision with advancement of a flap of mucosa to cover the defect. When the cancer involves no more than one-third of the lip, excision of a V-shaped segment including the lesion with adequate margins is all that is required. Simple approximation of the edges of the wound with closure usually leads to a satisfactory cosmetic result. Larger tumors require the use of flaps to close the defect created by removal of the cancer. A variety of ingenious techniques are available for repair and can lead to an acceptable appearance postoperatively. In the case of T3 and T4 lesions, irradiation is added to resection, the latter in the range of a 6000-cGy

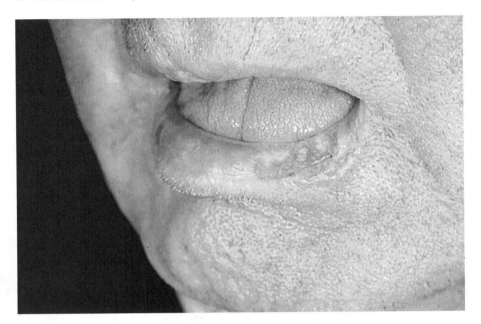

Figure 9 Squamous carcinoma of the lower lip.

tumor dose and 2500-cGy instital therapy. The neck dissection and irradiation of the neck are added even in T3 and T4 cases staged as N0. Resection of the primary site and nodes is done initially, followed by irradiation. In all cases when a margin containing cancer is discovered after resection has been done, irradiation is used as a salvage maneuver.

BUCCAL MUCOSA

Cancers originating in the mucous membrane of the oral cavity are almost all squamous carcinomas, the majority of which are raised above the surface. Many are preceded by white or gray precancerous leukoplakia seen most often in smokers. (Isotretinoin is reported to control precancerous leukoplakia and reduce the incidence of secondary cancer.) They may bleed and become painful, especially when the patient is eating. The extent and thickness of the lesions are correlated with prognosis. The lymph nodes in the upper neck can be involved, and selective neck dissection or irradiation is always included in the treatment of advanced T3 and T4 cancers. Primary T1 and T2 lesions can be treated successfully either with resection or irradiation, the latter being suitable only in superficial T1 and T2 cancers. Irradiation is especially suitable for cancers involving the commissures. Advanced cancer can extend into both or either alveolar ridge. Resection is the usual primary approach with removal of all structures invaded. This can include resection of a full thickness area of the cheek which then may require repair with flap or free graft using recent successful techniques. Irradiation may be a necessary addition subsequent to the operation.

ALVEOLAR RIDGE AND FLOOR OF THE MOUTH

The alveolar ridge has a basic bone structure including the teeth and overlying gingival mucosa. The upper ridge constitutes the outer inferior margins of the maxilla, and the lower ridge is the superior portion of the mandible. The retromolar trigone is located in the angle between the upper and lower portions of the ridge along the anterior margin of the mandibular ramus on either side. Cancers occurring in these locations occur more often in men and are predominantly squamous carcinomas and present as exophytic or ulcerating tumors, the latter more likely to be invasive. Lymphatic drainage is in the submental and upper anterior portion of the neck. Some of the common symptoms and signs consist of pain, bleeding at times, loosening of the teeth, and problems with wearing dentures. Size and extent of the tumor are related to the prognosis and likelihood of lymphatic invasion. These tumors are almost always treated by resection, although sometimes carcinoma of the retromolar trigone are treated by irradiation alone. If the patient is fortunate enough to have a lesion that will permit preservation of the integrity of the mandible, this is done. It is unfortunate that the cancer often has invaded sufficiently deeply to indicate a segmental mandibular resection and reconstruction. Because these neoplasms tend to spread to regional nodes, specific neck dissections, usually in regions I and II, frequently are indicated along with resection of the primary site. In the case of those classified as T3 and above, irradiation given after surgical resection is administered also. As is the case for other cancers of the mouth, the result of treatment depends in large part on the size of the primary tumor and extent of metastatic disease.

The floor of the mouth extends from the mandible laterally to the base of the tongue posteriorly. Cancer that appears there is most often squamous carcinoma. Neoplasms of salivary gland origin occur but are seen much more rarely. The tumors tend to be painful and invasive, extending to the lymph nodes in the superior and anterior neck, sometimes bilaterally. Surgical ablation is often used to treat these cancers, and the procedure may include partial resection of the tongue and mandible, depending on how far the malignant cells have invaded. In all cases, resection of regional nodes is considered. Irradiation can be used alone either combined with implantation therapy or using each type of therapy alone. The vocal cords and adjacent thyroid cartilage and the spinal cord must be shielded and compensatory fields designed when the neck is irradiated. The tumor dose used is in the region of 6000 cGy with

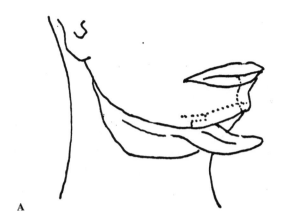

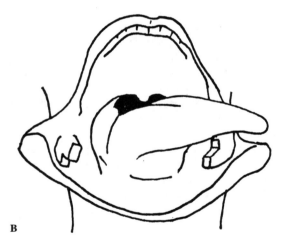

Figure 10 A. The dotted lines outline the incision when it is necessary to incise the lip for wider exposure of neoplasms in the oral cavity and the division of the mandible when wider exposure is necessary. Also illustrated is access to the mouth and neck through an inframandibular approach. B. Incision through lower lip and division of mandible for wider exposure of more distal posterior malignancies.

less in the lower neck and more when margins are found to contain malignant cells that justify additional radiation. Reconstruction following resection requires considerable skill but can be done with satisfactory obliteration of the defect and reasonable recovery of function. Lesions classified as T3 and beyond are usually treated by a combination of resection and irradiation with the latter following the surgical procedure. The results of treatment are related to the extent of the original disease.

TONGUE

Cancer of the tongue is more prevalent in the male population, and epidermoid carcinoma is the type encountered most frequently. Salivary gland tumors are seen much less commonly. Pain, bleeding, and some trouble with deglutition and speech accompany the disease as it progresses. The tongue extends from the floor of the mouth to the circumvallate papillae easily seen on the surface. The bulk of the organ is composed of the genio-, hyo-, palato-, and styloglossus muscles supplied by the hypoglossal nerves. The lymphatic drainage is abundant, with cancer cells migrating chiefly to regions I, II, and III. As in other regions of the oral cavity some of the malignant lesions exhibit surface ulceration and have a tendency to penetrate surrounding tissue more aggressively, whereas others are exophytic in appearance and not quite so aggressive.

Both surgical resection and irradiation constitute effective treatment for carcinoma of the tongue. The cancers originating in the tongue have a greater tendency to invade lymphatics earlier than those at other sites within the oral cavity. For that reason, most plans for therapy include either neck resection or irradiation of the nodal areas in the neck. Brachytherapy using iridium 192 or conventional teleroentgen therapy can be administered either alone or together. Resection frequently involves hemiglossectomy and may require removal of a segment of the mandible and appropriate neck dissection. The carrier for the iridium sometimes is placed at the time of operation and loading with radioactive isotope carried out later. The more advanced the cancer, the poorer the prognosis and the greater the need for combination therapy. Cancers classified as T1 and exophytic tumors classified as T3 and T4 can be treated with irradiation in doses as high as 5000 cGy supplemented by 3000 cGy of interstitial therapy. An operative approach can be used for both small and early cancers and those that are advanced. The usual approach is to include neck dissection, which gives access to the part of the tongue bearing the cancer and wide resection including block dissection of adjacent structures such as the mandible that have been invaded. Irradiation is usually added after the resection has been completed. Extensive experience over many years with both surgical and radiation therapy offers considerable reassurance to patients with carcinoma of the tongue. Even with extensive resections and radiation, functional recovery is usually achieved. Recurrence is usually within the lymph nodes, and additional irradiation is the most common approach to therapy.

BASE OF THE TONGUE

The base of the tongue extends from the circumvallate papillae to the epiglottis. Cancer of the base of the tongue consists principally of squamous carcinomas, with minor salivary gland tumors occurring much less frequently. The tendency for nodal metastases to be present is very great, and treatment usually includes irradiation or resection of cervical nodes even in T1 and T2 lesions. Grade T1 and T2 cancers can be treated either by resection or irradiation. Surgical procedures require access through the neck or by means of a midline incision in lip and tongue. Radiotherapy amounting to a tumor dose of 5000 cGy or more can be given through external ports supplemented by interstitial iridium 196 implants up to 3000 cGy. Treatment of nodal metastases is bilateral when the primary lesion is adjacent to or in the midline. Advanced cancer is treated by resection of primary lesion and appropriate groups of cervical lymph nodes followed by irradiation. When implants are used, split dosage is indicated at times. Also it may be necessary to do a laryngectomy, leaving the patient with a tracheostomy. Supraglottic resection is sometimes possible but not in those with respiratory problems. These more extensive operations are indicated because either the cancer has extended into the larynx or the removal of the cancer along with margins of tissue free of cancer will result in impairment of swallowing and initiate great problems with aspiration necessitating separation of digestive and respiratory tracts. Formerly a segment of mandible was removed in many of these cases, but this is rarely necessary with current surgical techniques and better knowledge of the patterns of invasion of cancer involving the base of the tongue.

OROPHARYNX

The oropharynx is composed of the base of the tongue, the soft palate, the tonsillar fossae, and the posterior pharyngeal wall. Etiologic factors and predominance in men correspond with these characteristics in other regions of the oral cavity. The neoplasms that occur in this region are squamous and adenocarcinomas of different types in approximately equal numbers. The N and M staging of these tumors is the same as for other tumors of the head and neck. The T staging appears below:

T1	Tumor ≤2 cm
T2	Tumor >2 to 4 cm
T3	Tumor >4 cm
T4	Tumor invades adjacent soft tissues and/or bone

Staging usually requires radiographic as well as physical examination. Lymphatic drainage is extensive to regions II, III, IV, and V and retropharyngeal nodes. Neck dissection or irradiation, therefore, is a frequent accompaniment of treatment of the primary cancer. Smaller and earlier lesions can be treated by resection with access provided by a lower central labial incision. Hemiglossectomy is often required along with neck dissection. Also, irradiation can be used to treat these lesions effectively. External beam dosage of between 5000 and 6000 cGy and interstitial iridium brachytherapy up to 3000 cGy have been used in combination. The treatment of larger and more advanced lesions classified as T4 present a greater challenge. When removal of the base of the tongue threatens problems with deglutition and aspiration, laryngectomy must be considered, especially in those with respiratory problems. Resection of the mandible is necessary infrequently. After initial treatment, when recurrence ensues, interstitial therapy, sometimes with split periods of treatment, is successful at times. Current surgical techniques to bridge defects resulting from resection have reduced the necessity of laryngectomy and have improved functional results. Also the radiologist has much more to offer in the way of advanced treatment plans than in former years.

HARD PALATE

Cancer of the hard palate can be superficial and localized or infiltrative, extending over a larger area than superficial examination suggests. The histologic types are divided between squamous and adenocarcinomas of salivary gland origin approximately equally. Surgical extirpation is suitable both for early and more advanced lesions. This involves a partial inferior maxillectomy requiring immediate prosthetic placement for providing adequate speech and maintaining deglutition when the defect created cannot be closed. Subsequent repair is sometimes possible. Radiotherapy is added to the plan of treatment at times when the margins for resection are questionable and there is nodal and/or neural involvement. Spread to regional lymph nodes is not encountered frequently. Irradiation can be used alone successfully when the cancer has extended to soft palate and retromolar trigone.

TONSILS, TONSILLAR PILLARS, AND SOFT PALATE

The tonsillar pillars, composed of the palatoglossal and palatopharyngeal muscles and overlying mucosa, enclose a fossa containing the tonsil. Most of the cancers are squamous carcinomas, but minor salivary gland tumors, lymphomas, and lymphoepitheliomas occur occasionally. Tumors in the tonsillar fossa are more apt to be advanced than those originating in other sites. Metastases are found in the lymph nodes of the upper cervical region including the retropharyngeal nodes. Because of the frequency of lymphatic spread, treatment usually includes therapy directed to appropriate groups of cervical nodes. When a decision is made to observe rather than to treat lymph nodes, it is usually when an early primary cancer originates in the soft palate. Either resection or irradiation can be used to treat small cancers detected early. External beam irradiation in combination with interstitial brachytherapy or the former can be used. Access can be gained by a lip-splitting incision if the approach is surgical. In advanced T3 and T4 cancers, resection of primary and metastatic sites is carried out initially. At times extension into the mandible necessitates partial resection. The surgical procedure is then followed by irradiation.

PHARYNGEAL WALL

The posterolateral aspect of the oropharynx has lymphatics draining into retropharyngeal and upper cervical lymph nodes. The cancers appearing in the wall are squamous carcinomas in most of the cases. An occasional minor salivary gland tumor may be seen in this location as well. Early T1 and T2 cancers can be treated either by resecting or irradiating them. The surgical approach is through the neck at the level of the hyoid and includes bilateral neck dissection. Problems with swallowing subsequent to treatment are more frequent following resection than when irradiation is used. Advanced T3 and T4 cancers are usually treated with resection, which often consists of pharyngolaryngectomy and almost always includes neck dissection. This is followed by irradiation therapy. Great care must be taken to shield the spinal cord adequately and to adjust ports and dosages to avoid any field having inadequate dosage. The resections of advanced cancers must include reconstructive procedures that may include musculocutaneous grafts, gastric mobilization and anastomosis, and either colojejunal interposition or free jejunal implants with microanastomosis. The multiple approaches to therapy of these somewhat inaccessible lesions used over the years are evidence for the difficulty they present for achieving early diagnosis and successful therapy. The percentage of success in treating cancer of the pharyngeal wall is gradually improving and doubtless will respond additionally to continued study and clinical trials.

NASOPHARYNX

The nasopharynx is situated between the antrum of the nasal cavity and the hypopharynx. The eustachian tubes are situated in the lateral wall and communicate with the inner ear. Most of the cancers appear in the lateral pharyngeal recess on either side. The mucosa is composed of mucociliary epithelium which is columnar and stratified. The three types of carcinomas appearing in the nasopharynx are classified by the World Health Organization as (1) keratinizing squamous carcinoma, (2) nonkeratinizing carcinoma, and (3) undifferentiated neoplasms often exhibiting an infiltrate of lymphocytes and called lymphoepitheliomas. The tumor staging used for the nasopharynx follows:

TX	Tumor not accessible
T0	No evidence of primary
Tis	Tumor in situ
T1	One locus
T2	> one locus
T3	Invasion of oropharynx and/or nasal cavity
T4	Invasion of cranial nerves and/or skull

Abundant lymphatic drainage of the nasopharynx provides the setting for spread of the cancers arising in the region to the regional nodes and beyond. In most cases this has occurred before the primary is detected, and often the first sign of malignancy is a mass in the neck. Spread to the retropharyngeal nodes and other loci is more easily detected by radiographic study than physical examination. Bilateral involvement of cervical nodes is not uncommon. Among other signs and symptoms associated with these neoplasms are pain, hearing impairment, tinnitus, otitis media, trismus, and involvement of cranial nerves (more often the first six).

Other than taking a biopsy, an operative approach to these cancers has only a minor role to play in therapy. Access is difficult, and complications have been discouraging in trying to combat larger lesions by this mean. There are occasions, however, when resection of a small tumor and recurrence limited in size is indicated. Irradiation is the most successful form of treatment and yields gratifying control in many cases of T1 and T2 cancer. Also it is possible to control disease in the cervical nodes with irradiation, although surgical resection, especially with recurrence, can be used as well. The dosage of irradiation often is in the range of 6500 to 7000 cGy or 5000 cGy plus 2500 to 3000 cGy interstitial irradiation. Multiple ports arranged as a three-dimensional approach to cross-fire the tumor has almost eliminated the problem of undertreatment of some areas of the target. Radiotherapy may include the traditional ports plus intracavitary irradiation to solve some of the problems presented by these tumors. Additional irradiation for recurrent disease can be successful. This can also include permanent iodine 125 implants for small foci of recurrent carcinoma. Chemotherapy at low dosage with such agents as 5-fluorouracil and cisplatin is used increasingly as radiosensitizers to improve the results of radiotherapy.

Chemotherapy constitutes an increasingly frequent addition to the treatment of nasopharyngeal carcinoma. Both single agents and combinations of agents have been used, but the number of cases is not great at the present time and many of the studies are not designed to study cancer in this location exclusively. Some of the agents that have been used are bleomycin, carboplatin, cisplatin, cyclophosphamide, doxorubicin, epirubicin, 5-fluorouracil, methotrexate, mitomycin, nitrosourea, vinblastine, and vincristine. So far, combinations with platinum compounds have yielded the best responses, and combinations have been superior to single drugs. Because of the limited information obtained so far from clinical trials, no conclusions concerning possible advantages of using induction or concomitant chemotherapy with irradiation are justified. Joining a group in a clinical trial is indicated at times as long as the patient understands the conditions for entering. Results using interferon-γ have not been very encouraging. It appears that chemotherapy will assume a standardized place in plans for treatment as more experience is acquired.

HYPOPHARYNX

The hypopharynx is situated above the esophagus and below the oropharynx and is behind or posterior to the larynx. Its component parts are the postpharyngeal wall, the lateral pyriform sinuses, and the postcricoid region. Approximately one-third of the cancers appear in each of the pyriform sinuses and the postpharyngeal and postcricoid regions combined, far fewer appearing in the postcricoid region. Almost all the neoplasms that appear in the hypopharynx are epidermoid (squamous) carcinomas, which frequently are poorly differentiated and resistant to treatment. Lymphatics are abundant in the hypopharynx, and approximately one-fourth of the primary neoplasms have spread to distant sites when first seen. Even among those patients exhibiting no evidence of nodal invasion at first, many are found later to harbor the neoplasm in the lymph nodes. The groups involved most frequently are those situated in regions II and III in the neck. In addition to the usual groups of cervical nodes, paratracheal, retropharyngeal, and thyroid gland sites also can be involved. Cancers appearing in the hypopharynx are often multiple and ulcerated and seem to develop in a widespread field of susceptible mucosa. They can invade the thyroid cartilage when originating in the pyriform sinuses or the cricoid when they appear in the postcricoid region. Although they are encountered less frequently in the postcricoid region than at other sites, cancers in that location can spread laterally and invade the fibers of the recurrent nerves and cause paralysis of the vocal cords. The submucosa and lymphatics provide available conduits for spread both upward and downward as high as the base of the skull and as low as the paraesophageal lymphatics. When the postpharyngeal wall and to a lesser extent when the postcricoid region is the primary site, the spread may be bilateral.

Alcohol intake and smoking are correlated with the appearance of these neoplasms, which also seem to occur more often in patients with iron-deficiency anemia (Plummer-Vinson syndrome) and those with nutritional problems including malabsorption of vitamin B_{12}. Although in proximity, cancers of the hypopharynx are usually more difficult to treat successfully than those in the larynx. In the United States these neoplasms appear more often in men in the upper hypopharynx and more often in women in the lower hypopharynx. Cancer of the hypopharynx is not visible when the usual physical examination is done, and this contributes to the characteristic late diagnosis of the tumors. Also the abundant lymphatic bed leading to the frequent and early spread of the disease, nutritional problems, poor physical condition of many of the patients, and multiple sites in some cases all contribute to the formidable problems cancer of the hypopharynx presents for effective therapy.

The staging of hypopharyngeal cancer is similar to staging of laryngeal cancer. The tumor designation is somewhat different, however, and appears below:

TX	Primary not accessible
T0	No evidence of primary
Tis	Carcinoma in situ
T1	Carcinoma, one locus
T2	Adjacent spread without fixation
T3	Adjacent spread with fixation
T4	Extensive invasion soft tissues, cartilage, and bone

Symptoms and signs that can appear with the advent of hypopharyngeal cancer are dysphagia, otalgia, hoarseness, pooling of secretions in the region, aspiration of secretions, and enlargement of cervical nodes. Some of the reasons that the diagnosis is made late in the course of the disease are: many symptoms and signs are caused by extension of the disease such as the hoarseness caused by invasion of the recurrent nerves, the patient may have problems resulting from other diseases or smoking too much or drinking alcohol in excess leading to numerous symptoms some of which are caused by the hypopharyngeal cancer but are attributed to the other problems, and symptoms such as pain in the ear can lead to an erroneous diagnosis. Visualization of the hypopharynx must be carried out to make a definitive diagnosis. This can be done with a flexible endoscope or with a light and mirror in the hands of a skilled examiner. Radiographic visualization with contrast material also may be useful. Biopsy and determination of the exact extent of the neoplasm and the general condition of the patient with correction of other problems insofar as possible are then necessary before treatment can begin.

Early and small cancers of the hypopharynx can be cured by either irradiation or resection. Unfortunately many cases are advanced when discovered with few in T1 or T2 groups, and therefore a combination of operative treatment with irradiation is the approach used most often. For example, invasion of cricoid or thyroid cartilages eliminates irradiation as the only therapy indicated. Operation precedes the treatment with irradiation unless there is some special reason for departure from this sequence. Any decision about the method of management requires consideration of the extent of the primary disease, the presence or absence of metastases and their location, whether and how much laryngeal invasion has occurred, and the performance status of the patient. Pharyngoscopy, laryngoscopy, and NMR examination usually help define the problem in anatomic terms. Use of 6000 to 7000 cGy of irradiation is within the usual range of radiotherapy. Exophytic tumors seem to respond best, but exophytic areas may be mixed with ulcerated areas in some tumors characterized by a less favorable response to therapy.

Most of the cancers of the hypopharynx have spread to cervical nodes by the time treatment is initiated, and this aspect of the problem must be addressed either by irradiation or specific neck dissection or a combination of both. Retropharyngeal cancers spread bilaterally most of the time. Decisions about plans for treatment require experience and careful evaluation. For example, when the primary cancer is small and secondary spread is much greater, irradiation can be done first with an appropriate type of neck dissection to follow. If no operation is planned, then the radiation dosage is usually higher. The operation then can be used only for salvage if the response to irradiation is not satisfactory. One paramount question to be answered is whether and how much of the larynx should be resected. When a postcricoid cancer is resected, a total laryngectomy is almost always done. Some small and thin cancers located in the postpharyngeal wall can be removed and the larynx remain. However this is not advocated for debilitated patients or those of advanced age. Large resections of the pharynx can lead to major difficulties in swallowing following the concomitant derangement in innervation. Partial laryngopharyngectomy is occasionally indicated, but unfortunately preservation of the larynx is not appropriate in most cases of hypopharyngeal cancer. Repair after resection (laryngopharyngectomy and laryngopharyngoesophagectomy) has been improved in recent years through the use of myocutaneous flaps, free jejunal grafts with microvascular anastomoses, gastric transposition, and colon-jejunal interposition. When irradiation is administered, the tumor dose is usually in the range of 5000 to 7000 cGy. Also the tracheostomy stoma must be irradiated over a period of about 2 months after laryngectomy with a dose of 6000 to 6500 cGy.

Chemotherapy has been used as one modality of combined therapy, but insufficient experience has been obtained for general conclusions to be drawn about how it may best be used in the treatment of hypopharyngeal cancer. With the passage of time, additional clinical trials should clarify the value of chemotherapy. Currently one of the problems is that trials in the past have not focused exclusively on cases of hypopharyngeal cancer alone.

Patients with cancer of the hypopharynx should not allow the difficulties in treating the disease to discourage them unduly. A great deal can be done to combat the disease. Lengthy experience with operative treatment and irradiation has clarified what each can offer singly and together. The techniques of both have been refined extensively into more effective weapons against this type of neoplasm. Many studies have revealed the nature and behavior of the cancers that arise in the hypopharynx, so the clinician is prepared to extend management to combat possible late complications. The response of early and localized cancer to current methods of management is gratifying in that cures occur in many cases, and much can be done with other patients who have more extensive disease.

LARYNX

Carcinoma of the larynx occurs in older age groups of patients and has been the subject of exhaustive studies on the best methods of management. It has become apparent that the exact site of any laryngeal malignancy affects the outcome of treatment, and therefore the anatomy of the larynx in relationship to the location of a malignancy must be known with precision. This relationship is also important in predicting possible lymphatic spread. The larynx is divided into the supraglottis consisting of epiglottis and false cords, the glottis consisting of the true vocal cords, and the subglottis. Cancer of the larynx appears to be associated with both smoking and drinking alcoholic beverages. The preponderance of the disease in men is gradually being erased, probably as a result of changing social habits. The association between cancer and imbibing alcohol is stronger for supraglottic than for glottic neoplasms. Other factors reported to be causal are asbestosis, gastric reflux, irritants causing chronic laryngitis, diet, irradiation, etc., but the most consistent etiologic relationship continues to be smoking and drinking alcohol.

The framework of the larynx is composed of several cartilages including the epiglottis, the thyroid cartilage, the paired arytenoids, and the cricoid. In addition, the small corniculate cartilages located within the posterior portion of the aryepiglottic folds articulate with the arytenoids and extend posteriorly and medially. Also the two cuneiform cartilages are located within the aryepiglottic fold anterior to the arytenoids. The aryepiglottic folds constitute the boundary between the larynx and hypopharynx, and neoplasms situated in this location are often called marginal tumors. Those lateral to the summit of the fold tend to have characteristics similar to those appearing within the hypopharynx, and those located medially within the endolarynx usually behave like supraglottic tumors. The true vocal cords, attached to the arytenoids, are adducted and abducted when these cartilages rotate horizontally in response to stimuli conducted by the recurrent nerves. The margin of the cords is covered by pseudostratified squamous epithelium with an underlying fibro-elastic and gelatinous lamina propria ideal for the fibration responsible for the voice. The remainder of the laryngeal epithelium consists of ciliated columnar cells. The presence of a neoplasm can easily impair endolaryngeal mobility of the vocal cords and give rise to symptoms quite early in the disease. For this reason greater numbers of early malignant and premalignant lesions are reported for the glottis than for lesions higher or lower in the larynx.

Lymphatics in the supraglottis are numerous and widespread and drain laterally and superiorly through deep cervical channels via the thyrohyoid membrane between the thyroid and hyoid cartilages, the latter being located just above the thyroid cartilage. As would be expected from this anatomic information, metastases from the supraglottic region are numerous. On the other hand, lymphatics in the glottis are scarce or nonexistent, and the presence of metastases, especially in early lesions, is not as great a possibility when the management of cancer in this location is planned. Lymphatics are profuse in the subglottic region, and metastases escape via the cricothyroid membrane spreading laterally and inferiorly into the deep cervical nodes. There is very little tendency for spread of metastases downward from the supraglottic region or upward from the subglottic region. Extension laterally from the primary site on one side to the other is not found very often in early tumors. Thus it is possible to consider the problem of treating cancers of the larynx a matter of separate compartments with some boundaries that are not breached in the ordinary course of events, especially in the cases of early and localized neoplasms. It has led to the practice of partial resection of the organ with the realistic anticipation of successful cure and more limited alteration in function.

Approximately 95 percent of neoplasms of the larynx are squamous cell cancers. Neuroendocrine tumors are diagnosed more frequently now than in former years, and adenocarcinomas along with sarcomas constitute most of the remaining malignancies. Much progress has been made in prognosticating the response of early and small superficial tumors from their anatomic appearance grossly and under the microscope. This is most useful in the case of glottic tumors. These tumors may be localized or can be diagnosed as dysplasia, carcinoma in situ, or invasive cancer. Also all three types can be found within one area at times. Supraglottic tumors tend to be more undifferentiated and both supraglottic and subglottic neoplasms are more difficult to treat. In general, the thickness of a neoplasm and the depth of invasion are related to its resistance to therapy and the presence of metastases.

Thorough examination of the patient and the larynx is essential before any treatment is even proposed. Not only the localization but the extent of a tumor and its extension can be determined with surprising precision. Examination of the larynx with the flexible laryngoscope is carried out with the patient awake in the sitting position. Detection of any alteration in surface contour, mobility, and the presence of tethering of the mucosal surface may require the use of the stroboscope. Invasion of cartilage and regional lymph nodes can be ascertained by the use of computerized tomography or nuclear magnetic resonance imaging. The presence of either or both alters planning of treatment. After diagnostic studies have been completed, staging can be determined and an overall plan of management delineated. The scheme for staging neoplasms of the larynx usually used is that outlined by the American Joint Commission on Staging, the salient features of which are outlined in the table below. The usual information about tumor (T), regional nodes (N), and distant metastases (M) is indicated.

TNM classification for laryngeal cancer

Supraglottis
Tis	Carcinoma in situ
T1	Localized, mobility unimpaired
T2	Glottis or adjacent spread, mobility unimpaired
T3	Limited to larynx with fixation
T4	Extralaryngeal spread

Glottis
Tis	Carcinoma in situ
T1	Cords invaded, mobility unimpaired
T2	Supra- or subglottic extension, mobility unimpaired
T3	Within larynx, cord immobile
T4	Extralaryngeal spread, thyroid cartilage destruction

Subglottis
Tis	Carcinoma in situ
T1	Subglottis only
T2	Extension to cords
T3	Cords immobile
T4	Extralaryngeal spread or cartilage destruction

Stage
I	T1	N0	M0
II	T2	N0	M0
III	T3	N0	M0
	T1, T2, or T3	N1	M0
IV	T4	N0, or N1	M0
	Any T	N2, or N3	M0
	Any T	Any N	M

Extensive experience has been acquired during years of management of laryngeal carcinoma with both surgical procedures and irradiation. More recently, a beginning has been made in evaluating the usefulness of chemotherapy in managing responsive tumors. In general, early and small neoplasms respond favorably both to resection and irradiation, but irradiation is seldom useful as the primary approach for treating larger and more widespread lesions. Comparisons of limited resections to total laryngectomy reveal that regional or limited resection can yield results that justify this more conservative approach, depending on the location and extent of the neoplasm being treated. Lateral and frontal vertical hemilaryngectomies, transverse hemilaryngectomy, partial pharyngolaryngectomy, and cordectomy all have a place in the armamentarium against this malignancy. The possible presence of involved lymph nodes must always be considered in management, and again the usual behavior of these tumors is helpful in making decisions about whether, where, and when neck dissection or the use of irradiation should be done.

Responsiveness to treatment of laryngeal carcinoma varies in the three major regions. Most cancers of the supraglottis originate in the epiglottis, and many times it is difficult to determine exactly the point of origin of larger neoplasms or whether they may have originated in the hypopharynx. Both irradiation and resection are effective in the successful treatment of smaller lesions. One question that always arises in these tumors is how to manage possible nodal involvement. Even when diagnostic studies fail to reveal cancer in the nodes, an aggressive approach is justified from past experience with failures resulting from inadequate control of nodal extension. An advantage of irradiation is that it can be used to treat both the tumor and regional nodes. However, failure means that surgical salvage may include total laryngectomy. In experienced hands, horizontal hemilaryngectomy not only can result in cures but also can preserve laryngeal function. When done, neck dissection and possible postoperative irradiation are additional necessities. The supraglottic or horizontal hemilaryngectomy is usually not considered in patients with pulmonary disease or in those who have had antecedent irradiation. Except in unusual circumstances, irradiation follows operation when both are used. Total laryngectomy combined with measures directed toward treating involved regional nodes is required for extensive malignancies. Radical neck dissection is no longer done with any frequency, and a regional approach to attack only those groups of nodes most apt to be involved is singularly appropriate for laryngeal cancers.

Carcinoma in situ of the glottis can be treated quite effectively with removal by means of scalpel or laser. They also can be cured with irradiation. Chemotherapy is useful at times to enhance the effect of radiotherapy. Larger lesions respond both to irradiation and vertical hemilaryngectomy. Lymphatic extension is much less likely because of the scarcity of lymphatics in this portion of the larynx. When irradiation is given, fraction sizes should be 200 cGy or greater. Superfractionation has yielded better results in the management of some of the larger tumors. Total laryngectomy is sometimes necessary when the more conservative measures have failed.

Subglottic cancer is most difficult to treat and often is extensive when first detected. At times these tumors even spread into the paratracheal nodes within the mediastinum. The wisest choice for management can be laryngectomy with tracheostomy, resection of regional nodes, and irradiation. Thyroidectomy can be indicated as well.

Chemotherapeutic agents such as cisplatin and 5-fluorouracil have been used as induction therapy, and doubtless many more clinical trials will be forthcoming to determine what chemotherapy can contribute to the control of laryngeal cancers. Planning the management of a laryngeal cancer requires extensive review of current results of clinical trials, and often the use of multiple modalities of treatment is indicated. Fortunately the types of cancer encountered most often, those of the glottis, are the ones treated most successfully; these arise where there are few lymphatics, they give rise to symptoms early in their course, and cures are achieved often without loss of function or undesirable cosmetic results. Even when laryngectomy is necessary, a tracheoesophageal prosthesis can provide adequate speech, tracheal airway, and satisfactory appearance.

TUMORS OF THE ENDOCRINE GLANDS

The endocrine gland tumors discussed in this section are those of the thyroid, parathyroid, and adrenal glands, carcinoids, pheochromocytomas, multiple endocrine neoplasms, and paragangliomas. The diagnosis of these malignancies includes a careful history to determine whether the characteristic clinical picture of signs and symptoms is present, physical examination, and biopsy providing a tissue diagnosis. Radiographic examination includes scans with appropriate isotopes, computerized tomograms, magnetic resonance imaging, ultrasound studies, and levels of specific electrolytes, hormones, and peptides in the blood and urine. The details of specific diagnostic studies indicated are included in the discussions of each type of these tumors.

Endocrine tumors of the pancreas are discussed in the section on the alimentary tract, those of the pituitary with tumors of the nervous system, and those of the prostate, testis, and ovary with tumors of the genitourinary tract.

THYROID

Nodules and enlargement of the thyroid gland include single and multinodular toxic and nontoxic goiter, thyroiditis, lymphadenoid goiter, adenomas, and carcinoma. Goiters occur most frequently in middle age, but those most likely to contain cancer appear at extremes of ages. Neoplasms are found two or three times more frequently in women than in men. Malignancies usually present clinically as a firm, sometimes fixed, mass in the neck which grows more rapidly than the usual goiter. There may be paralysis of the ipsilateral vocal cord with the passage of time as a result of paralysis of the recurrent nerve. Useful diagnostic measures are radionuclide scans using ^{131}I, which reveal the mass to be a nonfunctional or hypofunctional "cold" tumor and ultrasonography for distinguishing between cystic and solid tumors. (Usually cystic tumors are benign.) Cancer of the thyroid is found more frequently and accounts for more deaths than all other endocrine tumors. Assigning a specific cause in an individual case is usually not possible, but variation in risk is associated with sex, age, familial background, amount of iodine intake, the presence of nodular goiter, level of thyroid stimulating hormone, and exposure to radiation. Objective substantiation of the effect of irradiation has been obtained for populations such as those exposed to background emission in China, atomic bombing in Japan, and patients who had irradiation of the thymus, skin, and enlarged lymph nodes in the early part of the twentieth century in the United States. The K-*ras* oncogene seems to play a role in radiation oncogenesis. Thyroid cancer has been reported to follow a familial dominant pattern in some cases and to be found in conjunction with multiple endocrine neoplastic syndromes IIa and IIb. Microscopic and occult cancers of the thyroid often are found in the gland at autopsy after death from other causes.

Cancers of the thyroid vary widely in their appearance and behavior. The differentiated tumors may grow slowly with their malignant nature revealed only by invasion of capsule or extension via the bloodstream or lymphatic channels. Undifferentiated malignancies grow more rapidly and have an exceedingly poor prognosis. Papillary cancers constitute approximately two-thirds and follicular cancer approximately one-fourth of the malignancies of this organ and have the best prognosis. The former is more likely to spread through the lymphatics and the latter through hemovascular channels. The tall, columnar cell, and diffuse sclerosing types of papillary carcinoma constitute approximately 10 percent of papillary cancers and have a poorer prognosis than the remainder. Although follicular carcinomas constitute less than half as many differentiated carcinomas as papillary carcinomas, they account for twice as many deaths. The prognosis is worse in large tumors appearing in older age groups. Undifferentiated cancers of the thyroid constitute approximately 10 percent of the cases. The incidence seems to be declining, possibly because there has been greater success in differentiating them from other tumors such as lymphomas. The prognosis in these cases is very poor with median survivals of less than 1 year and 5-year survivals of less than 10 percent. Medullary carcinomas constitute approximately 5 percent of malignancies of the thyroid. They secrete calcitonin and other hormones. Determination of calcitonin level is a valuable means of detecting and identifying these tumors. By screening families with the dominant gene and those with either multiple endocrine tumors IIa or IIb, it is possible to detect medullary carcinomas quite early in their course. Primary malignant lymphomas and sarcomas also appear in the thyroid, and occasionally metastases from other organs such as breast and the gastrointestinal tract are deposited in the thyroid. The diagnosis of cancer of the thyroid gland is made most often by needle biopsy of nodules. Negative biopsies of nodules harboring cancer account for a very small percentage of negative biopsies. When a positive diagnosis for cancer or suspicion of cancer is reported, then the lesion should be removed immediately, the extent of resection depending on the specific type of cancer and its size. The detection of metastatic cancer is more difficult.

When a decision has been made for partial or total thyroidectomy, the neck is entered through a transverse "collar" (Kocher) incision which is carried downward through the platysma muscle which is usually somewhat rudimentary. A superior flap of skin and platysma is then developed upward. A midline incision is then made in the fascia, exposing the trachea and thyroid. At times it may be possible to complete the operation without dividing the sternohyoid and sternothyroid (strap) muscles, but usually they are divided between clamps to be left in place until the divided upper and lower margins are closed with a line of sutures after the thyroidectomy is complete. The superior pole is dissected free and the thyroid vessels divided and transfixed with nonabsorbable sutures. The recurrent nerve is visualized, and the blood supply to parathyroid glands preserved when the gland containing the cancer is elevated, and vessels are divided and ligated as they are encountered at the lateral and inferior margins of the gland. The isthmus and medial portion of the contralateral lobe are removed along with the specimen. When the recurrent nerve cannot be saved if adjacent tumor is removed, the surgeon may elect to leave that portion marked with clip(s) in place as markers for later irradiation. Total thyroidectomy consists of extension of the operative procedure described above for the contralateral lobectomy, removing the entire specimen as a single mass. When lymph nodes have been invaded, it may be necessary to extend the lateral limits resulting in an H-shaped incision. A median sternotomy is not necessary very often when a portion of the neoplasm is retrosternal. Careful hemostasis usually is all that is necessary to obviate the need for drains. Sutures in the skin can be removed on the second or third day with a scar that is minimal.

Complications following operation are hemorrhage, paralysis of the recurrent nerve(s), sympathetic nerve damage, paresis of the superior laryngeal nerve, and hypoparathyroidism. Great care to detect hemorrhage, cord paralysis, and hypoparathyroidism in the immediate postoperative period is mandatory. When total thyroidectomy is carried out, immediate thyroid medication is started. Also if a portion of the gland remains, thyroid hormone supplement may be required. Recovery is usually rapid, and adjuvant therapy can be started quite soon after the wound heals.

Except for small tumors confined to the thyroid, a total or almost total thyroidectomy with ^{131}I scanning to detect metastases and for therapy of recurrent cancer in some cases is the management usually advocated for papillary and follicular well differentiated neoplasms of the thyroid. Synthroid (levothyroxine sodium) is given in all cases for suppression of thyroid stimulating hormone. Resection of metastases and recurrences in the neck and distant metastases that are refractory to ^{131}I uptake is often the management method of choice in these cancers. Since so many follicular cancers of Hürthle cell type are benign, the above approach to therapy should not be initiated until an accurate diagnosis of malignancy is made. Doxorubicin has been the only type of chemotherapy that has induced some response of these well differentiated tumors.

Exploitation of the familial setting of medullary cancer, in which multiple endocrine neoplasms IIa and IIb and a dominant susceptibility gene play a role, may consist of repeated provocative testing with calcium and pentagastrin for high calcitonin levels. Total or almost total thyroidectomy should be done in the patients when the diagnosis of medullary carcinoma is made. Best results are obtained when medullary cancer is found without extension beyond the gland. Resection is less successful for extension to lymph nodes and distant metastases. Radiation therapy can be used, but this neoplasm is not very sensitive to irradiation. The use of sensitizers may lead to better results in the future. ^{131}I and ^{99m}Tc have been used to localize metastases and theoretically should be useful in therapy. When the size of metastatic disease is great, symptoms including debilitating diarrhea can be very troublesome as a result of the high levels of calcitonin. This can be alleviated by debulking the tumor mass. Medullary lesions are not very responsive to chemotherapy. Doxorubicin and 5-fluoruridine and dacarbazine have been reported to give some response.

Thyroid resection should be carried out for undifferentiated carcinomas only when they are small and localized. The prognosis is uniformly poor in more extensive disease. Irradiation of approximately 6000 cGy with doxorubicin as sensitizer has been used to treat these malignancies. The best responses have been obtained when doxorubicin or cisplatin has been used for chemotherapy. Other agents used with some suggestion of response are cisplatin with bleomycin; cisplatin, mitroxantrone, and vincristine; and bleomycin, doxorubicin, melphalan, and vincristine combinations.

TNM classification of malignant thyroid tumors (American Joint Committee on Cancer)

TX	Primary cannot be assessed
T0	No evidence of primary cancer
T1	Tumor ≤1 cm
T2	Tumor >1 to <4 cm
T3	Tumor >4 cm
T4	Spread beyond thyroid capsule
NX	Regional nodes cannot be assessed
N1	No nodal metastases
N1A	Local nodal metastases
N1B	Distant nodal metastases

(Continued)

MX	Distant metastases cannot be assessed
M0	No distant metastases
M1	Distant metastases

Staging cancer of the thyroid gland

Papillary or follicular carcinoma >45 years of age			
Stage I	T1	N0	M0
Stage II	T2	N0	M0
Stage III	T4	N0	M0
Papillary or follicular carcinoma <45 years of Age			
Stage I	Any T	Any N	M0
Stage II	Any T	Any N	M1
Medullary carcinoma			
Stage I	T1	N0	M0
Stage II	T2	N0	M0
	T3	N0	M0
	T4	N0	M0
Stage III	Any T	N1	M0
Stage IV	Any T	Any N	M1
Undifferentiated carcinoma			
Stage IV	All cases		

PARATHYROID

The usual number of parathyroid glands is four, but two, three, five, and six glands have been encountered. Also, much to the discomfort of surgeons, their location is not entirely predictable. Hyperparathyroidism with elevated serum calcium levels and concomitant clinical problems is the reason most patients seek medical help for carcinoma. Hyperplasia and adenomas cause the high levels of serum calcium as well. Previous irradiation of the head and neck increases the incidence of hyperparathyroidism, but the associated tumor is adenoma of the parathyroid rather than carcinoma. Single or multiple adenomas are responsible for 80 to 90 percent of cases, carcinomas for 1 to 4 percent, and hyperplasia for the remainder. Hypercalcemia also occurs in cases of multiple myeloma and metastatic disease in the bones. The classic clinical picture of carcinoma of the parathyroid is hypercalcemia, a mass in the neck, renal stones and calcinosis, and osseous decalcification with attendant problems. Serum alkaline phosphatase, urinary cyclic monophophatase, serum parathyroid hormone, and serum calcium are all elevated. Bones ache, the patient may have arthritic symptoms, later there may be abdominal and renal pain, and myopathy can appear later in the disease. Also anorexia, nausea, vomiting, depression, polyuria, and polydipsea are features at times. Carcinomas of the parathyroid occur most frequently during the fifth decade, and isolated cases with a familial pattern of inheritance have been reported. Possibly these may have been on the basis of antecedent hyperplasia, which is associated with multiple endocrine neoplasia syndromes MEN-I and MEN-IIa.

When carcinoma, adenoma, or hyperplasia is suspected, surgery should follow promptly. Preoperatively dehydration and electrolyte imbalance should be corrected with infusions and possibly diuretic administration and even hemodialysis may be required in some cases. It may also be advisable to give 1-alpha-hydroxy-cholecalciferol beforehand to combat possible tetany and hypocalcemia occurring immediately after the surgical correction of the hyperparathyroidism. Also, administration of methylene blue is helpful because it stains the hyperplasia, adenomas, and even malignancies of the parathyroid glands differentially. Otherwise preoperative localization studies are usually deferred until the patient has had at least one exploration of the neck.

The incision and approach to the parathyroid glands is the same as for the thyroid gland. The search for the diseased glands must be conducted with great patience, maintenance of careful hemostasis, and a methodical approach for possible sites where the disease may be localized. The recurrent nerve and inferior thyroid artery are identified and branches of the latter traced to parathyroid tissue which they usually supply. The thyroid is rolled forward gently for better visualization. In addition to the usual position for the four glands, exploration is extended to the tracheoesophageal groove, behind the esophagus, within the carotid sheath, in any groove in the thyroid, the thyrothymic ligament, and within the thymus, and these tumors have even been found within the thyroid. At a second operation a mediastinotomy and exploration may be necessary. Most carcinomas are whitish gray and attached to adjacent tissue. The entire mass including the adjacent thyroid lobe and the isthmus are removed en bloc. Also the ipsilateral lymph nodes are resected as well. External beam radiotherapy is advocated at times in the hope that it will help prevent recurrence. Operative mortality for operations on the parathyroid glands is less than 1 percent.

When the first operation has been unsuccessful, then preoperative localization should be considered before another exploration. It is unfortunate that these tests are expensive, many times equivocal, and require additional time for evaluation. The most successful is selective venous sampling from the superior vena cava, innominate, internal jugular, and small veins from the mediastinum and thyroid. Then each sample is tested for parathyroid hormone level. Unfortunately this test may not distinguish between a mediastinal tumor and one in the neck. Technetium 99m and thallium 201 can be used for obtaining an image of both parathyroid and thyroid glands. The use of ultrasound is much less expensive and can localize tumors in some positions but not in others. Computerized tomography and nuclear magnetic resonance imaging are somewhat limited for localization but can be helpful at times. After conclusion of tests for localization and preoperative preparation of the patient, a second exploration can proceed with a better chance of success.

Metastases from cancer of the parathyroid gland can appear in liver, bone, and lung. The treatment of recurrence and metastatic disease with irradiation has not been very successful. Chemotherapy with dacarbazine alone and combined with 5-fluorouracil and cyclophosphamide has resulted in some response in isolated cases. Debulking the cancer may help somewhat when the derangement in serum calcium is devastating and difficult to control. Early diagnosis and immediate treatment is the difference between success and the failure of delay.

ADRENAL

Hyperplasia of the adrenal glands associated with hypercortisolism is present in pituitary Cushing's disease and also when tumors such as oat cell carcinomas, carcinoids, pancreatic endocrine tumors, medullary thyroid carcinomas, pheochromocytomas, and ovarian adenocarcinomas produce an ectopic adrenocorticotrophic (ACTH) syndrome of hypercortisolism. Adenomas of the adrenal glands are usually less than 5 cm in size and are associated with hypercortisolism and hyperaldosteronism syndromes. Approximately half of the tumors occurring in the adrenal glands are benign and half are malignant. Great care must be taken to avoid missing the correct diagnosis of a malignancy masquerading as a benign adenoma.

Adrenocortical carcinomas occur at any age with peak incidences around age 5 and later in the fifth and sixth decades. More men than women develop nonfunctioning malignant adrenal tumors, and more women than men develop functioning malignancies. Most of these neoplasms have invaded locally or spread to distant sites when first diagnosed. However, they occur rarely, with an incidence of about two cases per million people. About half or more are palpable at the time of diagnosis when the abdomen is examined. Endocrine manifestations include Cushing's syndrome, precocious puberty, aldosteronism, feminization in men, virilization in women, and mixtures of these symptoms. Cushing's syndrome is the result of excessive amounts of glucocorticoids; among the symptoms that can follow are atrophy of the skin, acne, obesity of face and neck and trunk with typical "buffalo hump," osteoporosis, weakness, purple striae, poor healing of wounds, hypertension, edema, glucose intolerance, hirsutism of face, amenorrhea, and depression. Approximately half of adrenocortical carcinomas are functional tumors and half are nonfunctional. As a result of inadequate steroid production, nonfunctioning tumors and some functioning tumors are diagnosed late in the course of the disease when the tumors are very large and often have metastases. These large tumors may cause symptoms of abdominal pain, fatigue, and weight loss, and hemorrhage within them may result in fever, more severe pain, and even shock.

Among the tests in use to differentiate between Cushing's disease, ectopic sources of ACTH, adenomas, and carcinomas of the adrenal are determination of plasma ACTH, 24-h free unconjugated cortisol, single-dose overnight and low-dose dexamethasone suppression of cortisol secretion, and both 17-hydroxysterone and plasma ACTH after metyrapone. The most useful and widely used imaging technic for studying adrenal tumors is computerized tomography. Its use offers the detection of invasion and involvement of lymph nodes and liver, although differentiation between adenomas, carcinomas, hematomas, and lymphomas is not possible. The addition of selective angiography is sometimes helpful in determining operability. Magnetic resonance imaging is useful in determining whether there is invasion of adjacent vascular structures. Radionuclide imaging offers some additional diagnostic aid with and without catheterization of the adrenal vein. Also preoperatively it may aid in distinguishing carcinomas, pheochromocytomas, and adrenal metastases from adrenal adenomas, cysts, and lipomas. Some clinicians prefer to follow patients with tumors less than 3 cm in size with radiographic studies, advising operation only when growth occurs.

Resection of adrenal adenomas frequently results in cure. Since many are less than 4 cm in size, it may be possible to preserve some of the normal adrenal tissue at times. Obesity, hypertension, and temporary morbidity may persist after operation in those patients with Cushing's syndrome. Also, treatment with glucocortisol supplement may be necessary for some time. When hyperaldosteronism is present, the hypertension and metabolic derangements must be corrected preoperatively, monitored postoperatively, and adjusted thereafter when necessary. It can be difficult to distinguish between a benign adenoma and carcinoma, with invasion and metastatic foci the only gross distinguishing features. Any tumor larger than 6 cm is suspected to be malignant.

The only means available for curing adrenocortical carcinoma is surgical resection. Even if the resection is incomplete, operation can be beneficial, especially in the case of functioning tumors because of the resulting reduction in symptoms. Utilizing a transabdominal or thoracoabdominal approach, a radical resection, including adjacent invaded organs and lymph nodes, should be done when there is any chance of curative removal of the entire mass. This can include the vena cava if replacement can be accomplished as part of the procedure. Wedge resection of any hepatic metastases that are resectable should be done at the time of primary removal of the tumor mass. Steroid replacement therapy must be judiciously given as indicated.

Radiotherapy has been a useful adjunct for the relief of pain in bone containing metastatic tumor. Mitotane (*ortho,para*-DDD [*o,p'*-DDD]) has been used widely for the treatment of inoperable adrenocortical carcinoma, but the undesirable side effects of neuromuscular toxicity, gastrointestinal toxicity, and skin rash limit its usefulness. Results with other chemotherapeutic agents have been disappointing. A few complete and incomplete responses have been obtained with the use of suramin alone, cisplatin, cyclophosphamide, doxorubicin, and 5-fluorouracil alone and in combination, and bleomycin, etoposide, melphalan, Methyl-CCNU, and vincristine each in combination with other agents. Used most frequently are mitotane; cisplatin with or without etoposide; doxorubicin; and at times aminoglutethimide, ketoconazole, or metyrapone. Surgical cure is possible at this time only in patients with tumors confined to the adrenal gland in stage I and stage II. The 5-year survival of patients with stage I disease is not more than 50 percent. For those with local and distal spread the 5-year survival is approximately 10 percent. Adjuvant therapy is obviously needed for use even in early stage disease, but unfortunately none that is promising has been discovered up to the present time.

The two important malignant lesions of the adrenal medulla are neuroblastomas and pheochromocytomas. Neuroblastomas arise from neuroblasts in the adrenal medulla and in ganglia and appear within the first 5 years of life. They may appear as small tumors at times but can present as an extremely large retroperitoneal mass before being discovered. This malignancy invades the capsule and spreads along tissue planes and nerves usually without extending to adjacent organs early in the course of the disease. Distant metastases are found in bone including the orbit, bone marrow, liver, and less frequently the lungs with concomitant pain in bones and respiratory problems. Quite often the presence of an abdominal mass is the first indication of the problem. When the tumor secretes peptides that cause symptoms, it may be detected earlier than one that does not. Catecholamines are elevated in a large number of the cases, and "dumbbell" tumors invading the spine may cause neurologic problems. Diagnostic studies should include computerized tomography, bone scans, and radiographic views of the lungs and orbit. Also determination of serum levels of ganglioside GD_2, urinary catecholamines, and neurone-specific enolase offers some diagnostic help. Chromosomal abnormalities have been reported for a large number of these tumors and may affect the prognosis adversely.

Treatment of ganglioblastomas consists of following a careful plan combining operation, chemotherapy, and irradiation. Chemotherapy may be given first if there is some indication that it may improve the chance of successful operation. At times the initial operation consists of biopsy only, especially when prior needle biopsy has been unsatisfactory. A second operation is then considered when resection is indicated from evaluation of the results of all diagnostic studies, and any adjuvant therapy indicated is included in the plan of treatment. Of course the best outlook follows successful complete operative eradication of these malignancies. Radiotherapy is useful in the control of bone pain and in treating localized metastatic disease. It is also used for destruction of the patient's bone marrow when transplantation of bone marrow is planned. Chemotherapy has resulted in responses with the use of cisplatin, cyclophosphamide, doxorubicin, and teniposide. Usually the best response of adrenocortical neoplasms is treatment with mitotane; cisplatin with and without etoposide; doxorubicin; aminoglutethimide; ketoconazole; and metyrapone. When these tumors appear in infancy, the prognosis tends to be better than when first seen at an older age. Approximately 9 of 10 children in stages I and II and infants in stage III can be cured. Approximately three of four children in stage III and infants in stage IV can be cured, and only one in five of older children in stage IV can be cured by the combined therapy described.

TNM staging and classification of adrenocortical carcinoma

T1	No invasion		
T2	Invasion of adjacent fat		
T3, T4	Invasion of adjacent organs		
N0	No invasion of lymph nodes		
N1	Invasion of lymph nodes		
M0	No distant metastases		
M1	Distant metastases		
Stage I	T1	N0	M0
Stage II	T2	N0	M0
Stage III	T1	N1	M0
	T2	N1	M0
	T3	N0	M0
Stage IV	Any T	Any N	M1

International staging system for neuroblastoma

Stage I	Tumor localized to site of origin Gross excision without microscopic evidence of residual tumor Bilateral lymph nodes free of microscopic tumor cells
Stage IIa	Unilateral tumor with incomplete gross excision Bilateral lymph nodes negative microscopically
Stage IIb	Unilateral tumor complete or incomplete excision with positive ipsilateral invasion of lymph node(s) Contralateral lymph nodes negative microscopically
Stage III	Tumor extending across midline with or without infiltration of regional lymph node(s) Unilateral tumor and contralateral lymph node infiltration Midline tumor and bilateral lymph node infiltration
Stage IV	Tumor metastatic to other distant organs including lymph nodes, bone, bone marrow, etc.
Stage IVs	Stage I or IIa with spread limited to liver, skin, and bone marrow

CARCINOIDS

Carcinoids are APUDomas (amine precursor uptake and decarboxylation tumors) derived from enterochromaffin precursor cells. The tumors are found chiefly in the appendix, bronchus, jejunum, ileum, and rectum, but also can be found distributed to other widespread loci. Those in the bronchi are derived from the foregut, those in the appendix, jejunum, and ileum from the midgut, and those in the rectum from the hindgut. It is not possible to distinguish between benign and neoplastic lesions from their microscopic morphology, malignancies being distinguished by metastases to sites such as lymph nodes, liver, and bone. Their appearance can be confused with small cell neoplasms and adenocarcinomas. The characteristic carcinoid clinical syndrome is not present in all cases but is distinctive and impressive when it appears. It consists of flushing, facial telangiectasis, diarrhea, asthma, lesions of cardiac valves, and retroperitoneal fibrosis. Gastrointestinal peptides are responsible for the development of the syndrome, and numerous examples have been isolated from the tumors including pancreatic polypeptide, insulin, somatostatin, calcitonin, vasoactive intestinal peptide, neurotensin, and others. Often the carcinoids are designated with labels such as PPoma, insulinoma, and somatostatinoma, derived from the symptoms produced by the peptide. Serotonin levels tend to be high when the carcinoid syndrome is present and probably is responsible for diarrhea which can be relieved by serotonin antagonists. Also, asthma and fibrosis occur in patients with the syndrome, and most patients with hepatic metastases have the syndrome.

A great number of carcinoids are detected at autopsy and incidentally during the workup and treatment of other conditions. Most of those in the appendix are detected first at the time of appendectomy or other abdominal procedure. Those in duodenum and jejunum and ileum and in the rectum and colon may be found at the time of endoscopy and those in the bronchi and mediastinum at the time of radiographic examination of the chest. Those in the small bowel are associated with fibrosis which may lead to twisting and obstruction and associated symptoms. Larger tumors and metastases, especially in the liver, may be palpable. Tumors 1 cm and smaller are rarely malignant, whereas those greater than 2 cm in diameter are very likely to be malignant. Many carcinoids exhibit rather indolent growth patterns and may exist for several years without significant symptoms or obvious damage; asymptomatic tumors may have metastasized widely. The high levels of serotonin secreted by many of these tumors can be detected in the form of urinary 5-hydroxyindole acetic acid (5-HIAA). Determination of urinary 5-HIAA is the test most widely used to detect the carcinoid syndrome; other tests available are determination of human chorionic gonadotropin, chromogranin, and neuropeptide K in the plasma.

Numerous pharmacologic agents have been used to treat carcinoid tumors. They include chlorpromazine, corticosteroids, histamine receptor blockers, isoniazid, methysergide, and parachlorophenylalanine. The results have not been very successful, and side effects of the treatment have been great enough in many cases to discontinue therapy. The only chance of curing carcinoid tumors is resection, the extent usually varying with the size of the primary tumor. When tumors that are smaller than 1 cm are located in the appendix, appendectomy is all that is required. Larger neoplasms, 2 cm or greater, should be treated by a partial colectomy, including the appendix and terminal ileum and lymphatic and venous drainage. The management of carcinoids of the appendix between 1 and 2 cm in size is somewhat controversial. If the mesoappendix and adjacent nodes are involved, the same treatment as for larger tumors seems reasonable. However, some clinicians favor simple appendectomy for all tumors less than 2 cm in size. The tumors in the small bowel are more likely to be multiple. Most of the time resection of the bowel should be done. For tumors 2 cm and larger, wide removal of the specimen including the mesentery and regional lymphatics is advisable. Great care should be taken not to miss multiple tumors in the bowel. Tumors of the rectum and colon, unless small, should be treated by low anterior resection or abdominoperineal resection. Smaller tumors should be removed completely with wide margins. Carcinoid neoplasms of the bronchus should be resected with wide margins, usually requiring a lobectomy. More central tumors may require an operation with "sleeve" resection and reanastomosis of the bronchus. Peripheral carcinoids near the parietal pleura sometimes can be removed with a liberal wedge resection. Resection of hepatic metastases is useful since these tumors tend to grow slowly, and even if the operation is only a debulking procedure, the improvement or total relief of symptoms may be extended for a considerable length of time.

Additional therapeutic measures that are useful at times include arterial embolization, chemotherapy, human recombinant interferon alpha 2b, interferon-α, and leukocyte interferon alone or in various combinations. Hepatic artery ligation also has been used with some success with and without chemotherapy. In general, carcinoids are not very responsive to chemotherapy, but somatostatin may be effective in controlling the symptoms of carcinoid syndrome. Other agents that have elicited some responses at times are cisplatin, cyclophosphamide, doxorubicin, etoposide, 5-fluorouracil, and streptozocin. Various combinations of these and other pharmaceuticals have given no better results than those obtained with single agents alone. The results of treating carcinoids with external beam irradiation suggest that this modality gives best results when the objective is palliation of osseous and skin lesions. Also, a 5000-cGy tumor dose at the primary site has been used with some success to treat intraabdominal foci and intracranial and epidural lesions.

PHEOCHROMOCYTOMA

Pheochromocytomas are rather rare tumors that have an incidence of less than two per million people. Approximately 10 percent of these tumors are malignant. They are found in the distribution of the neural crest from the neck to the pelvis, and up to 90 percent of them originate in the adrenal medulla. They occur at any age with equal distribution between the sexes. The most striking feature of the tumors is the production of abnormally high levels of catecholamines (epinephrine and/or norepinephrine) resulting in secondary hypertension. The hypertension may be sustained or episodic and at times may be accompanied by severe headache, palpitations, tachycardia, tremor, anxiety, sweating, and seizures. If undetected and untreated, severe complications and even death may ensue. Several medications including those used in the course of giving a general anesthetic, may precipitate attacks, sometimes resulting in a fatal outcome. These tumors can be bilateral or even multiple and are usually 5 cm or smaller in size, weigh less than 100 g, and are seldom large enough to be palpable on physical examination. However, the liver can be palpable when metastases are present. The primary lesions can occur in a familial pattern alone or as part of the hereditary multiple endocrine neoplasia syndromes MEN-IIa and MEN-IIb. Also patients with pheochromocytomas have a higher percentage of neurofibromatosis than the population at large. Unexplained hypertension in children and young adults and occurring in a familial setting should lead to screening for this tumor.

Diagnostic studies always include computerized tomograms and measurement of 24-h urinary excretion of adrenaline, noradrenaline, and metabolites metadrenaline, normetadrenaline, and vanillylmandelic acid. At times, addition of an iodine 131 scan and measurement of plasma levels of catecholamines may be helpful. Provocative tests add considerable risk and usually are not necessary to establish the diagnosis. Nuclear magnetic imaging is expensive but can help localize single or multiple tumors and distinguish them from other masses. Also it is useful in situations such as pregnancy when irradiation is undesirable. It cannot be used to determine whether a tumor is benign or malignant. This distinction becomes evident only with extension of the tumor beyond the primary site and to liver, lungs, and/or bone.

Operation is the most successful treatment, but it should never be attempted without adequate preparation before and during the procedure with continued surveillance in the postoperative period. Otherwise the flooding of catecholamines from anxiety, the medications used by the anesthesiologist, and sudden fall in blood pressure at the time the tumor is removed can be preludes to disaster. Prophylactic management consists of administration of alpha and beta blocking agents a sufficient time beforehand for them to become fully active. For example, alpha blocking with phenoxybenzamine can be given 24 h before the anesthetic is initiated, followed by beta blockers such as atenolol or metoprolol. Effectiveness of the blockade then can be followed by monitoring vital signs, blood count, and estimates of circulating blood volume.

The choice of incision depends on the size of the tumor, its location, and whether more than one is present. Exposure can be obtained through vertical or transverse abdominal or thoracoabdominal incisions but rarely through a posterior route. Every effort should be made to remove the tumor completely and to remove as much as possible if complete excision cannot be accomplished. Fortunately up to 9 of 10 benign tumors can be cured. The 5-year survival is less than half of those who have a surgical resection for a malignant lesion. Irradiation has sometimes been successful for relieving bone pain from metastatic lesions. Also iodine 131 therapy has had some limited therapeutic usefulness. Chemotherapy has not initiated responses in many cases. Best choices for treatment are doxorubicin; 5-fluorouracil with and without streptozocin; dacarbazine; interferon alfa; cisplatin; cyclophosphamide; and octreotide.

MULTIPLE ENDOCRINE NEOPLASMS

Multiple endocrine neoplasia type I (MEN-I) is inherited as a dominant susceptibility gene on chromosome 11 and may result in as many as three endocrine glands being involved. It usually appears in middle age. Nine-tenths of patients with the trait have hyperparathyroidism involving hyperplasia of multiple parathyroid glands. Pancreatic endocrine tumors are present in approximately 80 percent of patients with MEN-I. They include insulinomas, gastrinomas, growth hormone releasing factor tumors (GRFomas), vasoactive intestinal peptide releasing tumors (VIPomas), and glucagonomas. Pituitary tumors occur about as frequently as pancreatic tumors. Endocrine secretions from these pituitary tumors include prolactin, ACTH, and growth hormone. Clinical features of the tumors are visual defects, Cushing's syndrome, and acromegaly. Hyperplasia, cortical adenomas, and carcinoma of the adrenal gland are found in about one-third of patients with MEN-I. Thyroid adenomas with hyperplasia also are found at times.

Medullary thyroid carcinoma is a constant feature of both MEN-IIa and MEN-IIb. Patients with MEN-IIa also have bilateral pheochromocytomas and hyperparathyroidism as features of the disease. The susceptibility gene is a dominant on chromosome 10. High calcitonin levels as a result of C-cell secretions in medullary hyperplasia, adenoma, and carcinoma are detectable by immunoassay following provocative testing using calcium infusion or pentogastrin injection. The determination of calcitonin level constitutes a useful marker for screening members of families with both MEN-IIa and MEN-IIb, leading to early diagnosis. Pheochromocytomas that occur with the MEN-II syndromes are rarely malignant. Scanning is suggested before an operation on the adrenal gland. Medullary hyperplasia is always present bilaterally even if a tumor is not found and the patient does not have symptoms of pheochromocytoma. Patients with MEN-IIb syndrome do not have hyperparathyroidism but have medullary thyroid carcinomas, pheochromocytomas, mucosal neuromas, prominent lips and jaw, abnormal dentition, medullated corneal nerves, and pes cavus. The dominant gene associated with the disease is also on the tenth chromosome but at a different locus.

The treatment of the hyperplasia causing hyperparathyroidism consists of removing up to all four glands with reimplantation of a portion of the tissue when all glands are resected. Recurrence indicates a second exploration. The treatment of pancreatic tumors is discussed under that heading. The transsphenoidal approach is indicated for resection if a pituitary tumor is found. The presence of medullary carcinoma should be treated with total thyroidectomy and central nodal resection. The abdomen should be explored for pheochromocytoma only with administration of alpha-adrenergic receptor blockade beforehand. All tumors should be removed. Whether bilateral adrenalectomy should be done is somewhat controversial. Because unilateral resection has resulted in prolonged survival in some cases, some clinicians favor unilateral resection in appropriate cases. Others advocate bilateral adrenalectomy in all cases because of the invariable hyperplasia. The results of a metaiodobenzylguanidine (MIBG) scan can be helpful in making the decision.

PARAGANGLIOMAS

Paragangliomas are unusual neuroendocrine tumors originating in the neural crest and secreting neuropeptides and catecholamines. The functional cell is the chief cell. The paragangliomas of greatest clinical significance are those tumors located in the region of the temporal bone, carotid body tumors, and those located elsewhere in the head and neck. Other sites are the viscera, retroperitoneum, mediastinum, and central arteries and veins. Paragangliomas are capable of secreting serotonin and catecholamines, including epinephrine. When stimulated by manipulation at the time of operation, secretion can be stimulated with disastrous results. The operator must be aware of the dangers and possess appropriate skill in vascular surgery in the case of carotid body tumors and in otology in the case of jugulotympanic tumors. For tumors that are inaccessible, radiation may be used, but this is often contraindicated in children. Malignant transformation has been reported to occur after irradiation, but the risk is considered to be small. The primary objective is reduction or elimination of function rather than absolute eradication of all tumor cells. When the tumors are small, operation is the treatment of choice; irradiation may be chosen when the size of the tumors is sufficiently great to increase the hazards of intra- and postoperative complications.

CANCER WITHIN THE THORACIC CAVITY

CARCINOMA OF THE LUNG (BRONCHOGENIC CARCINOMA)

Cancer of the lung is the cancer most frequently encountered in men, and the incidence continues to increase in women. Mortality is high with only about one-tenth of those affected surviving even with treatment. It is one of few neoplasms for which the etiology is known with some precision. Since the first report to the surgeon general on smoking and health, the importance of smoking as a prime agent causing the disease and responsible for a remarkable increase in occurrence has been accepted by all except groups financially dependent on income generated by tobacco. Workers such as table servers, drivers, construction workers, painters, and others with a tendency to smoke, along with shipyard workers, boiler makers, insulation workers, and others who are also exposed to various carcinogens have a greater chance of developing cancer of the lung than the population at large. Among carcinogens known to be responsible for pulmonary neoplasms are radon, asbestos, inorganic arsenic compounds, nickel, aromatic hydrocarbons, and chromium. They are active alone and enhance the carcinogenicity of tobacco tar.

The diagnosis of both bronchogenic and metastatic carcinoma of the lung requires bronchoscopic and/or percutaneous biopsy of the bronchus and pulmonary parenchyma, radiographic studies, and possibly magnetic resonance imaging. A history suggesting characteristics of the usual clinical course of the disease is useful in determining whether the tumor may be inoperable with invasion of the mediastinum, Pancoast's syndrome, and obstruction of the vena cava. At times mediastinoscopy also may be helpful in refining the

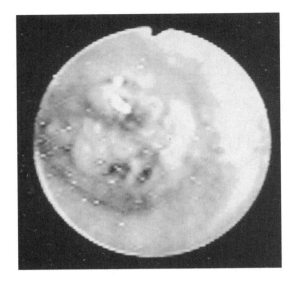

A

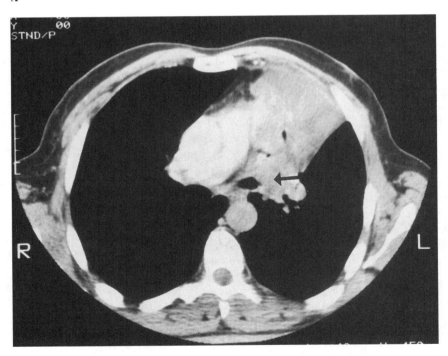

B

Figure 11 Bronchogenic carcinoma. A. Endoscopic view of bronchogenic carcinoma occluding the left main stem bronchus. B. Computerized tomogram of the same malignancy.

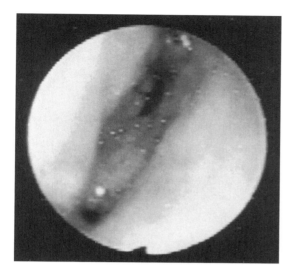

C

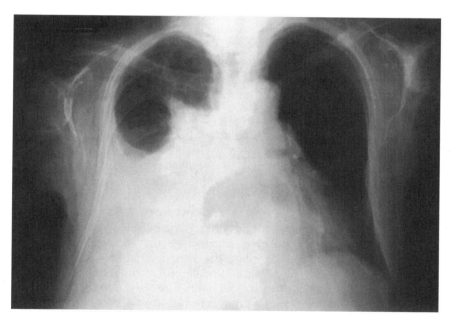

D

Figure 11 *(Continued)*
C. Endoscopic view of bronchus showing occlusion from external pressure of the enlarging cancer. D. Roentgen study of the neoplasm causing the compression.

diagnosis. When studied under the microscope, cancer of the lung is divided into four types:

1. Adenocarcinoma
    Bronchoalveolar
    Acinar
    Mucus secreting
    Papillary
2. Squamous cell
    Epidermoid
    Spindle cell
3. Large cell
    Clear cell
    Giant cell
4. Small cell
    Oat cell
    Intermediate cell
    Combined cell

Experience in the management of small cell lesions has led to a somewhat different approach than for the other types of cancer.

Bronchogenic carcinoma invades both lymphatic and vascular channels and extends to distant sites such as bone and brain as well as locally. The foci seen more peripherally at times are believed to have spread by dissemination through the bronchi. Although squamous carcinomas may grow relatively slowly, the advanced stage of the disease at the time of discovery doubtless affects the rate of control unfavorably. Cough, hemoptysis, pain, and wheezing appear relatively early to be followed by pleurisy, atelectasis, pneumonia, effusion, and dyspnea as the tumor grows and invades adjacent tissue. Malaise, weakness, anorexia, and loss of weight often are the symptoms bringing the patient to the physician the first time.

As the course of the malignant growth progresses, the vena cava may become compressed. The same problem can occur in the adjacent esophagus which may perforate when invaded. Hoarseness may occur as a result of invasion of the recurrent nerve. When the sympathetic nerves are affected Horner's syndrome ensues, consisting of ipsilateral smaller size of pupil, enophthalmus, and narrowing of the palpebral fissure. Pain related to invasion of brachial plexus and upper ribs is often referred to as Pancoast's syndrome. With the passage of time the neoplasm spreads to more distant sites as well as locally, although not in a consistent, regular pattern.

Extrapulmonary features of the disease include neuromuscular and skeletal manifestations such as peripheral neuropathy and osteoarthropathy including clubbing, vascular and hematologic abnormalities such as migratory thrombophlebitis and purpura, and dermatoses such as scleroderma. Paraendocrine phenomena respond as the tumor is treated successfully and represent an unusual altered function of some cells as they become malignant. Excessive quantities of hydroxycorticosteroids are present in the urine of some patients, especially those with small cell carcinoma. This leads to hypertension, characteristic facial appearance and other findings seen in Cushing's syndrome. There are other metabolic abnormalities in some bronchogenic carcinomas including hypercalcemia and ectopic gonadotropin. Presence of the latter can be associated with gynecomastia. Excessive antidiuretic hormone production can require intensive management of fluid and electrolyte abnormalities.

The diagnosis of bronchogenic carcinoma to be definitive must be based on microscopic examination of suspected tissue. Cytologic studies of sputum and aspirated specimens from the tracheobronchial tree are valuable aids. The relatively minor procedures of bronchoscopy and mediastinoscopy can be used to obtain specimens for examination. Also aspiration of pleural fluid and thoracoscopy may yield tissue for diagnosis. In addition, aspiration with a fine needle can be used for this purpose, but a negative biopsy does not mean that a neoplasm is not present. Approximately half of the cases of all except small cell cancers come to thoracotomy. Operability is the route to cure, but unfortunately about four-fifths of these patients are found too late for cure. Radiographic studies are most useful aids in making the diagnosis of cancer of the lung and following its course. Laminograms and computerized tomograms are quite helpful also, but nuclear magnetic resonance imaging has not added much in the way of unique diagnostic approaches. Biologic markers such as the ones mentioned in discussing metabolic abnormalities may suggest the correct diagnosis when they first occur. Scanning with radioactive isotopes such as cobalt and gallium may be used to localize metastases that would be undetected otherwise. Labeled monoclonal antibodies have not been as useful so far as hoped originally. After diagnostic studies have been completed, a thoracotomy should be done only when the neoplasm appears to be at least partially resectable.

Non–Small Cell Cancer of the Lung

The management of cancer of the lung depends on the histologic type of the neoplasm being treated. Small cell cancers have a poorer prognosis for equivalent stages when compared with non–small cell cancers. Adenocarcinomas and large cell cancers have a less encouraging prognosis than squamous lesions. Squamous cancers have the best prognosis and are found less frequently than adenocarcinomas. Large cell cancers occur less frequently and respond to treatment somewhat like adencarcinomas. The alveolar neoplasms are distinctive in their behavior pattern among the adenocarcinomas; non–small cell carcinomas usually are treated in a somewhat similar manner.

It is very important to obtain the best information possible about the extent of the disease before treatment begins. Occult carcinomas may be detected by screening methods consisting of radiographic studies of the chest, sputum examination of exfoliated cells, and bronchoscopy. These neoplasms are best treated by resection if the patient's condition permits or radiation therapy if operation is contraindicated. When the diagnostic work-up is complete, the stage can be determined. Management varies with the stage. The TNM staging for cancer of the lung appears below.

Several tests and procedures are useful in addition to a medical history and physical examination for determining the stage of the cancer. X-ray studies include those of the chest with anteroposterior, lateral, and sometimes oblique views; tomograms, consisting of computerized sections through the lungs, are most helpful. Nuclear magnetic imaging is expensive and has not proved to add measurably to information that can be obtained by other means. The use of radionuclide scanning has not been very useful, although labeled monoclonal antibodies may eventually add specificity to such tests, the lack of which now limits these studies. Bone scans are useful in localizing metastases; in the later stages of lung cancer brain scans are useful because of the high incidence of metastatic foci known to occur with this type of neoplasm. Fine needle aspiration guided radiography can provide positive biopsies of primary and metastatic lesions, but negative biopsies cannot be viewed as indicating the absence of neoplastic cells. A disadvantage of using needle biopsy is the possibility of pneumothorax, necessitating closed thoracotomy and drainage. Bronchoscopy with the flexible bronchoscope is a relatively benign procedure and along with mediastinoscopy is quite useful in staging the disease. Bronchoscopy is often the initial means for a definitive tissue diagnosis. The response to treatment may be anticipated to a certain extent by the presence of prognostic factors such as cancer genes (oncogenes), chromosomal abnormalities, growth factor receptors, neuroendocrine characteristics of the cancer, and specific blood group antigens in the tumor.

Surgical Resection for Cancer of the Lung

Surgical resection of stage I and II lung cancer offers the best chance for cure of the disease. As more experience has been accumulated over the years, it is apparent that a majority of the lesions can be treated with lobectomy with results comparable to pneumonectomy. However, the surgeon may find that the neoplasm is too extensive or localized in such a way as to make removal of the entire lung mandatory. In the case of some proximal lesions it is possible to remove the tissue involved including the bronchus and preserve more distant lobes by skillful plastic repair without jeopardizing the chance for cure. Lobectomy and at times segmentectomy can completely eradicate the cancer. Wedge resection or cautery excision is not indicated when there is a chance for a curative removal of pulmonary tissue containing the cancer and the patient's general condition permits. Mortality and morbidity from operations

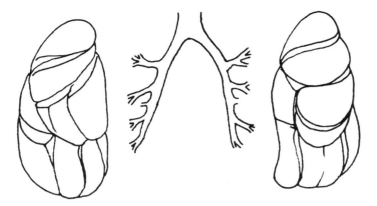

Figure 12 Diagram of segments of lungs and bronchial branches permitting lobectomy as well as pneumonectomy.

Right	Left
Upper Lobe	
Apical	Apical-posterior
Anterior	Anterior
Posterior	Superior lingula
	Inferior lingula
Middle Lobe	
Lateral	
Medial	
Lower Lobe	
Superior	Superior
Medial basal	Antero-medial basal
Anterior basal	Lateral basal
Lateral basal	Posterior basal
Posterior basal	

for pulmonary resection have steadily diminished with the passage of time, and problems are now more related to cardiovascular and pulmonary reserve than technical deficiencies. Careful preoperative analysis of cardiopulmonary disease in addition to the cancer, with correction of all the problems amenable to therapy prior to operation, is mandatory for avoiding preventable postoperative complications. When the cancer has progressed no farther than hilar nodes or visceral pleura, resection is the treatment of choice. Whether resection of mediastinal lymph nodes should be done routinely in addition is somewhat controversial. Certainly multiple samples of mediastinal nodes should be removed if for no other reason than making the staging of the disease more accurate.

In stage IIIA disease the tumor is locally advanced and may include nodal involvement classified as N2. These cancers frequently offer the possibility for complete resection, which is carried out *en masse*. Cure is possible even if the chest wall or diaphragm is involved. The prognosis is not as favorable when the invasion is in the direction of the mediastinum. However, cures have been obtained even when the apex of the lung and adjacent chest wall, including ribs and associated nerves, were invaded. The symptoms appearing when this type of invasion occurs are referred to as Pancoast's syndrome. If all the tumor cannot be removed surgically, supplemental radiotherapy is indicated. When the invasion of the mediastinum can be removed along with the tumor mass, cure is possible. Unfortunately vital structures may be invaded (T4 disease) along with N3 nodal invasion preventing the surgeon from removing all the cancer. If this status can be ascertained prior to undertaking operation, it is wise to do so. The more nodes involved, the poorer is the prognosis. It is wise in all cases that are associated with the questionable advisability of surgical intervention to have a surgical consultation to obtain the opinion of a practitioner with experience in actually undertaking the proposed procedure and information about current results of recent surgical approaches. Induction radiotherapy or chemotherapy at times has been helpful in aiding the surgeon by providing a resectable tumor. Resection of solitary metastases to brain, adrenal, and at a different site in the lung have resulted in cures. It is not often the only peripheral metastasis when only one site is discovered in bone, skin, or liver, however. Adjuvant chemotherapy is under investigation for stage IIIB disease.

Chemotherapy for Non–Small Cell Cancer of the Lung

The primary objectives of chemotherapy for non–small cell cancer of the lung is improving the quality of life and hopefully to extend survival; chemotherapy is used most often in the treatment of the later stages of this type of cancer. So far no regimen has led to cures, and this type of therapy is reserved for patients who can be treated while ambulatory. It is not suitable for patients with advanced disease of any major organ system and is best confined to those patients with a Karnofsky performance status equal or greater than 60 percent. Because of the superior rate of response to multiple agents, most therapy consists of two or more pharmaceuticals. Shortness of breath, cough, hemoptysis, pain, and loss of weight do respond to chemotherapy; it is important to begin treatment sufficiently early before collapse of segments of the lung, pneumonia, obstruction of vena cava, and other complications less responsive to treatment occur. Complications of chemotherapy specifically depending on the agents being used are alopecia, constipation, peripheral neuropathy, sloughing of skin and soft tissue, infections as a result of leukopenia, bleeding as a result of thrombocytopenia, hemolytic anemia, renal damage, nausea, and vomiting. Tests to monitor the occurrence of these problems are used throughout the period of treatment and management altered in response to side effects.

Both paclitaxel plus cisplatin or carboplatin and vinorelbine plus cisplatin are accepted currently as standard therapy. Other combinations of useful drugs are mitomycin, vinblastine, and cisplatin (MVP); mitomycin, ifosfamide, mesna, and cisplatin (MIC); and gemcitabine with and without cisplatin. Other programs that have been used for the treatment of this type of cancer are vindesine and cisplatin; etoposide and cisplatin; vindesine and mitomycin; vindesine, cisplatin, and mitomycin; and cyclophosphamide, doxorubicin, and cisplatin. Other drugs of promise are docetaxel, irinotecan, bisacetamide, gemcitabene, hexamethylene, ifosafmide, vinorelbine, and taxol. The most promising combinations are constantly being revised as the results of ongoing clinical trials become available.

Irradiation Therapy for Non–Small Cell Cancer of the Lung

The use of irradiation therapy for cancer of the lung is used primarily to render a lesion operable or to be used in cases with contraindications for operation related to the presence of other medical problems or refusal of the patient to have an operation. Limitations of irradiation are undesirable side effects of irradiation dermatitis, nausea, effects on tissues not involved with the neoplasm being treated such as the spinal cord and danger of pneumonia, esophagitis, and difficulties in adapting the field of irradiation to the contours of the tumor. The maximum tumor dose with acceptable side effects is not always easily determined. Great care must be taken in determining the length of treatment, the dosage for each session, and the number, size, shape, and placement of the fields to be irradiated. It is necessary to be certain that the position of the patient in relation to the therapy machine is constant throughout each treatment. To reduce the dosage of irradiation to which normal tissue is exposed, the beam of irradiation is cross-fired from separate ports at the tumor target which then receives the sum of all the irradiation, whereas the tissues outside the target receive only the dose through a single port. Three-dimensional models are devised for each patient to take into consideration the amount of total irradiation received by the tumor. The somewhat complicated calculations take into consideration the effect of the irradiation not only at the site of entrance and depth of the tumor but also at the point of exit. Irradiation is effective at the local site of delivery in contrast to chemotherapy, which is distributed throughout the circulatory system.

Postoperative irradiation is useful when resection has not been complete and microscopic examination of any margin reveals tumor cells. This brachytherapy can be done by the use of special cones adapted for delivery of irradiation or seeds containing radioactive isotopes implanted at the time of operation. When delivered after closure of the chest wound, clips left by the surgeon for orientation and x-ray studies of the chest can be used as guides for teletherapy with the hope of eradicating remaining cancer cells at the margins of the resection. The use of irradiation directed to metastatic sites is most successful for those in bone and for hemoptysis, and less successful for atelectasis as a result of bronchial obstruction and pleural effusion. It is indicated more frequently in cases of spinal cord compression than is operative decompression, and has a place for whole brain irradiation because of the high percentage of cases ultimately having the tumor spread to this site. In recent years neutron irradiation has been used at times to treat tumors thought to be hypoxic because this type of treatment does not depend on the presence of molecular oxygen in contrast to the mechanism of damage to cancer cells attributable to gamma and other types of irradiation. The usefulness of sensitizing agents such as cisplatin to enhance the effect of irradiation on tumor cells has not been proved in clinical trials up to this time. A large body of evidence has accumulated about the effect of variations in dosage and methods of administration alone and with different combinations of irradiation with operative intervention and chemotherapy without the emergence of any new regimen clearly superior for the management of carcinoma of the lung using irradiation.

Management of Small Cell Cancer of the Lung

Small cell cancer of the lung, formerly referred to as oat cell carcinoma, exhibits a clinical course and response to treatment at variance with the other types of cancer of this organ. It comprises not more than one quarter of the neoplasms originating in the lung and arises from basal neuroendocrine cells. Cushing's syndrome (increased secretion of cortisone), symptoms similar to myasthenia, low sodium from antidiuretic hormone, sensory impairment, retinal degeneration, and ataxia are associated with the presence of this cancer. A simple staging used in the Veterans Administration studies is often used. Limited disease consists of tumors within one hemithorax and nodes draining this region, and extensive disease is defined as spread outside the location of the limited disease. The usual diagnostic studies useful in staging can be curtailed when extensive disease is verified by distant metastases including bone, brain, cord, abdominal organs, and lymph nodes. Levels of CEA (carcinoembryonic antigen) and neuron-specific enolase have been reported to correlate with size of the tumor and response to chemotherapy.

The use of resection for small cell carcinomas has been uniformly disappointing even when combined with chemotherapy. Currently the rare case with a small coin lesion detected radiographically with no evidence of lymphatic invasion or spread elsewhere is the only situation for which a surgical approach is considered routinely. In recent years operation has gained favor as an option because operative mortality is low and recurrence is often local, suggesting that reducing the tumor load may make chemotherapy more effective. Information about the usefulness of preoperative as well as postoperative irradiation remains somewhat equivocal. On the other hand, a combination of irradiation and chemotherapy has proved to be effective in eliciting a gratifying response including both local control and survival in cases of limited disease when concurrent radiotherapy and chemotherapy are used. Hyperfractionation of dosage seems to enhance the effect of irradiation. Alternative chemotherapy-irradiation must be done with minimal intervals. Chemotherapy is more effective with multiple than with single agents. Combinations that have produced gratifying responses are cisplatin and etoposide (PE), as well as carboplatin and etoposide (PE), and combinations of two and three additional agents with cyclophosphamide including doxorubicin and vincristine (CAV) and doxorubicin and etoposide (CAE).

Other useful compounds and combinations are paclitaxel with or without carboplatin and/or etoposide; ifosfamide, mesna, carboplatin, and etoposide (ICE); etoposide, ifosfamide, mesna, and cisplatin (VIP); etoposide; gemcitabine; topotecan; and docetaxel, Doxorubicin, and vincristine, and etoposide, and methotrexate, lomustine, and vincristine also have been used. Chemotherapy may be administered in successive courses over a period of many months, and various methods and combinations have been devised to improve results of long-term therapy. So far chemotherapy is not curative, and long-term survival is rare, with survival of those with limited disease at approximately 25 percent and with extensive disease, 5 percent of the original group at the end of 5 years. Relapsing disease has been treated both with chemotherapy and at times with radiotherapy, but results have been disappointing.

TNM staging of cancer of the lung

I	T1-2N0M0
II	T1-2N1M0
IIIA	T3N0-1M0
	T1-3N2M0
IIIB	T4 or N3M0
IV	M1
Tumor	
TX	Malignant cell
T1	<3 cm
T2	>3 cm
T3	Pleura, pericardium, diaphragm, chest wall <2 cm from carina
Nodes with Cancer	
N0	None
N1	Ipsilateral hilar or bronchopulmonary
N2	Ipsilateral hilar, subcarinal, or supraclavicular
N3	Contralateral hilar, subcarinal, or supraclavicular

(Continued)

Metastases	
M0	None
M1	Present

MALIGNANT MESOTHELIOMA

The majority of tumors of the pleura are mesotheliomas. They are tumors of serosal surfaces and arise in the pleura, periotenum, pericardium, tunica vaginalis of the testes, and atrioventricular node of the heart and less frequently in the adrenal, liver, and mediastinum. They occur much more frequently in men than in women. The incidence increases with age, and mesotheliomas are usually discovered in the fifth through the seventh decades. Approximately 80 percent are the result of domestic or occupational exposure to asbestos. Many others are the result of exposure to irradiation, and no causal factors are apparent in the remainder. Chrysotile asbestos fibers are serpentine or curly and represent a lower risk than the crocidolite and amosite rodlike amphiboles. The latter fibers may contaminate chrysotile asbestos, and some investigators believe that they are the major reason for the development of asbestosis when there is contamination. Asbestos has the unusual property of being able to introduce DNA into cells, but chromosomal abnormalities occur much less frequently in mesotheliomas than in such neoplasia as bronchgenic carcinomas. Erionite is present in local rocks in one region of Turkey and is responsible for malignant mesotheliomas in that region. The use of asbestos in commerce and construction is now illegal in the United States, and ultimately this should reduce the numbers of these malignancies. Mesotheliomas are epithelial or sarcomatoid tumors or a mixture of the two. The diagnosis is sometimes difficult to make and can be confused with adenocarcinomas arising in the bronchus and other sites. Therefore it is imperative that an accurate diagnosis is reached before definitive therapy is undertaken. Material from pleural and peritoneal effusions, bronchial and pleural biopsies, and cell blocks of tissue obtained at thoracotomy and abdominal exploration can yield an accurate assessment of the diagnosis with the use of histochemical techniques and electron microscopy.

Symptoms and signs of mesothelioma include pain in the chest wall unlike that of pleurisy, dullness to percussion of the thorax, pleural effusion, dyspnea, fatigue, and loss of weight. When the malignancy invades the pleura and adjacent structures, additional symptoms and signs may appear including fever, sweating, anemia, thrombophlebitis, Horner's and superior vena caval syndromes, spinal cord compression, and hypercalcemia. Spread to lymph nodes of the mediastinum and occasionally to cervical nodes along with hematogenous dissemination occurs rather late in the typical course of the disease.

Symptoms and signs of primary malignant mesotheliomas of the peritoneum are pain, increase in girth, fluid wave associated with ascites, loss of weight, the presence of palpable tumor(s), amyloidosis, clotting abnormalities, achalasia, and intestinal obstruction. The use of computerized tomography and nuclear magnetic resonance visualization has improved the accuracy of the location and extent of these malignant mesotheliomas arising both in the thoracic and abdominal cavities. In addition to the usual complete blood count, blood chemistry, electrocardiogram, and blood typing when thoracotomy is planned, bronchoscopy, mediastinoscopy, and pulmonary function testing should be considered. Forced expiratory volume greater than 2 L is desirable. An abnormally high value for carcinoembryonic antigen usually suggests the presence of a neoplasm other than malignant mesothelioma. When the primary cancer arises in the peritoneum, obtaining sufficient material from aspiration of ascitic fluid is successful in less than 10 percent of cases, and peritoneoscopy or open biopsy must be done to obtain sufficient tissue for the necessary histochemical and electron microscopic studies required for accurate diagnosis. Also, the latter procedure yields a reliable assessment of the extent and amount of disease.

Benign mesotheliomas are encountered occasionally and can be excised with success. Multilocular peritoneal cysts or benign mesotheliomas appear within the peritoneal cavity; unless they are growing, excision is not urgent. Primary malignant mesotheliomas that occur in the pericardium and tunica vaginalis of the testes are quite rare.

Malignant mesotheliomas that are localized in the pleura or peritoneum give the best chance for cure, but unfortunately most patients present with a more advanced stage of the disease. Tumors confined within the parietal pleura or stage I disease may be treated successfully with pleurectomy performed through a posterolateral thoracotomy incision. The parietal, pericardial, and diaphragmatic pleura are stripped away followed by decortication if indicated. After closure the wound is drained with one or two tubes for removal of fluid and care of bronchopleural fistulas if they occur. This operation provides the answer to pleural effusion and in some cases results in removal of the entire neoplasm. When the malignancy has invaded the pleura and surrounding structures, a more extensive procedure is indicated at times for ipsilateral disease. The extrapleural pneumonectomy can be a formidable procedure. Although it is not always necessary, a thoracoabdominal incision is indicated for adequate exposure in other cases. The periphery of the diseased tissue is excised, and the pericardium is opened early in the course of the operation to facilitate exposure of the stem bronchus within the pericardial cavity where it can be clamped, divided, and sutured. It is frequently necessary to remove the diaphragm. Then the abdominal cavity can be inspected and any extension there removed if possible. Then the diaphragm is replaced with a graft of material such as Gortex. In the usual case no drains are necessary when the abdomen is closed. Some of the complications known to occur after this operation are chylothorax, empyema, broncopleural fistula, vocal cord paralysis, and respiratory insufficiency. When the lung cannot be mobilized and the neoplasm is extensive, removal of a portion for additional laboratory studies and debulking, when practical, and immediate closure of the chest wound is the wise course to follow.

Mesotheliomas arising in the abdominal cavity exhibit peritoneal foci, masses sometimes with contained hemorrhage, mesenteric thickening, and ascites. Hematogenous spread to bone, brain, and liver occurs quite late or not at all, but a large number of the cases feature pleural plaques at the time of diagnosis. Operation can reduce the tumor load, correct any problems of impending or actual intestinal obstruction, and alleviate the problem of ascites by shunts or appropriate use of catheter drainage. The modalities available for palliation are radiotherapy and chemotherapy which are being revised constantly in an attempt to avert the usual final outcome of the disease as a result of hypoxia, respiratory infection, intestinal obstruction, or pericardial involvement.

Chemotherapy with single agents has been disappointing, and many trials with combinations of such agents as cisplatin, cyclophosphamide, doxorubicin, 5-fluorouracil, mitomycin C, and vindesine have been reported. Responses in larger randomized trials tend to be no more than 14 percent or only about one-fourth as great as those reported in smaller trials. There is a tendency not to report the result of trials when the rate of response has been low. Greater success seems to attend the combination of operation, chemotherapy, and sometimes irradiation. Intraoperative chemotherapy and brachytherapy at times reduce pleural and peritoneal effusions with some destruction of the cells nearest the surface when agents such as cisplatin and iodine 125, phosphorus 32, and iridium 192 have been used. The prognosis is less favorable in cases with nodal involvement and sarcomatoid histology. Unfortunately adjuvant therapy singly or combined does not often extend survival.

Over the years irradiation has been used as the primary treatment of malignant mesotheliomas, for spot therapy of localized disease, to treat tumors that have been debulked, and to prevent the seeding of neoplastic cells in abdominal and thoracic wounds after thoracoscopy and peritoneoscopy. One of the difficulties has been potential damage to various organs in the field and how to protect them with shielding, appropriate reduction in dosage, methods of administering external beam therapy such as rotating arc fields, and appropriate combinations of therapy with electron beams and radioactive isotope brachytherapy. Tumor dosages have ranged from 2000 to 7000 cGy. Unfortunately there has been no extensive objective clinical trial for reference establishing effective and safe dosages and methods of administration. In more recent years radiation therapy has been combined with chemotherapy which usually has reduced the dosages used for concomitant irradiation. Complications that can follow irradiation are epidermitis, malaise, nausea, vomiting, pneumonitis, reduction in pulmonary function, pulmonary fibrosis, hypoxia and dyspnea, pericardial effusion, esophagitis, hepatitis, and myelitis, representing powerful reminders to adjust dosages, shielding, combinations af therapy, and methods of administration in an effort to eliminate all but temporary effects such as nausea, vomiting, and epidermitis following the therapy. The use of brachytherapy to treat malignant mesotheliomas with agents such as colloidal radioactive gold (^{198}Au) or phosphorus (^{32}P) has been most effective when residual tumor is microscopic, since the dosage declines rapidly with the depth of the tissue being radiated. By alternating the usual photon treatment with electron beam therapy the dosages of the former appear to be effective in a much lower range of dosages. Using three successive sessions, fractionating 2000-cGy therapy for a final tumor dose of 6000 cGy has been reported to yield palliative results with reduced rate of complications. Currently, most radiologists are adjusting dosages, fractionation, and methods of administration with the objective of achieving at least the palliation of pain and dyspnea. Reports of trying cobalt 60 irradiation, fast neutrons, and exploitation of photolumenescent compounds have appeared as well. Many patients are now receiving both irradiation and chemotherapy in cooperative and planned programs, including operation when the extent of the cancer permits.

TNM classification of malignant mesothelioma (International Union against Cancer)

TX	Primary tumor not assessed
T0	No evidence of primary tumor
T1	Primary tumor parietal and visceral pleura only
T2	Invasion ipsilateral lung, pericardium, diaphragm, endothoracic fascia
T3	Invasion ipsilateral chest wall, ribs, and mediastinum
T4	Extension to contralateral lung and pleura, peritoneum and contained organs, and cervical tissue
NX	Nodes not assessed
N0	No nodal metastases
N1	Metastases to ipsilateral hilar nodes
N2	Metastases to ipsilateral mediastinal nodes
N3	Metastases to contralateral mediastinal, scalene, or supraclavicular nodes
MX	Distant metastases not assessed
M0	No distant metastases discovered
M1	Distant metastases

TUMORS OF THE MEDIASTINUM

A diverse group of tumors occur within the mediastinum, and they tend to be found individually within the same compartment of the space. The mediastinum is located within the thoracic inlet above, the diaphragm below, and the medial surfaces of the parietal pleura laterally. Its superior compartment is situated between the sternum anteriorly and the pericardium posteriorly. The middle or visceral compartment is the central space containing the heart, great vessels, trachea, central bronchi, and esophagus. The posterior compartment is the remaining prevertebral space and that in the paravertebral gutters. The tumors found most frequently in the anterior compartment are thymomas, lymphomas, and germ cell tumors. Cysts are the most common tumors found in the visceral middle space, and neurogenic tumors appear with approximately the same frequency as cysts in the posterior compartment.

When a tumor of the mediastinum is found or suspected from symptoms or radiographic studies, the question arises immediately about whether it is a neoplasm or vascular lesion or the spinal canal is involved. For help in making an accurate diagnosis clinicians have a number of techniques at their command. In addition to the usual radiographic visualization, computerized tomography indicates the homogeneity of the mass and whether it may consist of multiple nodes and also the presence of cysts and metastatic foci. Ultrasonography and nuclear magnetic resonance imaging clarify the presence of cystic structure(s) without exposure to radiation. Venograms and angiograms with contrast material can clarify the presence of obstruction or vascular abnormalities including aneurysms. Fluoroscopy of the diaphragm can determine the functional status of each phrenic nerve, and a myelogram may be useful in planning the treatment of certain neurogenic tumors. Tumor markers are available for diagnosing and following the response of some tumors to therapy. Beta-chorionic gonadotropin (beta-CGT) may be elevated in the presence of choriocarcinoma and to a lesser extent with embryonal carcinoma, seminoma, and yolk sac tumors. Also the level of alpha-fetoprotein in the serum can be elevated in patients with hepatocellular carcinoma, embryonal carcinoma, and yolk sac tumors.

Aspiration with a fine needle is a valuable aid in making the diagnosis of many of the tumors occurring in the mediastinum. The risks of bleeding and pneumothorax have not been a major problem. Mediastinoscopy is useful in establishing the nature of lymphatic tumors but probably should only follow fine needle aspiration to avoid biopsy of a blood vessel masquerading as a lymph node. The value of thoracoscopy has not been established at the present time. Mediastinotomy is always available for diagnostic studies and resective therapy for lesions located in the anterior compartment. Diagnostic studies must be done with great precision before planning any operative management of neurogenic lesions of the posterior compartment, since a combined thoracic and neurosurgical procedure requires advanced planning for both.

Staging of mediastinal tumors

Stage I	No microscopic invasion of macroscopic capsule
Stage II	Microscopic invasion or macroscopic invasion into fat or pleura

(Continued)

Stage III	Macroscopic invasion of pericardium, great vessels, pleura
Stage IVA	Pericardial or pleural disease
Stage IVB	Lymphatic or hematogenous dissemination

Neoplasms of thymic origin constitute approximately half of the tumors found in the anterior compartment and are found elsewhere infrequently. In addition, thymic cysts and hyperplasia occur in children. Other tumors are thymic carcinomas, thymic lymphomas, Hodgkin's disease, and carcinoids. Thymomas are often classified into four groups depending on the content of epithelial cells and lymphocytes as follows: (1) predominantly epithelial, (2) predominantly lymphocytic, (3) mixed lymphoepithelioid, and (4) spindle cell. Also they are sometimes classified as cortical, medullary, and mixed based on immunohistochemical analysis. Usually thymomas are not found in children younger than the mid-teens, most of the time occuring in adults during the sixth through eighth decades. Various immune disorders accompany the neoplasms. The one found most frequently is myasthenia gravis, which affects at least one-third of patients with these neoplasms. Antibodies to acetylcholine act on receptors at the myoneural junction resulting in weakness of the voluntary muscles and fatigue. Red cell aplasia is an autoimmune disorder occurring in up to half of patients with thymomas. Remission follows resection of the tumor in some cases. Another condition that occurs in about 10 percent of patients with thymoma in hypogammaglobulinemia for which resection also can be beneficial. Cushing's syndrome can be associated with carcinoids. Other symptoms encountered in some patients are cough, dyspnea, chest pain, respiratory infections, fever, and venous obstruction. Medical therapy includes prostigmine hydrobromide and steroids when necessary. Also plasmapheresis elicits some response and is included on several alternate days in the preoperative preparation of patients. Most often it is possible to be certain of the diagnosis without needle biopsy which carries the danger of disseminating the neoplasm along the needle tract. Steroids are discontinued well before operation is scheduled, and antecholinergic medication is stopped about 12 h beforehand. A pulmonary function test also should be done preoperatively, and radiation may be considered initially to reduce the size of a large tumor, especially when it is causing obstruction of the superior vena cava.

The chest is opened through a median sternotomy, and the neoplasm is widely excised to obtain margins free of tumor. Both pleural cavities are opened, and the pleura, lungs, and phrenic nerves inspected carefully. Wedges of lung containing portions of the tumor as well as sections of peridardium are removed if necessary. Also one phrenic nerve can be sacrificed if the necessity arises. Involvement of the veins including the superior vena cava may require longitudinal removal of a portion of the wall affected, with repair, or resection and replacement with a vascular graft. Radioopaque clips placed at the margins of dissection aid the radiologist in outlining appropriate ports for adjuvant radiotherapy. Decision about the necessity for postoperative irradiation can be reached after pathologic study of the specimen(s) removed. Survival for 5 years after operation in stages I and II has been reported to be greater than 90 percent, but recurrence is high in cases of stages III and IV leading to recommendation for postoperative irradiation as part of the plan for treatment. Resection of recurrent tumors of the thorax may also be indicated at times.

Thymomas usually respond to irradiation, and it constitutes adjuvant therapy, which is valuable in prolonging survival as much as 5 percent. However, there is some controversy about whether it should be used after enucleation of noninvasive encapsulated tumors. For invasive neoplasms and those incompletely resected, it is mandatory. It is administered as external beam therapy in divided tumor dosages up to 5000 cGy with ports arranged to avoid injury to the spinal cord. The area covered by ports is sufficient to cover the entire thymus in the protocols of some radiologists. Higher dosages can be associated with complications of pneumonitis, mediastinitis, pericarditis, and myocarditis. The moving strip technique may reduce the danger of injury to the lungs.

Single chemotherapeutic agents proven active in treating thymomas are cisplatin, vincristine, doxorubicin, some alkylating agents such as cyclophosphamide, and corticosteroids. The compounds have been used in various combinations as well, as both adjuvant and neoadjuvant therapy. Some of these combinations are cisplatin, epirubicin, and etoposide; cisplatin, cyclophosphamide, epirubicin, and etoposide; cisplatin, cyclophosphamide, doxorubicin, and vincristine; and cisplatin, cyclophosphamide, doxorubicin, and prednisone. Needed are more clinical trials to provide objective evidence about the comparative effectiveness of the various agents and methods of administration.

Thymic carcinomas arise from thymic epithelium, but they are much more malignant than the thymomas from the same source. These tumors contain spindle and squamous cells and may be quite undifferentiated. The lymphoepitheliomas bear some similarity to those that are found in the nasopharynx, and an etiologic relationship to Epstein-Barr virus is suspected. Because of their usual pattern of behavior, therapy must be intensified and aggressive for success. Responses have been achieved with various combinations of chemotherapeutic agents including bleomycin, cisplatin, and vinblastine and etoposide.

Carcinoids constitute rare malignancies among the group of endocrine tumors found in the mediastinum, including parathyroid cancers. Usually they are not encapsulated, may be invasive, and can be distinguished from thymomas by using electron microscopy and immunohistochemical studies. These neoplasms can metastasize to lymph nodes and bone and are classified as one of the amine precursor uptake and decarboxylase tumors (APUDomas).

They can elaborate elevated levels of adrenocorticotropic hormone (ACTH) resulting in Cushing's syndrome, calcitonins, prostaglandins, kinins, peptides, and amines. Treatment consists of wide resection of the entire thymus gland containing the tumor and adjuvant radiotherapy and sometimes chemotherapy.

Hodgkin's disease and non-Hodgkin's lymphomas occur in about equal numbers in the mediastinum, which is not usually the only site of these diseases. If no tissue is available elsewhere for biopsy, it is mandatory to biopsy the mediastinal nodes. Fine needle biopsy does not yield an adequate specimen very often, although it can eliminate mistaking a blood vessel for a lymph node. Mediastinoscopy or median sternotomy are the routes for making a definitive diagnosis. The type of Hodgkin's disease encountered most frequently is the sclerosing variety which spreads to adjacent nodes in centripital fashion. The diffuse large cell or lymphoblastic lymphomas spread centrifugally with skipped regions giving a characteristic pathologic appearance. Non-Hodgkin's lymphoma is usually treated with chemotherapy, but when the mass is small, irradiation alone can be tried. Masses of larger size require both irradiation and chemotherapy.

Germ cell tumors constitute about one-tenth of all mediastinal tumors, and they occur at any age from childhood to the fifth decade. Those found in the mediastinum are similar to those occurring in the testes, and the chance that they are metastatic from testis or ovary must be kept in mind. Confirmation that the primary site is not in the mediastinum requires biopsy of the testis only if a palpable tumor, positive ultrasound study, or indication of retroperitoneal or abdominal mass or enlarged lymph nodes is made from computerized tomograms. Germ cell tumors are classified into seminomas and nonseminomatous tumors. The latter include teratocarcinomas, embryonal carcinomas, choriocarcinomas and endodermal sinus (yolk sac) tumors, all of which may have seminomatous portions.

Approximately half of all germ cell tumors are seminomas (germinomas, dysgerminomas) occurring in men during the third and fourth decade and seldom in women. When some of these tumors have other components, alpha-fetoprotein and/or beta-chorionic gonadotropin are elevated. Only a fraction of the tumors can be completely resected, but they are radiosensitive. Tumor doses as high as 4500 cGy are used by some radiotherapists, whereas others use lower dosages. Lymph nodes from the cervical chain to the level of the diaphragm are included in the ports. Extending the field of irradiation to the upper abdomen is controversial. These neoplasms can metastasize not only to lymph nodes but also to liver, bone, brain, and other sites. Regimens of chemotherapy with cisplatin include such combinations as bleomycin, cisplatin, and vinblastine with and without doxorubicin; the one usually used to elicit responses even in advanced disease is bleomycin, cisplatin, and etoposide. Schemes such as neoadjuvant chemotherapy followed by surgical resection for locally advanced disease, resection and irradiation for limited disease, and neoadjuvant chemotherapy and resection, with chemotherapy to follow for advanced disease have all been tried. Only about 20 percent of these tumors can be completely excised, and some therapists are reluctant to advocate resection to reduce the size of the tumor mass.

Nonseminomatous germ cell tumors are either pure tumors predominantly of one type or mixed. The constituents are seminomatous, teratomatous, embryonal, trophoblastic (choriocarcinomatous), and endodermal. Benign and malignant teratomas occur in approximately equal numbers. Teratocarcinomas usually contain elements of embryonal cell carcinoma. Other components can include sarcoma, adenocarcinoma, and squamous cell carcinoma. Gynecomastia occurs in up to half of males with choriocarcinoma. Elevated levels of alpha-fetoprotein, and beta-chorionic gonadotropin are found in many of these tumors and are useful in confirming the diagnosis and following the response to therapy. If elevated levels are found, it is permissible to omit biopsy before beginning therapy at times for a rapidly growing tumor. Carcinoembryonic antigen levels also may be elevated in some patients. Symptoms may include chest pain, cough, dyspnea, fever, hemoptysis, and loss of weight. Small tumors can be treated by resection followed by radiation therapy. Cisplatin is usually the principal constituent of chemotherapy for malignant nonseminomatous tumors. Resection is instituted when residual tumor persists after chemotherapy. Almost two-thirds of patients who are responders to chemotherapy survive 5 years. Patients with negative levels of serum markers frequently require more intensive therapy. Even in the presence of metastatic disease, cisplatin therapy has resulted in some long-term survivors. Intensive treatment with bleomycin, cisplatin, and vinblastine with or without doxorubicin followed by resection of residual neoplasm has been used, but probably used most frequently at the present time is BEP (bleomycin, etoposide, and cisplatin). Choriocarcinomas and pure endodermal sinus tumors are the most refractory to this approach to treatment. Prognosis is poorest when complete excision of the tumor is not possible and when the tumor markers do not subside to normal levels after chemotherapy.

Neurogenic tumors arise chiefly from autonomic ganglia and nerve sheath (Schwann) cells and appear most frequently in the paravertebral gutters. Found less frequently are pheochromocytomas, paragangliomas, and neuroectoderma tumors. Autonomic ganglion tumors are found in children and adolescents. Benign ganglioneuromas are rarely symptomatic and rarely produce catecholamines. The two malignant varieties are neuroblastomas, occurring mostly in children under 3 years of age, and ganglioneuroblastomas in older children; both are associated with calcification and bone destruction. Symptoms include cough, dyspnea, chest pain, dysphagia, Horner's syndrome, and if catecholamines are elaborated, flushing, sweating, and diarrhea. The objective of therapy for all neurogenic tumors is complete removal of the lesions. This can be done with satisfactory frequency in benign ganglioneuromas, but survival for 5 years after treatment of malignant tumors declines to 30 percent with only children younger than 2 years having 5-year survivals as high as 90 percent. When these tumors extend through the intervertebral neural foramen and assume a dumbbell shape, a single-stage combined thoracic and neurologic operation is required with visualization of the spinal cord throughout the procedure to lessen the possibility of injuring the cord. Compression of the cord and uncontrolled bleeding can occur if a portion of the tumor remains. Paragangliomas behave somewhat like carcinoids. Those in the paravetebral gutters appear in young adult patients, and approximately half of the tumors secrete catecholamines. Those in the anterior compartment appear in older patients and are more invasive; about half lead to the demise of the patient. The tumors grow slowly but can metastasize or recur after many years. Therapy consists of resection as complete as possible. Recurrence may respond to irradiation.

Nerve sheath tumors occur chiefly in young adults; approximately one-tenth of them are malignant. Neurilemmomas occur more frequently than neurofibromas. The latter are encapsulated and may be multiple in von Recklinghausen's disease. They involve the intervertebral neural foramen more frequently than do autonomic ganglion tumors. The approach to therapy for these tumors is enucleation of the benign tumors and complete resection of the malignancies with clear margins when possible. The prognosis is good for the benign lesions, but survival of patients with malignant lesions is not good, with few surviving more than 1 year.

Approximately one quarter of all mediastinal tumors are cysts. They consist of foregut cysts (bronchogenic from the tracheobronchial tree and enteric duplication cysts from the esophagus), mesothelial cysts (originating from pericardium or pleura), and rare neurenteric and gastroenteric cysts associated with abnormalities of the spinal column and sometimes communicating with the infradiaphragmatic gastrointestinal tract. Among complications that may occur are malignant changes, infections, hemorrhage into the cyst, and erosion into adjacent structures. Because of these possibilities, the management indicated is removal of the cyst even if it is asymptomatic.

Numerous types of other tumors are also found in the mediastinum. Teratomas appear with equal frequency in young adult males and females. About one quarter of these tumors contain calcium and are composed of various fractions of tissues derived from endoderm, mesoderm, and ectoderm. Most are asymptomatic unless they have reached a large size. They are usually resected through a median sternotomy incision from the superior anterior compartment where they usually occur. Approximately half of the connective tissue tumors appearing in the mediastinum are malignant. They can be excised if benign, and many mesenchymal tumors respond to various combinations of resection, irradiation, and chemotherapy. Benign mediastinal lipomas are in the anterior compartment, and the malignant lesions are usually in the posterior compartment. Diagnosis can be made by means of computerized tomography. Resection of the malignancies as well as removal of lymphangiomas may be difficult. Also mesotheliomas present technical problems when they are invasive. Hemangiomas usually grow slowly, and a decision to resect them is viewed with some apprehension by surgeons because of the danger of bleeding, and operation is not justified unless the amount of bleeding becomes an emergency.

CARCINOMA OF THE ESOPHAGUS

Carcinoma of the esophagus constitutes little more than 1 percent of malignancies. It is found with greater frequency among populations in some parts of Africa and China, but wherever it occurs the disease proves exceptionally difficult to treat successfully. Symptoms are sufficiently subtle in the beginning to provide no urgent warnings to the patient to seek medical help, and the extent of the disease represents a major problem when first discovered. This involves dysphagia, first when solid food is ingested and then even with liquids. There may be pain, cough, pulmonary infection, perforation into the trachea, regurgitation, weight loss, involvement of mediastinal structures such as the recurrent nerve(s), and eventually spread to lungs, liver, regional lymph nodes, and even to brain. Smoking and drinking are prominent in patients with this cancer even in primitive societies. Most of the cancers are epithelial squamous carcinomas, localized at first and later spreading to cover as much as 6 cm of the length of the esophagus. Adenocarcinomas are rather rare, although in the type of esophageal epithelium found in organs referred to as Barrett's esophagus, the lower end of the organ is paved with columnar glandular epithelium. This may become metaplastic and give rise to epidermoid lesions, but adenocarcinomas occur in the esophagus as well. Many years ago when the ingestion of lye was a frequent cause of burns of the esophagus, carcinomas appeared in the scarred areas.

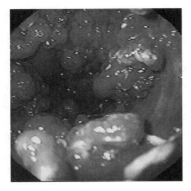

Figure 13 Papillomas of the esophagus.

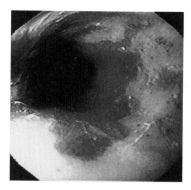

Figure 14 Barrett's epithelium of the lower esophagus.

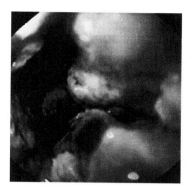

Figure 15 Adenocarcinoma of the esophagus.

The objective of surgical management of this type of cancer can be curative or palliative. Preoperative diagnostic studies including radiographic studies of the chest, esophagrams with contrast medium, cytologic studies of aspirate, hepatic scan, and esophagoscopy-bronchoscopy are used to confirm the diagnosis, assess the extent of the disease, and estimate the likelihood of effective treatment. Most operations resecting the involved esophagus consist of resection of the cancer followed by some type of mobilization of the stomach or colon with attached blood supply to reestablish the continuity of the gastrointestinal tract. A personal preference is to use an interposition of right colon with a small segment of attached distal ileum (or left colon if technically more desirable) between the upper esophagus and the stomach and then resect the thoracic esophagus containing the cancer through a right thoracotomy incision. Although originally done in two stages, the procedure can now be done in one. If the abdominal portion of the procedure reveals metastases, then the cancer is irradiated. In any case, the colon is passed upward through the anterior mediastinum, and the upper anastomosis is done in the neck and the cologastrostomy in the abdomen. When an interposition operation is done in this manner, patients do not have the problem of obstruction of the alimentary tract during the remainder of their lives and can eat; many complications are averted as a result, even if the lesion cannot be eradicted completely. The procedure is applicable to lesions at any level, even in the cervical region. The operation most widely used at the present time is anastomosis of the stomach and the remaining upper esophagus after the esophageal neoplasm is resected. Early diagnosis and more effective therapy are needed to improve the low rate of survival. Perhaps continued extensive investigation will yield improved methods for single or combined management.

Carcinomas of the esophagus do respond to irradiation therapy, but there is no encouraging evidence that this type of treatment alone is the answer to

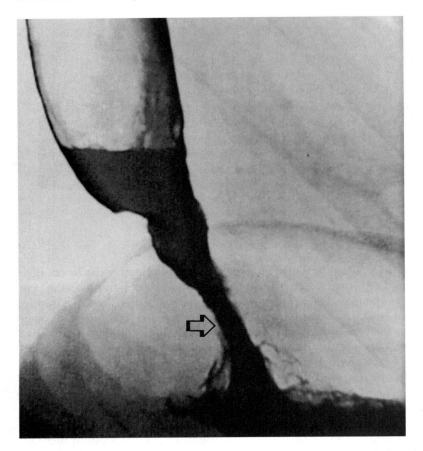

Figure 16 Roentgen study showing carcinoma of the esophagogastric junction.

curing the disease. In a group of 722 patients with esophageal carcinoma composed of both urban and rural dwellers in Africa treated only with irradiation and studied personally, half survived only 2 months and only 1 percent lived longer than 1 year. There were no cures. The results are somewhat better in the United States currently, probably because patients coming to treatment are not so far advanced. Radiotherapy has been used both preoperatively and postoperatively with and without chemotherapy. So far the results are insufficient to give a valid answer about the best use for this modality.

Chemotherapy has been administered to many patients with esophageal carcinoma. Possibly chiefly because the numbers of cases are relatively small in Western populations, the accumulation of information is less than desired at the present time. Chemoradiotherapy preoperatively followed by resection is being examined along with other approaches. Those agents most favored

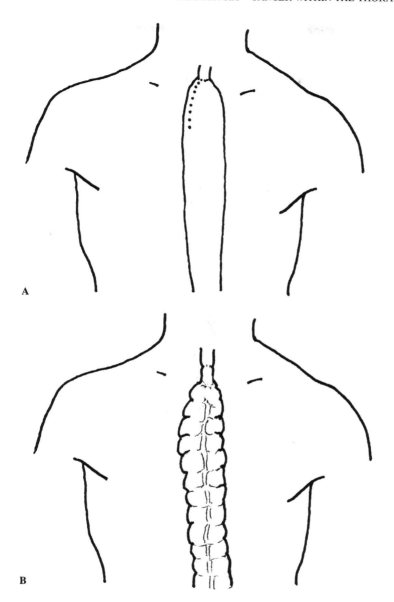

Figure 17 Reestablishment of continuity of the alimentary tract. Following esophagectomy or as a palliative bypass. A. Cervical esophagogastrostomy. B. Use of a segment
of left colon or proximal colon and terminal ileum.

as components of chemotherapy are cisplatin and 5-fluorouracil. Others that have yielded some responses are paclitaxel, mitomycin, Adriamycin (doxorubicin), bleomycin, and methotrexate. Perhaps good advice to the patient is to enter a well controlled study designed to compare different types of treatments, although this type of investigation is not always easily available. It is important in such case-control studies to investigate the relative place of specific types of surgery, chemotherapy, and radiotherapy in a coherent and carefully constructed total regimen. Otherwise for most patients reliance must be placed in the judgment of their surgeon, radiotherapist, and medical oncologist to devise the most promising combined approach to individual problems.

CANCER WITHIN THE ABDOMINAL CAVITY

STOMACH

Gastric cancer was probably known to Hippocrates. It accounts for less than 3 percent of neoplasms in the United States with one-fifth of patients surviving 5 years. In most countries except Poland and Japan the incidence appears to be diminishing slowly. In the United States, Great Britain, and Japan the relative percentage of the primary tumors in the proximal stomach has increased, although more of the total are located distally. Also the lesions in the fundus are more likely to be invasive than those located distally. The disease is responsible for the greatest mortality from cancer in Japan and occurs very frequently in countries located elsewhere in Asia, Europe, and South America. In Japan it is responsible for approximately one-half of the deaths from cancer in men and one-third of those in women.

Antecedent polyps, atrophic gastritis and metaplasia, hyperplasia associated with Menetrier's disease, ulceration, infection with *Helicobacter pylori,* and prior gastric operation have all been implicated with an increase risk of gastric cancer. Also there is an apparent increased incidence of gastric cancer in identical twins and some families. Individuals with the A blood group have a slightly higher risk for the more diffuse type of gastric cancer. Also there is increased risk for gastric cancer in individuals with pernicious anemia, hypogammaglobulinemia, and those engaged in fishing, painting, metal working, ceramic occupations, and printing. Nitrosamines are carcinogenic for laboratory animals and probably are carcinogenic for humans as well. Various dietary habits such as the ingestion of smoked meats have been implicated, but these conclusions remain somewhat controversial.

There are three gross types of gastric carcinomas. The superficial spreading configuration including linitis plastica infiltration is found least commonly,

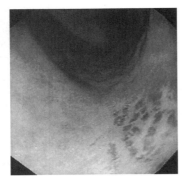

Figure 18 Kaposi's sarcoma of the stomach.

appearing in less than 10 percent of patients with cancer of the stomach. In the United States at least half of these tumors have metastasized at the time of discovery. Nodular, polypoid, fungating, ulcerating tumors account for about one-tenth of cases and tend to have the best prognosis. Fifty percent or more of patients with gastric cancer have sessile tumors that are sometimes mistaken for gastric ulcers. The microscopic appearance of these cancers can be classified according to the relative amounts of mucosal and muscular invasion for use in estimating the prognosis. Multiple primary lesions constitute between 5 and 10 percent of the neoplasms appearing in the stomach.

With the increasing use of endoscopy, a classification in addition to the TNM classification and staging is often used for early gastric cancer. This and the TNM table are given below. Overlapping types occur as would be expected and can include types I and IIA, types IIA and IIC, and types IIC and III. Types I and IIA are classified as intestinal and types IIC and III as infiltrating when examined microscopically. The distribution of the various types of cancer in the Japanese population has led to the speculation that the distribution is unique with the types having the best prognosis appearing more frequently than in other countries. This remains somewhat questionable. Certainly screening with endoscopy and air contrast radiographic examination has been more successful in Japan and is rarely attempted where the incidence of the disease is much lower.

Classification of early gastric cancer

Type I	Protruding
Type II	Superficial
A	Elevated
B	Flat
C	Depressed
Type III	Excavated

TNM classification and staging of gastric cancer

Primary tumor
T0	No primary tumor
TX	Involvement unknown
Tis	Tumor in situ
T1	Mucosal involvement only
T2	Tumor in all layers of mucosa
T3	Serosa invaded with or without extension beyond
T4	Diffuse involvement of wall of stomach

Lymph node involvement
T0	None
NX	Nodal involvement unknown
N1	Adjacent perigastric nodes
N2	Nodes involved in both curvatures or beyond

Metastases
M0	No distant metastases
M1	Distant metastases

Stage 0	Tis	N0	M0
Stage IA	T1	N0	M0
IB	T2	N0	M0
IC	T3	N0	M0
Stage II	Any T	N1	M0
Stage III	Any T	N2	M0
Stage IV	Any T	Any N	M1

It is unfortunate that the symptoms and clinical signs of gastric cancer usually do not appear very early in the disease, and the majority of patients have had symptoms for 6 months or more before the proper diagnosis is made. The earliest symptoms are those of indigestion and sometimes mild abdominal discomfort frequently attributed to peptic ulcer or some other problem. Symptoms can include fulness after meals, dysphagia, nausea, vomiting, weakness, anorexia, flatulence, and pain in the upper abdomen. Also weight loss, melena, anemia, a palpable mass, or enlarged lymph nodes palpable around the umbilicus and left supraclavicular fossa may appear. The patient may become jaundiced, the liver may be palpably enlarged, a mass may be palpated in the pelvis, and ascites can be present late in the course of the disease. Carcinoembryonic and oncofetal antigens may be elevated, achlorydria may be present, and blood may be detected in the stools, but positive tests are not always obtained or can be the result of other conditions as well. Also cytologic study of gastric washings may reveal malignant cells in the presence of cancer. A definitive diagnosis is usually reached after endoscopy and/or radiography with barium contrast medium. In Japan air contrast studies are used more

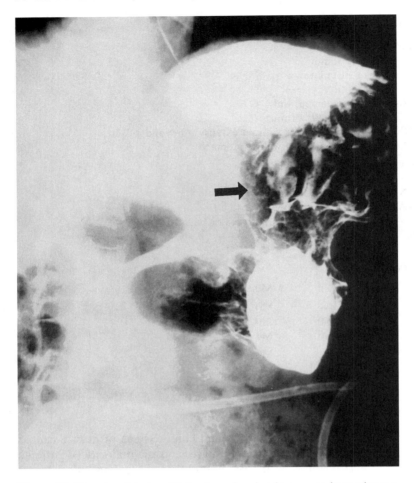

Figure 19 Roentgen study with barium showing large gastric carcinoma.

frequently than elsewhere. The addition of ultrasonography, computerized tomography, and nuclear magnetic imaging enables the radiologist to determine the extent of the disease beyond the stomach as well. The cells may invade the liver, pancreas, spleen, ovaries (Krukenberg's tumors), and pelvis (producing a Blummer's shelf). Determination of nodal involvement by means of endoscopic lymphangiography, ultrasonography following the ingestion of an emulsion of oil and water, and other means have not been of great practical value.

The first successful surgical treatment of gastric cancer is attributable to the careful preliminary examination of clinical records and trial of possible operative techniques in the laboratory by Theodor Billroth and

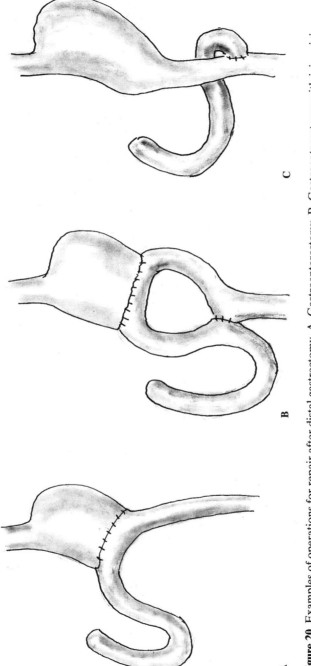

Figure 20 Examples of operations for repair after distal gastrectomy. A. Gastroenterostomy. B. Gastroenterostomy with jejunojejunostomy. C. Gastroenterostomy with Roux-en-Y jejunojejunostomy.

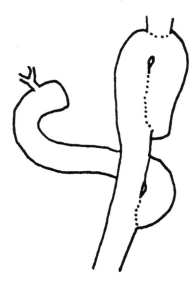

Figure 21 Construction of a jejunojejunostomy pouch below an esophagoenterostomy following total gastrectomy.

colleagues. The first resection of a gastric cancer and reanastomosis of the remaining proximal stomach to the duodenum with survival of the patient was in 1881. The patient later died from extension of the disease beyond the stomach. The operation was called a Billroth I procedure. Later, Billroth closed the duodenum and used a proximal segment of the jejunum for constructing a gastrojejunostomy. This Billroth II procedure was the antecedent of many variations of gastrectomy with restoration of the gastrointestinal tract including operations by Polya and Hofmeister similar to the Billroth II procedure, partial closure of the proximal stomach before the anastomosis, dividing the jejunum so as to leave a short segment for anastomosis lower down (end-to-side jejunojejunostomy) providing a longer segment to bring up and anastomose to the remaining stomach constituting a Roux-en-Y procedure, and the formation of a pouch from the open arm of the Roux-en-Y jejunal segment and anastomosing the pouch to the esophagus after total gastrectomy. The repair done most frequently is closure of the duodenum followed by bringing up a loop of proximal jejunum either anterior or posterior to the transverse colon and anastomosing it to the remaining stomach. After total gastrectomy the anastomosis is done in the same way with the addition of a side-to-side jejunojejunostomy below the esophagojejunostomy to form a pouch. The extent of resection necessary

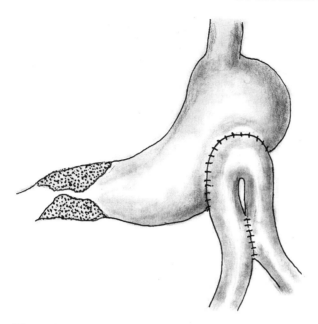

Figure 22 Palliative gastrojejunostomy for advanced distal gastric neoplasm.

beyond the stomach has received a great deal of attention. In Japan gastrectomies are classified according to whether no nodes are resected (R0), the perigastric nodes are resected (R1), or an extensive resection of nodes and adjacent tissue is carried out, removing as much *en bloc* as possible (R2), and sometimes the spleen and pancreas (R3). The operation that has usually been done elsewhere in the past has included removal of omentum but less extensive resection of more distal structures, although partial hepatectomy for localized metastatic disease is sometimes advantageous. Some surgeons believe that their experience does not indicate that the more radical R2 and R3 procedures add to the number of cures and that the incidence of complications is increased. Continued examination of comparative results is obviously indicated. Operative mortality has decreased with experience and now is less than 2 percent. Operative palliation consisting of anastomosing a proximal loop of jejunum to the proximal stomach is usually limited to those cases of advanced cancer with obstruction when other methods of treatment are not successful. Bleeding is seldom sufficiently difficult to necessitate palliative operative intervention.

Radiotherapy has been used for treating gastric cancer in combination with surgical therapy with some response, although these tumors are more resistant to irradiation than many others. It has been utilized intraoperatively when the target can be determined more accurately and, at times, preoperatively to reduce the bulk of the tumor mass. The danger of damaging adjacent structures and lack of knowledge about the extent of the cancer limit the use of radiotherapy as a preoperative measure, however.

Neoadjuvant (preoperative) and adjuvant chemotherapy has been tried extensively to treat gastric cancer with some responses. There is no evidence that is not controversial to indicate that survival is affected. It is usually accepted that combinations of chemotherapeutic agents yield better results than chemotherapy with one alone. 5-fluorouracil with or without leucovorin is chosen by many chemotherapists for initial treatment. Others that have been used in various combinations with some success are Adriamycin (doxorubicin), cisplatin, etoposide, 5-fluorouracil, mitomycin, and semustine. The regimen selected must always be altered when hematologic, gastrointestinal, or other toxicities from treatment become too great. When this occurs, acceptable practice is to substitute appropriate single or multiple agents that have not been used previously. Results of chemotherapy generally have been disappointing. Response rates are low, and responses are of brief duration. The overall status of the patient must be taken into consideration when deciding whether to attempt palliative therapy.

PANCREAS

Cancer of the Pancreas

Cancer of the pancreas is the second most common neoplasm of the gastrointestinal tract occurring with approximately one-fifth the frequency of colorectal cancer. The disease is diagnosed in older age groups usually beyond the fifth decade. Reports of incidence of the disease at times show the number of men having the disease is twice that of women. No specific susceptibility genes are known, but Polynesians and those in the black population of the United States are known to have a high incidence of pancreatic cancer. Unfortunately clinical management of the disease including all modalities yield 5-year survivals as low as 3 percent.

A number of factors have been related to the onset of the disease. Experimentally the disease has been induced in hamsters and rats with nitrosamines and azaserine, respectively, and workers having an industrial exposure to benzidene, naphthylamine, and petrol have a higher incidence of the cancer than those in the population at large. Factors reported to increase the risk of the disease are smoking cigarettes, chronic pancreatitis, diabetes mellitus, and a high intake of dietary fat.

Symptoms bringing the patient to a physician are pain in the upper abdomen radiating through to the back somewhat relieved by change in posture and progressing insidiously, jaundice, loss of weight, and depression. Additional clinical findings may be bleeding, palpable enlarged liver and gallbladder, pancreatitis, diabetes mellitus, upper abdominal mass, polyarthritis, subcutaneous nodules, migratory thrombophlebitis, and ascites. Computerized tomography and endoscopic ultrasound are quite useful in delineating pancreatic cancer and metastatic foci in lymph nodes, liver, peritoneum, and omentum. Also nuclear magnetic resonance imaging has been used selectively. Often a valuable aid in delineating smaller lesions is endoscopic examination with cholangeopancreatography. If not successful, the percutaneous route may be used for visualizing hepatic and pancreatic ducts with the concomitant danger of seeding cancer cells along the needle tract. Chronic pancreatitis, sarcoidosis, and tuberculosis can be confused with cancer of this organ. Serum markers that may be elevated in cancer of the pancreas are carcinoembryonic antigen (CEA, a glycoprotein found in fetal tissue) and antibodies developed against cell lines of human colonic cancer (CA 19-9 and CA 195), human ovarian cancer (CA 125), and human pancreatic cancer (SPAN-1 and DUPAN-2). Their reliability as indicators is reduced because of lack of specificity and positive results appearing more frequently late in the course of the disease and seldom when the cancers are early, small, and curable. Positive diagnoses always are based on results of examining biopsies. However, in certain situations such as trying to differentiate between chronic pancreatitis and cancer, surgery is acceptable rather than additional delay. When the results of computerized tomography, laparoscopy including peritoneal washings, and angiography are negative, approximately three-fourths of the patients are found to have resectable cancer of the head of the pancreas. When the biliary tract is partially or completely obstructed, a decision about decompressing it must be made. If possible, decompression should be done endoscopically, leaving a stent in place to maintain its patency. Percutaneous decompression can be done if the endoscopic route is not accomplished successfully but carries with it more complications. The time of survival is sufficiently brief after palliative resection and the absence of evidence that hormonal, chemotherapeutic, and radiologic adjuvant therapy seldom prolongs survival additionally to make the indication for pancreaticoduodenectomy acceptable only when the disease is thought to be in stages TI or TII.

Benign tumors of the pancreas

Epithelial tumors	
Adeoma	Insulinoma
Acinar cell adenoma	Oncocytoma
Acinar cell cystadenoma	Papilloma
Cystadenoma	Polyp
Cystic papilloma	PPoma
Gastrinoma	VIPoma
Glucagonoma	

(Continued)

Nonepithelial tumors	
Hemangioma	Lymphangioma
Leiomyoma	Neuroma
Lipoma	Somatostatinoma

Malignant tumors of the pancreas

Epithelial tumors	
Acinar cell carcinoma	Insulinoma (malignant)
Adenocarcinoma	Islet cell carcinoid
Adenosquamous carcinoma	Islet cell carcinoma (inactive)
Cystadenocarcinoma	Microadenocarcinoma
Gastrinoma (malignant)	Mucinous carcinoma
Glucagonoma (malignant)	PPoma
Giant cell adenocarcinoma	VIPoma

Nonepithelial tumors	
Fibrosarcoma	Lymphangiosarcoma
Hemangiopericytoma	Lymphoma (malignant)
Hemangiosarcoma	Neural Tumor (malignant)
Histiocytoma (malignant)	Plasmacytoma
Leiomyosarcoma	Rhabdomyosarcoma
Liposarcoma	Somatostatinoma

The experience of the surgeon assigned to operate is a major factor in obtaining optimal results. The mortality following the exercise of good judgment and skillful resection and reconstruction is approximately 5 percent and quite acceptable for such a major procedure as pancreaticoduodenectomy. The surgical procedure currently done in most centers is an operation very similar to the first one done by Whipple in 1935. A variation that does not alter mortality is preservation of the antrum and pylorus of the distal stomach and the first few centimeters of the duodenum, which should reduce the chance of ulceration and postgastrectomy nutritional problems and syndrome. The first objective after opening the abdomen is careful assessment of resectability and confirmation of the diagnosis. However, if a diagnosis from tissue samples could not be reached preoperatively and cannot be obtained expeditiously intraoperatively, the procedure continues. The duodenum and head of the pancreas are mobilized, biopsies of any lymph nodes suspected of harboring metastases are taken and reviewed, and the possibility that adjacent blood vessels and tissues are invaded is eliminated, then the definitive procedure is initiated. The operation consists of resection of the head of the pancreas, cystic and common ducts, gallbladder, and duodenum. Then reconstruction is carried out to ensure the continuity and patency of the alimentary and biliary tracts. Operative variations which do not seem to affect survival favorably are total pancreatectomy and extending the margins of resection including removal of a segment of the portal vein and portions of mesenteric arteries.

Those patients who are not found to be resectable may have partial or total obstruction of the biliary tract and/or the gastrointestinal tract. A decision must be reached about the necessity for relief by means of a surgical procedure. Biliary obstruction can be relieved by choledochoenterostomy or endoscopic or percutaneous placement of a stent left in place. Gastric or duodenal obstruction can be relieved by a gastroenterostomy.

At the time of resection, those patients who have retroperitoneal neural invasion with pain may warrant chemical neurolysis, using alcohol or phenol. Also, endocrine therapy for those who have unresectable tumors is reported to yield extended median times of survival.

Although more than 40 chemotherapeutic agents have been used alone or in various combinations to treat adenocarcinoma of the pancreas, gemcitabine and 5-fluorouracil are agents known to yield the best results in terms of palliation and have been used extensively alone and with other agents. Among many other chemotherapeutic agents and various combinations that have elicited responses are ifofamide; mitomycin C; streptozocin; Adriamycin, 5-fluorouracil, and mitomycin C; adriamycin, 5-fluorouracil, and cisplatin; and cyclophosphamide, 5-fluorouracil, methotrexate, mitomycin C, and vincristine. Chemotherapy has had little impact on survival from carcinoma of the pancreas, and many oncologists recommend that patients who are candidates for chemotherapy enroll in an ongoing clinical trial.

Adjuvant radiotherapy has been used for many years in the treatment of cancer of the pancreas. It is unfortunate that many trials have been confined to relatively few cases, and results have been somewhat conflicting. Radiotherapists have many techniques at their command; some have proved more useful than others. External beam high-energy photons have been used most widely. Others are electron beam therapy, charged particle irradiation (negative pi mesons, helium atoms), high linear energy transfer (LET), and radioactive isotopes such as iodine 125. Irradiation has been given as neoadjuvant (preoperative) therapy, intraoperative therapy, and therapy both postoperatively and in cases that are not resectable. Also it has been combined with chemotherapy in some trials. It is quite clear that so many factors affect the outcome of treatment that each case must be treated individually, taking into consideration the size of the tumor, the extent of invasion and spread, the stage of the disease, the nutritional status of the patient, previous medical history, and susceptibility of adjacent organs to possible damage by irradiation. Although theoretical advantages of some of the types of energy transfers justified trials in the treatment of pancreatic carcinoma, high linear energy transfer has not been successful in the limited experience recorded despite the fact that the amount of oxygen available to treated cells does not affect the results, whereas responses to photons are reduced by lower oxygen tension. Also charged particle irradiation has not been effective in limited trials although the entire

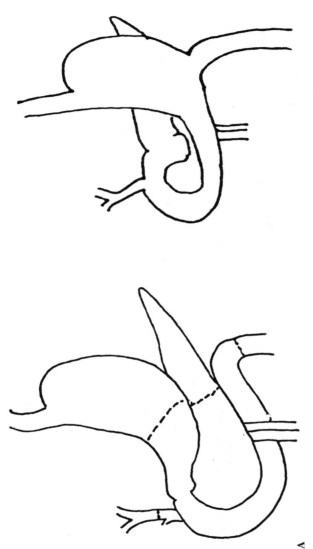

Figure 23 Pancreatic resections for malignant disease. A. Whipple procedure for carcinoma of the head of the pancreas. B. Resection of the tail of the pancreas with splenectomy for more distal neoplasms.

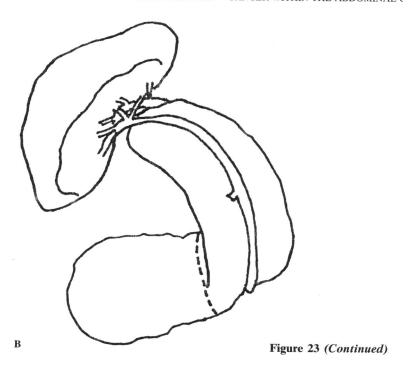

B

Figure 23 *(Continued)*

field exhibits uniform dosage. External beam high-energy radiation, electron beam therapy and radioactive isotope interstitial brachytherapy continue to be features of adjuvant radiotherapy.

Neoadjuvant radiotherapy has been used for cases of localized disease. It has been used with and without chemotherapeutic agents such as 5-fluorouracil and mitomycin C. Radiotherapy has been given in tumor dosages from 5000 to 6500 cGy, and results suggest that the chance of resectability may be increased and survival affected favorably. Intraoperative therapy has the advantage of permitting greater effective dosage of radiation, sparing adjacent organs an undesirable amount of irradiation, and more accurate delineation of the target field. Orthovoltage photons, electron beam therapy, and interstitial implantation of radioisotope (usually ^{125}I) have all been administered intraoperatively, and results suggest prolonged relief of pain and perhaps longer survival after electron beam therapy.

Islet Cell Tumors of the Pancreas

Five different types of cells are known to constitute the islands of Langerhans, each with a specific secretory product. Alpha cells secrete glucagon, beta cells produce insulin, gamma cells excrete somatostatin, F cells produce pancreatic polypeptide (PP), and enterochromaffin cells secrete serotonin. These neuroectodermal cells are also capable of producing other material such as adrenocorticotropin, gastrin, growth hormone, neuron-specific enolase, and vasoactive intestinal peptide (VIP). The polypeptides produced are detectable by immunoassay leading to the clinical diagnosis. Islet tumors may be single or multiple and disseminated throughout the pancreas and may be present in conjunction with multiple endocrine neoplasia.

Islet cell tumors of the pancreas consist of functioning and nonfunctioning tumors. The nonfunctioning tumors cause obstructive or other symptoms as a result of the enlarging mass. They are larger than functioning tumors when discovered and are malignant more often. When found, they are treated as malignant neoplasms and surgical resection is indicated when feasible. The diagnosis is confirmed by the presence of neurone-specific enolase in the tissue. Functioning islet cell tumors may be detected by specific secretory activity and array of symptoms. Those encountered most frequently are insulinomas and gastrinomas. Found less frequently are glucagonomas and VIPomas. Somatostatinomas have rather nonspecific symptoms and are encountered rarely, usually incidentally during an unrelated procedure, with about half of the tumors located outside the pancreas. They are removed when present.

Insulinomas are the pancreatic neuroendocrine tumors appearing most frequently. The local effects of these tumors usually are minor compared with those related to hyoglycemia. At times the patient may have been misdiagnosed as having a neurologic or psychiatric problem. Symptoms found frequently are weakness, lethargy, visual and motor problems, anxiety, confusion, and sweating occurring most commonly after meals. Patients may gain a considerable amount of weight because they eat frequently to avoid the undesirable symptoms. Characteristically hypoglycemia is found along with inappropriately high levels of insulin produced by fasting and/or exercise. Usually hypoglycemia occurs after fasting within 72 h and almost always when exercise is added. An immunoreactive insulin level >20 mU/mL is diagnostic of the presence of an insulinoma. Normally this level falls to <7 mU/mL with fasting. Almost all malignant insulinomas have high levels of proinsulin as well as insulin.

TNM classification of cancer of the pancreas

T1	Neoplasm Confined to Pancreas
T1a	Tumor <2 cm
T1b	Tumor ≥2 cm
T2	Spread to bile duct, duodenum, stomach only
T3	Advanced direct extension, nonresectable

(Continued)

N0	Regional lymph nodes not involved
N1	Regional lymph nodes involved
M0	No distant metastases
M1	Distant metastases
TNM X	Not assessed

Staging carcinoma of the pancreas

Stage I	T1-2, N0, M0	No direct extension, nodes not involved
Stage II	T3, N0, M0	Direct extension adjacent tissues, nodes not involved
Stage III	T1-3, N1, M0	Regional nodes involved, with or without direct extension of neoplasm
Stage IV	T1-3, N0-1, M1	Distant metastatic disease

Usually it is possible to control the levels of glucose satisfactorily with medical management until desirable preoperative diagnostic studies have been completed. Frequent small feedings may be all that is necessary. If not, diazoxide can be used to suppress the release of insulin. Also somatostatin analogue has been used for the same purpose. If a patient has hypercalcemia, parathyroidectomy should precede exploration of the abdomen. Methods used to localize insulinomas preoperatively are ultrasonography, computerized tomography, and selective arteriography. Also transhepatic portal venous sampling has been useful in experienced hands.

Most insulinomas are solitary but a few are found in multiple loci and may be combined with multiple endocrine neoplasia type I. Malignant insulinomas are usually larger than benign tumors, and approximately half of them have spread beyond the pancreas at the time they are discovered, usually to the surrounding tissue and liver. Diffuse microadenomatosis can be encountered and is usually seen only in children. Resection should be done and is beneficial whatever the type of presentation, single, multiple, diffuse, with or without metastases, or combined with multiple endocrine neoplasia type I.

Operation should include enucleation of the adenoma(s), complete anatomic exposure of the pancreas to permit bimanual examination, removal of all gross tumor masses, and wedge resection of hepatic metastatic disease sparing the hepatic artery for possible chemotherapy. If no tumor can be found at operation, then the body and tail of the pancreas are removed in serial segments (preserving the spleen), with the pathologist examining each during the operation. Postoperative chemotherapy using 5-fluorouracil and streptozocin elicits complete responses in about one-third of cases with modestly improved survival. Recommended for chemotherapy are streptozocin and doxorubicin or fluorouracil, dacarbazine, interferon alfa, and chlorozotocin. Some of the patients develop diabetes postoperatively. If the tumor(s) cannot be localized either preoperatively or intraoperatively and diazoxide therapy fails to control clinical symptoms, an intensive effort to locate the source of the disease should be reinstituted.

The neuroendocrine tumor of the pancreas that ranks second in terms of prevalence is the gastrinoma. The symptoms of peptic ulcer disease refractory to ordinary treatment and the clinical syndrome these tumors produce were first pointed out by Zollinger and Ellison. In addition to pain similar to that of ordinary peptic ulcer disease, patients may have diarrhea and esophagitis along with hyperacidity, which is in response to gastrin produced by the tumor. Hypercalcemia is frequently present. The disease may be familial. The secretin stimulation test usually causes the gastrin level to rise >200 pg/mL. immediately. Fasting gastrin levels of 500 pg/mL and greater suggest the presence of the disease as well. The presence of G-cell hyperplasia results in exaggerated response to test meals, which is not a feature of the clinical syndrome associated with gastrinomas. Gastrinomas may be accompanied by multiple neuroendocrine neoplasia type I, may be solitary or multiple, and may present as microadenomatosis of the duodenum. Many of the lesions are malignant and are found in the area around the head of the pancreas designated the gastrinoma triangle, including lymph nodes as well as the pancreas.

H2 receptor antagonists and omeprazole may help control the peptic effects of gastrin and with the usual measures to combat hyperacidity allow sufficient time for diagnostic localization of the tumor(s). Preoperative diagnostic studies should include dynamic computerized tomographic scanning, selective arteriography, and (when available in expert hands) transhepatic venography. Ultrasonography is useful intraoperatively as well as preoperatively. The perfection of radioimmunoassay has increased the chance of detecting gastrinomas earlier in the course of the disease.

Because of the possibility of malignancy and metastases, patients with a diagnosis of gastrinoma should have an abdominal exploration with enucleation of all tumors in head and body of the pancreas. Dissection should be sufficiently extensive to expose the entire pancreas and allow bimanual examination of body and tail. The distal portion of the pancreas can be removed, preserving the spleen. All nodes in the gastrinoma triangle should be removed. If no tumor is found, then the duodenum is opened and searched for microadenomas. Fortunately resections that are curative now approach 50 percent.

Glucagonomas induce a clinical syndrome of mild diabetes and a necrotizing erythematous dermatitis and may include glossitis, loss of weight, anemia, and tachycardia. Concentration of glucagon may reach levels >50 pg/mL. Somatostatin analogues can palliate the rash by inhibiting the release of glucagon. Treatment of the diabetes with insulin as required, hydration, amino acids, glucose, and prednisone are measures that can control distressing symptoms until diagnostic studies to localize the tumor(s) are completed. Operation to remove the source of the problem is then indicated.

VIPomas are associated with achlorhydria, flushing, watery diarrhea, and hypokalemia. Vasoactive intestinal peptide produced by these tumors is a neurotransmitter and hormone that induces the bowel to produce cyclic adenosine monophosphate (cAMP) stimulating the secretion of water and electrolytes in huge amounts. The disease has often been designated as pancreatic cholera. Therapy while diagnostic studies are completed consists of replacing fluid and electrolytes and the use of somatostatin analogues and indomethacin to inhibit the diarrhea. A few of these tumors are found in neural tissue beyond the pancreas, but most are in the pancreas. VIPomas are solitary lesions in most patients but may be multiple in approximately one-fifth of the cases. About one-half of these tumors are malignant, and all require removal. The operative management is similar to that described for insulinomas.

Tumors of the pancreas listed that have not been included in the discussions above are encountered rarely or do not present a clinical problem of importance. Earlier detection of all the types of tumors discussed is a goal which should improve the rather discouraging results of treatment. Carefully planned clinical trials should be continued to assess the value of various methods to diagnose and cure the disease.

LIVER

Hepatocellular carcinoma is the type of cancer found most frequently throughout the world in some Western populations and in broad geographic areas in both Asia and Africa. The incidence of this type of neoplasm in the United States is approximately one-tenth of that in continental China, and those appearing in the Occident seem to be less aggressive than those seen in the Orient. Wherever rates of endemic hepatitis are high, the prevalence of hepatocellular cancer is high as well. Carcinogenic hydrocarbons such as 20-methylcholanthrene are known to cause cancer of the liver in rodents, but none are thought to be a major factor in the appearance of human hepatomas. Hepatocarcinogens elaborated by bacteria, fungi, and vegetation such as senecio and cycad plants are ingested in many parts of the world. This neoplasm also is associated with consumption of alcohol and the concomitant development of cirrhosis and exposure to aflatoxin. Inoculation with hepatitis B virus results inevitably in hepatocellular carcinoma in transgenic mice and is thought to be the primary cause of most of these neoplasms in endemic areas. Other than transplantation, surgical resection is the treatment of choice but is hampered by the cirrhosis frequently present. Possible widespread prophylactic management with viral vaccine has been frustrated by the indifference of populations where the disease is most common.

Late clinical signs of hepatic cancer are jaundice, ascites, bleeding from esophageal varices, and enlargement of the liver or the appearance of a palpable tumor. Jaundice occurs when the bile ducts are invaded and obstructed. Ascites appears when the portal vessels are compressed and occluded, and hematemesis and melena ensue when the hepatic veins are obstructed. Alphafetoprotein is elevated in many cases but not in all. Routine screening for the disease usually includes ultrasonography and determination of alphafetoprotein, the former being more reliable. Intraoperative ultrasonography has been very helpful in localized hepatocellular cancer and in delineating the course of hepatic veins, which is useful to the surgeon in preventing loss of blood during resection and facilitating balloon dilation. Enhanced computerized tomograms are more accurate than preoperative sonography, and magnetic resonance imaging is quite useful in accurately detecting metastatic cancer of the liver and hemangiomas. The use of arteriography is the best means for identifying vascularized malignancies, but nuclear scanning has not been a very consistent aid in distinguishing benign from malignant tumors. Endocyanine clearance has been advocated as a means to predict the safety of hepatic resection but has not been used widely. Carcinoids, glucagonomas, VIPomas, insulinomas, leiomyosarcomas, and similar tumors signal their presence by releasing secretions such as insulin whose effects reveal their identity in the liver and other loci. Biopsies before celiotomy risk dissemination of neoplasms and hemorrhage from hemangiomas and other vascular tumors. Fortunately the results of imaging studies are sufficiently reliable to make biopsies preoperatively rarely urgent unless neoadjuvant therapy is planned.

Benign neoplasms of the liver frequently occur and include hemangiomas, cholangioadenomas, and focal nodular hyperplasia. Cholangioadenomas and focal nodular hyperplasia require no treatment. Hepatic adenomas can become malignant. All patients with this diagnosis receiving estrogen therapy should have the tumor removed by enucleation if growth does not cease within a few weeks after cessation of estrogen. If the tumor stops growing or regresses, follow-up studies with ultrasonography should continue for no less than 1 year. Cystadenomas are benign lesions and should be removed by enucleation only if the tumor causes compression sufficient to result in jaundice or other symptoms. Cystadenocarcinomas occur very rarely and can be cured by removal. Hemangiomas larger than 8 cm in diameter require operative management because of the danger of rupture even though it rarely occurs spontaneously. The extent of the tumor can be ascertained by ultrasonography, and removal need consist only of enucleation. These tumors seldom recur. Angiosarcomas, fibrosarcomas, and rhabdomyosarcomas are the principal types of primary sarcoma found in the liver. Angiosarcomas are associated with a history of exposure to arsenical pesticides, testosterone given to boys with Fanconi's syndrome, vinyl chloride used in the manufacture of plastics, and the well publicized past use of Thorotrast as a radioactive contrast medium.

Angiosarcomas constitute formidable clinical problems without successful approaches to therapy to date. In contrast, both fibrosarcomas and leiomyosarcomas respond to resection and chemotherapy. Also, they may be detected earlier than they would be otherwise by the associated hypoglycemia they induce. Cystadenocarcinomas are sometimes confused with hepatocellular adenocarcinomas. Their principal clinical manifestations arise from obstruction of the bile ducts. Definitive treatment consists of balloon "thrombectomy" of the ducts involved and resection of the hepatic parenchyma invaded in those cases without overwhelming multicentric lesions.

Cancers metastatic to the liver occur far more frequently than primary hepatic neoplasms. Major sources are cancers of the colon and rectum, pancreas, stomach, bronchi, and esophagus. The prognosis depends on the size and extent of the malignancies, the degree of differentiation, and the portion of the liver occupied. Metastases from neuroendocrine tumors make their presence known by secreting vasoactive substances and peptides, which usually brings about earlier detection. As growth of the neoplasm progresses, clinical symptoms and signs begin to appear. Those that may occur are malaise,

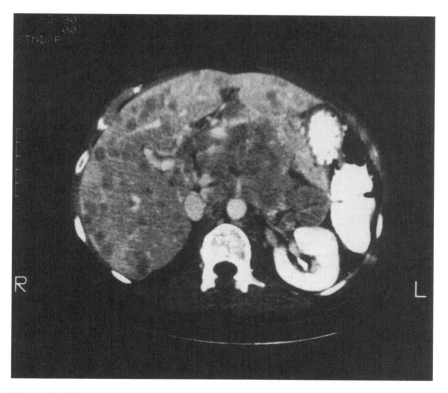

Figure 24 Computerized tomogram showing multiple hepatic metastases.

pain, fever, jaundice, pruritis, ascites, the presence of a palpable mass, and enlargement of the liver. Also the levels of carcinoembryonic antigen and serum alkaline phosphatase are elevated. The same imaging methods used to detect primary cancer are available and used for detection of metastatic disease.

More optimism about the justification of treating patients with hepatic metastatic disease is prevalent today than in the recent past, and most patients have the benefit of careful and extensive evaluation to determine whether operation on the primary neoplasm and/or the metastatic site(s), arterial embolization, radiotherapy, and chemotherapy and biotherapy are justified. If metastatic cancer from the pancreas, esophagus, or stomach are detected preoperatively, justification for resection is seldom present. Metastatic cancer from colon, rectum, and neuroendocrine tumors grow relatively slowly compared to neoplasms arising from other sites. Also, even partial destruction of the neuroendocrine neoplasms can relieve the distressing symptoms often for quite an extended period.

Possibly the unique feature of the hepatic parenchyma is its ability to regenerate over a postoperative period of up to 1 year even in the adult, recalling the legend of avian destruction of Prometheus' liver with regeneration each night, permitting the same horrible event to recur each day. This property of the liver and the somewhat surprising lack of major destruction by most metastatic tumors allows the resection of as much as three quarters of the organ. The anatomic structure of the liver, consisting of a dual blood supply from the portal venous system and the hepatic arteries and drainage by the hepatic veins along with a triad of artery and veins and biliary duct within a hilar sheath at the apex of each of eight lobes that are separable, affords the surgeon sufficient landmarks to control the flow of blood and bile during ablative operations. The clinical work-up in preparation for resection usually includes prothrombin time, partial thromboplastin time, complete blood count, the usual blood chemistry, alpha-fetoprotein level, carcinoembryonic antigen determination, hepatitis serology, typing and cross-matching, and B_{12} determination in addition to using various imaging techniques described above. A vertical abdominal incision with optional sternal splitting extension has almost completely replaced the thoracoabdominal approach to hepatic resection except in cases of primary or metastatic neoplasms located posteriorly, which are not approachable otherwise. Currently, morbidity and mortality associated with these operations has been reduced to acceptable levels. Cancer of the colon and rectum metastatic to the liver as well as primary hepatocellular adenocarcinoma can be treated successfully by hepatic resection. Even when there is a recurrence of the metastatic disease, it is worthwhile to consider a second operation. Many physicians do not advise resection of hepatic metastases from cancers of the lung, pancreas, and stomach because of the poor prognosis based on prior experience. To be an acceptable candidate for operation, a patient must be in good physical condition, and the primary lesion

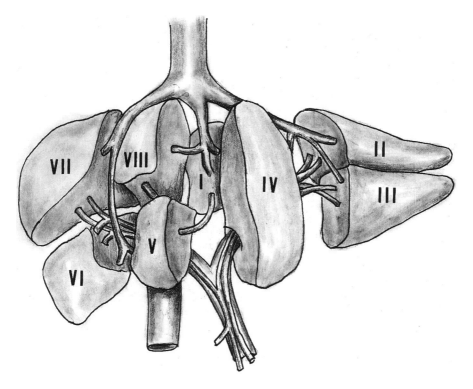

Figure 25 Diagram of segments of the liver permitting resection alone or in various combinations.

and/or metastases must offer the possibility of resection when their location and extent are considered. An additional approach to therapy is embolization. It is possible to cannulate the celiac axis, entering through the femoral artery and advancing the catheter into the arterial branches supplying vascular and neuroendocrine malignancies and then injecting alcohol, coils of fine steel wire, or gelfoam. This type of embolization can be very effective, occasionally completely destroying the tumor.

Orthotopic transplantation should always be considered as a possible means for managing primary cancer of the liver. Also transplants of liver lobes from living donors is sometimes advocated, relying on the powers of regeneration characteristic of this organ. More adequate immunosuppression with the advent of cyclosporin and monoclonal antibodies and extensive experience with the technical procedure have made hepatic transplantation for malignant disease no longer investigational, and approximately one-third of patients now survive 5 years. The preoperative preparation at times must include exploratory operation to determine whether metastatic disease is pres-

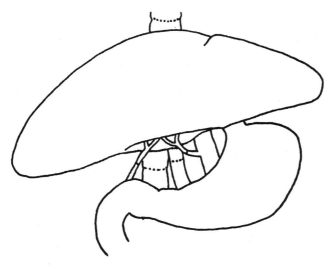

Figure 26 Diagram of hepatic transplantation with sites for anastomosis of inferior vena cava above the liver and, from left to right, the hepatic duct, the inferior vena cava, the portal vein, and the hepatic artery below the liver.

ent. The choice of which situation warrants the operation is currently highly selective. Contraindications are primary and secondary cancer external to the hepatobiliary system, advanced cardiac and pulmonary disease, AIDS, alcohol or drug abuse, and extrahepatic infections when severe. Extensive biliary surgery, positive hepatitis B antigen, age over 65, portal thrombosis, and renal failure are relative contraindications. Patients over 65 whose physical condition and laboratory studies are adequate are now considered candidates at times, thrombosis of hepatic and portal veins can now be corrected by using vein grafts, and experience with patients in renal failure including hepatorenal transplantation suggest that it is possible to manage these patients satisfactorily.

Most favorable results of transplantation have been for small hepatomas in cirrhotic livers and fibrolamellar neoplasms that grow slowly. Primary malignancies of the liver in both right and left lobes and less extensive neoplasms with cirrhosis sufficient to prevent resection are usually candidates unless one of the contraindications above is present. About half of those transplanted have recurrence of the cancer within the first year. Cholangiocarcinomas have a less favorable prognosis than other types of hepatic cancer. The infusion of preservation solution and cooling of the donor organ extends the time for grafting to 24 h. The operation itself requires an average of approximately 8 h. Cost of the procedure currently is $100,000 to $200,000, and the number of grafts continues to be limited by the number of donors. Until xenografting is possible and the cost is reduced, the numbers of these operations will continue to be restricted.

Radiation has been used at times for the relief of pain with temporary success. However, the primary problem with this method of adjuvant therapy is that there is a limit beyond which radiation hepatitis is induced. The effective dosages for adequate responses of hepatic neoplasms may be much greater than the sensitivity of hepatic cells to irradiation. Biliary ductal epithelium has a somewhat greater tolerance than the hepatic parenchyma. When irradiation is given, the total tumor dose in relation to the amount of irradiation in each fraction and the numbers of treatments must be calculated carefully.

Numerous trials of chemotherapy have resulted in 5-fluorouracil and fluorodeoxyuridine maintaining their position as the most effective drugs eliciting responses of colorectal neoplasms. The responses are enhanced by giving the chemotherapy intraarterially through the hepatic artery even though the metastases reach the liver via the portal system. Responses occur in approximately one quarter of the cases of metastatic cancer of the colon, but there is no convincing evidence of prolonged survival following this type of treatment.

Trials of many single drugs, the most common being cisplatin, 5-fluorouracil, doxorubicin, neocarzinostatin, and VP-16, have been uniformly disappointing in terms of responses and survival when they are given alone or in combination systemically for the treatment of primary cancer of the liver. This experience has produced little justification for systemic chemotherapy at the present time. On the other hand, regional administration of chemotherapy has elicited more favorable responses. When the neoplasm involves both major lobes, they are treated in alternate separate sessions. Neoadjuvant therapy is sometimes advocated to reduce the tumor mass before resection, using agents such as cisplatin and doxorubicin. Hepatoblastomas seen in childhood are known to respond to vincristine, 5-fluorouracil, and carboplatin; cisplatin and doxorubicin; and etoposide. The addition of embolization to chemotherapy has been used extensively in the Orient, but additional complications associated with the procedure suggest some caution when considering this technique. Studies based on the presumed effect of hormones on hepatic cancer, including treatment with tamoxifen and antiandrogens, have not led to any consensus about the value of this approach to treatment.

Both primary and metastatic cancer of the liver continue to offer one of the greatest challenges for the oncologist. Remarkable progress has been made in surgical therapy including orthotopic transplantation, diagnostic tests, and clinical management of the disease. New effective agents are needed for systemic chemotherapy as well as more effective agents for regional treatment. Much needs to be done to capitalize on the effect of hormones on these cancers and the usefulness of various biologic approaches to therapy.

TNM classification of hepatic cancer

TX	Primary cannot be assessed
T0	No primary tumor
T1	Single tumor ≤2 cm, no vascular invasion
T2	Single tumor >2 cm, no vascular invasion Single tumor ≤2 cm, vascular invasion Multiple tumors ≤2 cm, vascular invasion, one lobe
T3	Single tumor >2 cm, vascular invasion Multiple tumors ≤2 cm, vascular invasion, one lobe Multiple tumors >2 cm, one lobe, with or without vascular invasion
T4	Multiple tumors more than one lobe, or involvement major branch or portal or hepatic veins
Nx	Lymph nodes cannot be assessed
N0	No metastatic disease regional nodes
N1	Metastatic disease regional nodes
MX	Distant metastatic disease cannot be assessed
M0	No distant metastatic disease
M1	Distant metastatic disease

Staging of hepatic cancer

Stage I	T1	N0	M0
Stage II	T2	N0	M0
Stage III	T1	N1	M0
	T2	N1	M0
	T3	N0	M0
Stage IVA	T4	Any N	M0
Stage IVB	Any T	Any N	M1

GALLBLADDER AND BILE DUCTS

Cancer of the gallbladder is associated with symptoms that are rather nonspecific and include nausea and vomiting, anorexia, pruritus, jaundice, and upper abdominal pain in the later stages of the disease when an abdominal mass may be palpable as well. Usually early disease is found incidentally. By far most of the lesions are mucinous, papillary, signet-ring cell, or tubular adenocarcinomas. Squamous and adenoacanthomatous neoplasms are encountered much less frequently, and carcinoids, clear cell malignancies, malignant melanomas, and spindle cell neoplasms are rarely found. Adenomas, adenomyomatosis, mucosal dysplasia, and polyps may be present in gallbladders containing neoplasms. Cancers of this organ spread by direct extension and venous, perineural, and lymphatic routes, each reducing the chance of controlling the disease. Several staging systems are being used in classifying carcinomas of the gallbladder. The TNM classification and staging of the American Joint Commission on Cancer and International Union against Cancer and the Nevin system of staging appear in the accompanying tables below.

The stage of cancer of the gallbladder is associated with the presence and the size of gallstones, increasing age, the anatomic structure of common and pancreatic ducts allowing mixing of bile and pancreatic secretions, and employment in the automobile, metal, rubber, and wood structural industries. Cancers of the gallbladder and cystic ducts have been induced in laboratory animals exposed to 20-methylcholanthrene and other carcinogenic hydrocarbons. This type of cancer is seen most often in people from the United States, Mexico, Israel, and some parts of Europe. It is seen least in black natives and migrants from Africa.

Both ultrasonography and abdominal computerized tomography are useful in making the diagnosis of cancer preoperatively. The most accurate test for assessing operability and making the diagnosis is capitalizing on the vascularity of the neoplasm by injecting contrast material into the superior mesenteric artery and obtaining a computerized portogram. Resection is the only means for curing cancer of the gallbladder; unfortunately no more than one-third of cases are resectable at the time of operation. The type of operation carried out ranges from cholecystectomy with hepatic wedge resection to cholecystectomy, right hepatectomy, pancreaticoduodenectomy, and nodal resection extending to and including paraaortic nodes. Support for more radical resections is limited to occasional reports of cures but without proof from any objective clinical trial with appropriate numbers of cases and controls. Extending the procedure is accompanied by increased morbidity and mortality, and comparisons of results after radical and conservative operations show no appreciable differences in survival. Carcinomas of the gallbladder found incidentally and limited to the mucosa have an excellent prognosis with cholecystectomy. If the neoplastic cells have extended to and beyond the serosa, the outlook is much less favorable.

External beam supervoltage irradiation of 5000 cGy has been used in advanced disease for the relief of pain and pruritis and has been found quite useful. Also brachytherapy with iridium 192 introduced into the common duct may relieve symptoms. Irradiation given intraoperatively has the advantage of localizing the irradiation accurately, reducing the amount of irradiation to tissues uninvolved and shielding adjacent organs. Unfortunately there does not appear to be any dramatic extension of survival, although combination of radical operation with postoperative irradiation has given slightly better figures for survival in a limited number of cases.

Adjuvant chemotherapy has been administered systemically, utilizing numerous agents alone and in various combinations such as cyclophosphamide, etoposide, 5-fluorouracil, tegafur (Ftorafur), semustine (methyl-CCNU), mitomycin C, and streptozocin with mean rates of response less than 20 percent. Best responses have been obtained with fluorouracil with and without leucovorin; fluorouracil, doxorubicin, and mitomycin (FAM), and cisplatin. When suitable agents are administered through the hepatic artery, the mean responses can be more than doubled. Also rates of response to chemotherapy vary widely depending on the extent of the neoplasm being treated from approximately 50 percent for lesions of the mucosa to less than 10 percent for those extending to serosa and lymph nodes with little response when the disease invades the liver.

Carcinoma of the gallbladder can be cured only by resection in favorable cases. Extending the operation for advanced disease to one of the more radical procedures has not yielded any convincing change in the rate of cures, which continues to be around 5 percent. Radiation therapy can give some palliative relief, and adjuvant chemotherapy has yielded responses that encourage some continuation of administration via the hepatic artery. Limited disease is best treated with cholecystectomy with postoperative irradiation when indicated. Removal of the gallbladder, if possible, with some type of biliary bypass can be appropriate management in advanced cancer of this organ.

Primary cancers of the extrahepatic biliary tract are primarily adenocarcinomas occupying the wall of the duct and sometimes extending into the lumen. Some are less well differentiated than others and can be diffuse. They appear late in life and are found more often in men than women. It is important to separate them from neoplasms in the intrahepatic ducts, pancreas, ampulla of Vater, and gallbladder and cystic duct. The lesions appearing in the proximal tract including the common hepatic duct and bifurcation into the hepatic ducts are found more frequently than those located at a lower level in the common duct and level of the junction with the cystic duct. The percentage of lesions resectable in the distal portion of the ductal system is approximately double that for lesions in the proximal portion.

TNM classification of the stages of cancer of the gallbladder

Tis	Carcinoma in situ
T1	Neoplasm in mucosa or muscle only
T1A	Mucosa
T1B	Muscle
T2	Transmural invasion
T3	Transmural, lymphatic, or <2 cm hepatic invasion
T4	Invasion of two or more organs or >2 cm of the liver

(Continued)

Stage 0	Tis	N0	M0
Stage I	T1	N0	M0
Stage II	T2	N0	M0
Stage III	T1	N1	M0
	T2	N1	M0
	T3	Any N	M0
Stage IV	T4	Any N	M0
	Any T	Any N	M1

Nevin staging for cancer of the gallbladder

Stage I	Intramucosal invasion only
Stage II	Invasion of mucosa and muscularis
Stage III	Transmural invasion
Stage IV	Metastases to cystic duct and lymph nodes
Stage V	Metastasis

Cancer of the biliary tract is often confused with benign disease with cocomitant delay in treatment. Often jaundice is the first clinical sign bringing the patient for medical help. Loss of weight and abdominal pain accentuate the need for immediate diagnostic and therapeutic decisions. Also pruritis may be the complication that makes the patient most miserable. The best procedure for obtaining the diagnosis and localizing the cancer(s) is endoscopic cholangiopancreatography. Less desirable but useful is transhepatic cholangiography. Often the diagnosis is made at the operating table in which case intraoperative cholangeoscopy should be done along with cholangeography. The operation can be executed more expeditiously with knowledge obtained from preliminary cholangeoscopy whether the diagnosis is or is not known preoperatively.

The operative procedure, which offers the only cure for the disease, is more successful for cancer of the distal lesions, which permits removal of twice as much of the duct when compared with only about one-third of the tissue in proximal neoplasms. The operation must also include the construction of an anastomosis between the proximal hepatic duct(s) and the alimentary tract to reestablish drainage of the biliary system. This may also be done by tubal drainage of the biliary obstruction in cases that are not resectable. Whether radical resection is justified in advanced disease is not clear, but more extensive procedures are being undertaken now than formerly. Currently the survival of patients with cancer of the proximal biliary tract is unusual. The 5-year survival of patients operated on for more distal malignancies is less than 10 percent. Sufficient palliation from both chemotherapy and radiotherapy justify continued adjuvant therapy for the management of residual cancer and lesions that are not resectable.

SMALL INTESTINE

The small bowel constitutes approximately 75 percent of the total length of the intestinal tract. No more than 6 percent of tumors of the bowel are found in the small intestine, about a quarter of which are found in the duodenum, the shortest portion. Some of the reasons that have been assigned for this relatively low incidence of tumors are rapid transit time, fewer bacteria in this portion of the bowel, the presence of enzymes capable of destroying carcinogens, and the presence of immunoglobin A (IgA) and other immune factors. Several symptoms are associated with tumors of the small intestine at times. Bleeding is found more often in the duodenum than elsewhere, sometimes with hematemesis and, if profuse, melena. Obstruction, both incomplete and complete, is found and at times is the result of volvulus or intussusception. Jaundice and pancreatitis may follow the growth of a benign tumor or invasion of a malignancy at the ampulla. Perforation also may be one cause of the patient's symptoms. Cafe au lait spots may signal the presence of neurofibroma(s), mucocutaneous pigmentation accompanies Peutz-Jeghers syndrome, and telangiectasias occur in the Osler-Render-Webber syndrome.

Appropriate diagnostic studies include radiographic examination of the abdomen along with computerized tomography and at times nuclear magnetic resonance imaging and barium studies of the small bowel. Ultrasound studies can be useful, and angiography of the mesenteric vessels can localize the site of some lesions as well as suggest the appropriate diagnosis. Endoscopy with biopsy is often the most useful of all the diagnostic tests. Many of these tumors are discovered at the time of operation. Transillumination may aid in discovering the exact site(s) involved.

Benign tumors found in the small bowel most frequently are leiomyomas, lipomas, adenomas, and hemangiomas. The remainder such as lymphangiomas, pseudolymphomas, and ganglioneuromas are found infrequently. Hamartomas occur somewhat at random throughout the entire gastrointestinal tract. Malignant tumors of the small intestine include fibrosarcomas, liposarcomas, adenocarcinomas, angiosarcomas, lymphangiosarcomas, lymphomas, neurofibrosarcomas, and carcinoids.

Benign Tumors

Benign epithelial tumors can be very troublesome when located in the duodenum where they occur most often. Tubular adenomas are usually polypoid; villous adenomas are sessile and are more likely to become malignant. Removal of these tumors endoscopically should not be attempted if they are 2 cm or larger. Resection with wide margin is more easily carried out in jejunum and ileum, whereas even a benign tumor may occlude the ampulla with jaundice and/or pancreatitis. When local excision is done, then endoscopic follow-up must be a mandatory part of management. Because adenomas can become malignant, they should be removed. Familial polyposis such as Gardner's syndrome may include tumors in the small as well as the large bowel. Brunner's gland adenomas occur in the duodenum and may be polypoid, nodular, or diffuse. Since they rarely become malignant, some practitioners prefer to follow their course with endoscopic examinations rather than removing them, especially in the case of diffuse lesions that would require an extensive procedure. Inflammatory polyps are resected, or a sleeve resection of the bowel is performed. The polyps are multiple in Peutz-Jeghers syndrome, which is inherited as an autosomal dominant. It is usually discovered in the first three decades of life and consists of the appearance of polyps throughout the gastrointestinal tract and mucocutaneous pigmentation of face, lips, buccal mucosa, and at times the palms and soles. Malignancies occur more frequently in the duodenum than elsewhere and appear in about 5 percent of patients with the disease. Management consists of local resection when indicated and careful follow-up, usually with multiple operations required in the usual course of the disease. There is increased risk of malignancy of the small bowel in Crohn's disease and tropical sprue (celiac disease), and the clinician treating patients with these diagnoses must always be alert to the possibility and act definitively to remove any neoplasm when it appears. Rare polyposis syndromes are juvenile polyposis and the Cronkite-Canada syndrome. The former consists of polyps of the large as well as the small bowel; these are benign tumors. The latter features polyps in the entire gastrointestinal tract and ectodermal changes including pigmentation of the skin, alopecia, dystropy of nails, steatorrhea, and diarrhea.

Staging cancer of the small bowel (Blackledge)

Stage I	Neoplasm within gastrointestinal tract
Stage II	Local mesenteric node metastases
Stage III	Neoplasm perforating bowel
Stage IV	Metastases paraaortic nodes and beyond
Stage V	Metastases in viscera or bone marrow

Staging cancer of the small intestine (Ann Arbor)

Stage I	Metastatic disease single site or nodal group (IE)
Stage II	Metastatic disease same side of diaphragm of more than one nodal group or single extranodal site and one or more nodal groups (IIE)

(Continued)

Stage III	Metastatic disease, both sides of diaphragm with or without cancer in extranodal sites (IIIE), spleen (IIIS), or both (IIIES)
Stage IV	Metastatic disease, viscera or bone marrow

Lipomas are found most frequently during the sixth and seventh decades, and often occur in the ileum. Intralumenal, extralumenal, and intramural presentations are found, and they can grow to large size and may be palpable on abdominal physical examination. Complications can include volvulus, perforation, intusussception, bleeding, and intestinal obstruction, but many are asymptomatic. Surgery is usually not necessary unless symptoms or the size of the tumors make removal necessary.

Smooth muscle tumors (leiomyomas) usually appear in the jejunum and ileum late in life from the fifth decade. They can become malignant, and they are removed when the diagnosis is reached or suspected. Complications include volvulus, obstruction, perforation, and hemorrhage. Fibromas are not found in the small intestine very often. Approximately one-quarter of patients with the neurofibromas of von Recklinghausen's disease have lesions in the gastrointestinal tract. Bleeding and obstruction can occur, and resection of the affected bowel is indicated. Schwannomas, gangliocytic neuromas, and paraganglioma are not encountered very often. They are usually removed in the process of making the diagnosis. Capillary and cavernous hemangiomas and telangiectasia of the bowel may require operation and mesenteric vessel angiography and transillumination to locate the sites of the disease and hemorrhage. Lymphatic cysts, lymphangiomas, and lymphangiectasis of the small bowel may lead to hypoproteinemia and require resection. Hamartomas are lesions where there is overgrowth of the normal tissue at the site; they rarely require removal.

Duplications and Heterotopic Tumors

Conditions that may be mistaken for tumors are duplications of the small bowel as well as heterotopic tissue and endometriosis localized in the small intestine. Congenital duplications are either cystic or tubular, the latter opening into the normal intestine. One of the difficulties in dealing with the abnormality is the common mesenteric blood supply of the duplication and the normal bowel. Treatment is resection of the duplicated segment if possible. However, it may be possible to anastomose the duplicated segment only to the normal bowel or core out the mucosa. If the segment is not extensive, then the duplicated segment can be resected in its entirety. Heterotopic tissue such as gastric mucosa and pancreatic tissue are usually not disturbed unless complications of bleeding, obstruction, or perforation occur. Resection of the segment containing the offending tissue is then carried out. When in the vicinity of the ampulla in the duodenum, removal without current symptoms may be wise because of the likelihood of biliary obstruction. Cases of endometriosis affecting the small bowel are not encountered very often and usually are diagnosed at the time of operation. If limited, resection of the segment of small bowel affected can be done.

Adenocarcinoma

Adenocarcinoma is the neoplasm of the small bowel that occurs most frequently and is located more often in the duodenum and jejunum than in the ileum. It leads to the most difficult problems when originating in the first and second portion of the duodenum. Pancreaticoduodenectomy and regional resection of the lymphatic drainage is the procedure advocated for removal of the neoplasm and metastatic spread when there is a reasonable chance for a successful technical procedure. Unfortunately the results have been very discouraging after many years of experience. The regimen of chemotherapy used most frequently is combinations including 5-fluorouracil. In those lesions that cannot be resected, irradiation therapy may be useful in helping control bleeding. For adenocarcinomas below the second portion of the duodenum, resection of the bowel and wide resection of the mesentery and regional lympatic drainage is the best approach.

Carcinoids

Carcinoids constitute approximately one-third of the malignancies found in the small intestine. They are indolent neoplasms that grow slowly. The appendix is the most common site, but they appear elsewhere including the duodenum. As many as one-third of the tumors may be multicentric, which must be kept in mind in planning therapy and delineating the extent of the lesion. They are included as one of the APUDomas, or tumors that feature amine precursor uptake and decarboxylation. Those tumors derived from the midgut can secrete high levels of serotonin. Also several peptides can be secreted including glucagon, gastrin, and somatostatin. In almost all cases the serum levels of hydroxyindoleacetic acid (HIAA) are high. The clinical syndrome of carcinoid includes flushing in the area of the head and neck and upper chest which can be initiated by ingestion of foods containing pyramine such as chocolate, asthma, valve disease, diarrhea, abdominal pain, and ileus. An intense desmoplastic reaction occurs in the vicinity of these lesions causing kinking of the bowel, shortening of the mesentery, and mesenteric ischemia. Although many of the tumors are not symptomatic, this is not true of those found in the duodenum where most of them cause symptoms of jaundice, ulcer, obstruction, intususception, and vasopressor effects of glucagon, gastrin, and somatostatin. Almost all tumors larger than 2 cm have metastasized. Those in the liver may be quite large.

Diagnostic studies should include computerized tomography and at times nuclear magnetic resonance studies and mesenteric arteriography. Treatment varies from wide local excision to pancreaticoduodenectomy and resection of terminal ileum and ascending colon, depending on the location and multiplicity of the lesions and including the draining lymphatics in the mesentery and region involved. Care in handling the tissue is essential, since the pressure may elicit an intense vasospastic reaction. Reduction in the size of the tumor mass is important in controlling symptoms associated with the carcinoid syndrome, and dearterialization and partial resection are worthwhile even though the entire mass cannot be excised. The somatostatin analogue SMS-201 can control symptoms in some patients. Chemotherapy that has been most effective is fluorouracil with and without streptozocin and doxorubicin along with cisplatin; cyclophosphamide; dacarbazine; and interferon alfa. Interferon-α and mitomycin C have been used as well. The success of treatment appears to be correlated with the size of the tumor and metastatic mass, ploidy of the primary neoplasm, and whether the patient is a female or had no symptoms.

Primary Lymphoma

To make the diagnosis of primary lymphoma of the small bowel, the possibility that it is part of disseminated disease must be eliminated. There should be no peripheral or mediastinal lymphadenopathy or involvement of liver or spleen, and the peripheral blood differential and leukocyte counts should be within normal limits. Modified classifications of these lymphomas of the small intestine are summarized in the accompanying tables. The four types are Mediterranean, Western, Hodgkin's, and juvenile. The most common of these lymphomas in the Middle East and Africa is the Mediterranean disease, which features clubbing of the nails, diarrhea, and pain. The lesions characteristically extend throughout the small intestine and include the nodes in four-fifths of cases. Diagnosis is usually made by endoscopic biopsy of the thickened and nodular bowel wall. Treatment consists of chemotherapy with no more than one quarter of the young adults who have the disease surviving more than 5 years. Western lymphomas, the most frequently encountered of all those in the small bowel, occur in older patients, predominantly in males. The lesions are found most often in the lower bowel and may be sufficiently large to be palpable and sometimes perforate. The usual management of the disease is an exploratory celiotomy with wide resection of the segment of intestine involved and the draining lymphatics in the mesentery along with affected regional nodes. Adjuvant chemotherapy has been valuable adjunctive therapy, although some clinicians do not advocate it after complete resection. Median survival after resection and chemotherapy is around 3 years. Adjuvant radiotherapy has been used, but many oncologists prefer to rely on operation plus chemotherapy. Hodgkin's disease rarely occurs in the small intestine and is treated by resection followed by systemic chemotherapy. Juvenile lymphomas are similar to Burkitt's tumors and are treated by surgical resection and adjuvant systemic chemotherapy with survival of approximately 75 percent.

Sarcoma

Sarcomas of the small intestine are sometimes classified as stromal (leiomyosarcomas and leiomyoblastomas) and autonomic nerve sarcomas. They may present as a palpable mass and/or cause bleeding, obstruction, and perforation. These tumors are vascular and present as either an exoenteric or endoenteric mass. Treatment consists of wide excision including adjacent tissue. Duodenal lesions may require pancreaticoduodenectomy. These tumors usually have not spread to adjacent lymph nodes at the time of discovery, and it is necessary to resect widely only the mesenteric drainage of the specimen being removed. Peritoneal and hepatic metastatic disease responds to both adjuvant radiotherapy and chemotherapy. Evidence that adjuvant therapy extends survival is equivocal.

Metastatic Cancer

Metastatic cancer of the small bowel can originate in numerous primary sites, the most frequent being melanomas. Other primary cancers known to metastasize to the small bowel are those spreading from abdominal organs transperitoneally and on contact and those elsewhere such as neoplasms of lung, breast, and thyroid. Operative intervention for bleeding, perforation, and/or obstruction may be necessary.

APPENDIX

Patients with tumors of the appendix may not have symptoms characteristic of acute appendicitis, and very often the diagnosis is made as a result of findings at the time of operation for another problem. Even when the focus is on the appendix as the cause of the difficulty, the diagnosis may not be made at the time of the first operation because of the time required for microscopic examination of the specimen. Therefore, appropriate therapy often requires a second operative procedure. Also a second malignancy may be present or may develop subsequently with sufficient frequency to justify careful and prolonged follow-up.

Almost 9 of 10 primary neoplasms of the appendix are carcinoids with adenocarcinoids, mucinous adenocarcinomas, and adenocarcinomas similar to those in the colon constituting up to 15 percent of these tumors. Approximately half of all carcinoids are localized in the appendix with a preponderance of female patients. The carcinoid syndrome is rarely associated with tumors in this site, and quite often the symptomatology does not suggest a problem with the appendix. Some of these tumors secrete serotonin, which can be detected by the presence of 5-hydroxyindole acetic acid in the urine. Other types of appendiceal neoplasms do not have a preponderance in either sex. Appendiceal adenocarcinoids exhibit a more aggressive behavior than that of carcinoids. They spread throughout the appendix and beyond and may be the primary lesion in Krukenberg tumors. A mass in the right lower quadrant and symptoms suggesting acute appendicitis are features of mucinous cystadenocarcinomas. At operation the tumor appears as a mass invading the wall of the appendix and may be associated with ascites, pseudomyxoma peritonei, intraabdominal metastases, and intestinal obstruction. It may be difficult to distinguish benign mucinous cystadenomas from mucinous cystadenocarcinomas based on gross inspection alone. Microscopic study of mucinous cystadenocarcinomas demonstrates appendiceal invasion by glandular arrangements of cells and malignant atypical cells within mucinous deposits on the peritoneal surfaces not present in mucinous adenomas. Adenocarcinomas arising in the appendix frequently are symptomatic, suggesting acute appendicitis and at operation may present as a mass at the base of the appendix. These carcinomas behave very much like those in the colon with invasion and metastases. They may be diagnosed intraoperatively, but the diagnosis often may not be known until pathologic examination is complete.

When localized in the appendix, carcinoids are frequently treated by appendectomy, but, when the lymphatics of the mesoappendix and beyond contain metastases, right hemicolectomy is indicated. A personal preference is to include a short segment of the distal ileum as well as the colon along with the lymphatic drainage of the bowel being removed. When localized, treatment results in almost all patients surviving 5 years. With invasion and metastases in the liver and elsewhere, resection and debulking may be indicated. Additionally, arterial embolization and recombinant Interferon alfa-2a and Interferon-α are sometimes useful. Somatostatin can be effective in controlling the carcinoid syndrome. Occasionally responses follow treatment with cisplatin, cyclophosphamide, doxorubicin, etoposide, 5-fluorouracil, and streptozocin alone or in various combinations. Irradiation to cerebral, intracranial, dermal, and osseous foci may result in some palliation.

Patients with the rare adenocarcinoids have a relatively good prognosis when localized, four out of five surviving 5 years, but the prognosis is much worse for those with lesions that have spread beyond the appendix. Most of these tumors require right hemicolectomy. Also oophorectomy is indicated and should be discussed with the patient preoperatively. [In any case of Krukenberg tumor(s) with the primary source unknown, the appendix should be removed since it may arise from an occult appendiceal adenocarcinoid.] Experience with radiotherapy and chemotherapy has been limited because these tumors occur so infrequently; but, in general, experience with carcinoids may be used as a guide to therapy.

Mucinous adenomas can be treated successfully with appendectomy. Right hemicolectomy is the usual treatment for mucinous cystadenocarcinomas, since the long-term survival of patients thought to have the neoplasm localized in the appendix and treated with appendectomy is about half that when right hemicolectomy has been done. When there is extensive spread of the disease, debulking is worthwhile along with omentectomy, oophorectomy, and drainage of accumulations of mucin. Multiple palliative operations may be more successful than chemotherapy and/or radiotherapy. However, radiotherapy and chemotherapy with agents such as cisplatin, chlorambucil, 5-fluorouracil, melphalan, mitomycin C, and thiotepa are sometimes used alone and in various combinations with some responses.

Adenocarcinomas occur in older patients in contrast with mucinous and other tumors of the appendix, which occur in younger patients. The diagnosis is almost never made preoperatively, but sometimes is made at the time of operation. When it is made postoperatively, then a second operative procedure is imperative. It is unfortunate that most of these tumors are advanced when they are recognized, and many are in Dukes' stage C. Right hemicolectomy is done along with oophorectomy in postmenopausal women. The results are the same as for this type of cancer appearing in the colon. Resection of limited metastases such as solitary lesions of the lungs and limited spread to liver can be justified. Although total abdominal radiotherapy is associated with too many undesirable side effects, radiotherapy can be used to treat isolated foci. Also 5-fluorouracil, the most effective chemotherapeutic agent, cisplatin, levamisole, and mitomycin C as well as leucovorin and interferon-α are used alone or in various combinations with some success.

LARGE INTESTINE

Cancer of the colon and rectum is the neoplasm of the alimentary tract most frequently encountered. Approximately half of patients with the disease can be cured by surgical resection with the best prognosis in those with tumors that are most localized. Irradiation is used preoperatively fairly frequently in cases of cancer of the rectum and at times postoperatively as well. Adjuvant chemotherapy is useful, and less frequently biologic therapy is indicated. The chemotherapeutic agent that continues to be the most effective is 5-fluorouracil. It is often administered in combination with other chemotherapeutic agents and with biologic substances such as leucovorin and interferon-α. The presence of carcinoembryonic antigen and blood in the stool are of limited usefulness in detecting the disease early. Also periodic barium x-ray studies and colonoscopy increase the chance of discovering precancerous lesions of the colon in older patients. A digital rectal palpation should always be included in any physical examination.

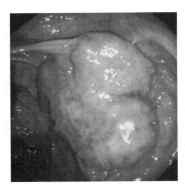

Figure 27 Endoscopic view of adenocarcinoma of the cecum.

Susceptibility to cancer of the colorectum is greater in both males and females past 40 years of age. Adenomas of the colon may become malignant, and hereditary polyposis syndromes have been well documented. Cancer of the colon appears more frequently in Crohn's disease, late inflammatory disease of the colon, sporadic polyposis, and after the appearance of an initial carcinoma of the colon. Mutations of various tumor suppressor genes have been associated with the stepwise development of colon cancer, and these neoplasms also have been attributed to a Western type diet based on the lower incidence of colon cancer among populations such as the Japanese and a few religious groups and the discovery of carcinogenic mutagens in the stool. The adenomatous polyposis coli (APC) and mutated in colon cancer (MCC) genes associated with heritable cancer of the large bowel have been identified and localized in the 5q21 region. Although not found in large numbers, almost all patients with the autosomal dominant gene for familial adenomatous polyposis (FAP) syndrome will develop colon cancer. The Gardner syndrome, another autosomal dominant condition, is found less frequently and is characterized by development of cancer following the appearance of adenomatous polyps in both large and small bowel along with other tumors such as sebaceous cysts and tumors of connective tissue. Also carcinoma of the colon occurs occasionally in the presence of the Turcot and Oldfield syndromes. Hereditary nonpolyposis colon cancer (HNPCC) is a feature of both Lynch I and Lynch II autosomal dominant syndromes which are characterized by multiple colon cancers at an early age, the Lynch II syndrome exhibiting widespread early carcinomas of other organs as well as the colon.

Staging of Carcinoma of the Large Intestine

The Dukes' system of staging carcinoma of the large bowel is based on the extent and spread of the disease with the survival of patients decreasing

Dukes' A to Dukes' C neoplasms. The A lesions are confined to the mucosa and submucosa of the bowel. B1 lesions have entered the muscularis but have not reached the serosa. B2 malignant tumors have reached the serosa and may have extended through this layer and involved the surrounding fatty tissue. Lymph nodes have been invaded with malignant cells in C neoplasms. Sometimes those without involvement of apical node are designated C1 lesions and those with penetration of the serosa and nodal involvement designated C2 cancers. The more detailed International Union against Cancer-American Joint Committee on Cancer TNM staging of colorectal cancer is considered more useful than the Dukes' system by many clinicians and investigators. Designations of primary tumors in this system are: TX, cannot be assessed; T0, no evidence of tumor; Tis, carcinoma in situ; T1, tumor invades submucosa; T2, invades muscularis propria; T3, invades subserosa or nonperitonealized pericolic or perirectal tissue; T4, perforates peritoneum or invades other structure or organs directly. Designations for regional lymph nodes are: NX, cannot be assessed; N0, no nodal metastases; N1, metastases in 1 to 3 pericolic or perirectal nodes; N2, invasion of four or more pericolic or perirectal nodes; N3, invasion of any node along a vascular pathway. Designations for distant metastases are: MX, cannot be assessed; M0, none; M1 distant metastases. The two systems are compared in the following table.

Staging of colorectal cancer

Stage 0	Tis	N0	M0	
Stage I	T1	N0	M0	Dukes' A
	T2	N0	M0	Dukes' A
Stage II	T3	N0	M0	Dukes' B
	T4	N0	M0	Dukes' B
Stage III	Any T	N1	M0	Dukes' C
	Any T	N2, N3	M0	Dukes' C
Stage IV	Any T	Any N	M1	

Surgical Management of Colorectal Carcinoma

The presence of a malignant tumor of the large bowel requires surgical resection for cure. When polyps are discovered, the possibility that one or more harbor malignant cells must always be kept in mind. When polyps are removed endoscopically, the base must be examined microscopically, and follow-up with colonoscopy is indicated even when there is no evidence of cancer or residual cancer. Unless there is an adequate margin free of neoplastic cells, the segment of colon containing the polyp(s) must be removed. Because of the possibility that neoplastic changes have occurred

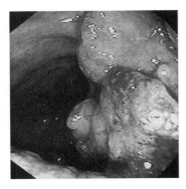

Figure 28 Endoscopic view of adenocarcinoma of ascending colon.

elsewhere in the large bowel, appropriate diagnostic study of the entire bowel consisting of colonoscopy or double contrast barium enema should always be done prior to exploratory operation. Staged operations may be indicated in the presence of intestinal obstruction with a preliminary diverting ileostomy or colostomy. However, it may be possible to carry out the procedure in one stage in selected cases without undue risk. Preliminary cleansing of the bowel and administration of antibiotic is always desirable. Also diagnostic studies such as ultrasound of the liver and computerized tomograms to obtain any evidence possible for metastatic disease are useful to the surgeon in suggesting the most expeditious procedure in the operating theater.

The operating surgeon may wish to ligate the bowel proximally and distally to stop additional intraluminal spread of cancer cells during the unavoidable manipulation of the bowel even though it is minimal. It is equally important to ligate the blood supply of the bowel to be removed to eliminate the problem

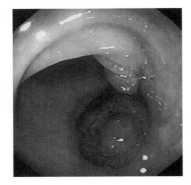

Figure 29 Polyp of descending colon with twisted pedicle.

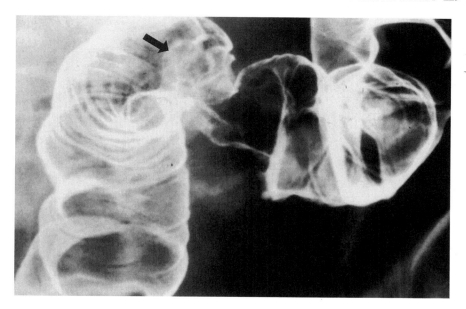

Figure 30 Barium air contrast demonstration of sigmoid adenocarcinoma.

of intravascular dissemination of malignant cells. The proximal and distal sites of division of the intestine should be several centimeters beyond the proximal and distal edges of the tumor. It may be necessary to resect even more of the bowel to ensure that the lymphatic and venous drainage of the site of the neoplasm is included in the resection of the mesentery with contained blood supply and lymphatics. Careful and thorough exploration of the abdominal cavity is done to exclude local extension to the body wall, to peritoneum, to lymph nodes, and to liver. The cecum, transverse, and sigmoid colon may be completely covered with a peritoneal sheath, but the remainder of the bowel wall may be in direct contact posteriorly with adjacent tissue and represent a greater possibility for local extension. When a preliminary ileostomy or colostomy has been done, the definitive operation for removal of the neoplasm proceeds as described. After the proximal and distal ends of the bowel remaining after resecting and removing the specimen containing the tumor are anastomosed, reestablishing the continuity of the lumen, the ileostomy or colostomy proximal to the resected neoplasm can be taken down and the bowel reanastomosed at that site, or this can be left for a later time, depending on the judgment of the surgeon.

When it is found that there is spread of the cancer to lymph nodes, locally, or to distant sites such as liver and lung, the operating surgeon can resect local recurrences, metastases to the peritoneum, to lymph nodes, to adjacent organs, and to the liver. Although removal of metastatic cancer is usually only

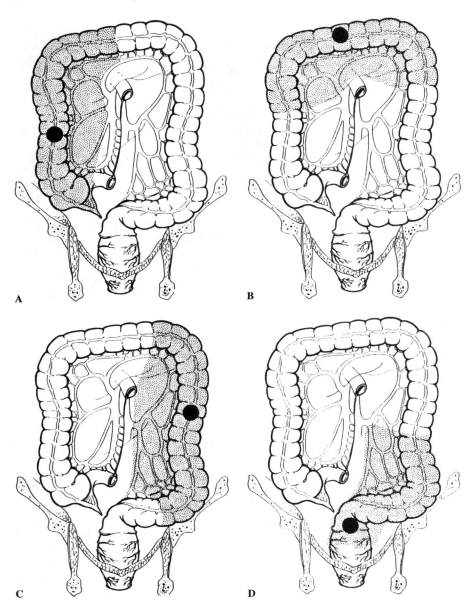

Figure 31 Extent of Resections for colonic cancer. A. Ascending colon. B. Transverse colon. C. Descending colon. D. Rectosigmoid colon. E. Low end-to-side anastomosis after resection of rectosigmoid colon with preservation of the anal sphincter. F. Extent of resection for adenocarcinoma of the distal sigmoid colon requiring distal colectomy and colostomy.

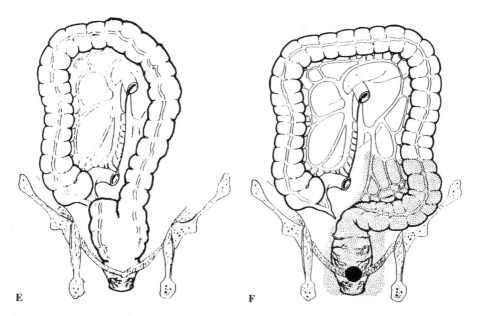

E   F

Figure 31 *(Continued)*

palliative, resections of limited spread to the liver and to the lung at times yield cures. Before operating, the surgeon should obtain permission for ovarian resection from postmenopausal women because of the predilection of cancer of the large bowel to spread to that organ. (Even though the ovaries appear grossly to be normal, many clinicians advise ovariectomy when an operation to remove a colorectal carcinoma is done.) In the case of premenopausal patients who wish to have children, agreement must be reached between the surgeon and these patients about whether an ovary that does not have a normal appearance is to be removed.

After operation, CEA titers must be determined every 2 to 3 months for 3 years, colonoscopy should be done annually, and careful follow-up physical and laboratory examinations including radiographic studies of the chest, ultrasound study of the liver, and scans of liver, spleen, and bone should be done when indicated. Whenever there is an indication of recurrence, then an additional "second-look" exploratory operation should be considered, since resection can offer a chance for cure in this disease. The number of patients surviving 5 years following a second resection is not great, but amply justifies considering the procedure. When hepatic metastases are found, radiotherapy can give temporary relief, cryotherapy has been substituted effectively for resection in some cases, and systemic chemotherapy can be helpful when there is bilobar involvement. Surgical resection can be effective treatment, especially when the metastatic disease is confined to one lobe. When discovered at the original exploration, it is sometimes wise to do the hepatic resection as a second stage.

When it is not possible to resect the neoplasm either at a first or second operation then a bypass procedure is carried out to prevent subsequent obstruction. Abdominoperineal resections of the distal colon, rectum, and anus for distal lesions low in the pelvis leaving the patient with a permanent colostomy are done much less frequently now than in the past. The technique of resecting low-lying lesions followed by successful anastomosis has improved, and combined irradiation and chemotherapy of anal lesions has been more successful. Even recurrent carcinoma of the rectum has been resected successfully. When the distal rectum and anus are preserved, a margin of at least 2 cm of normal tissue should extend beyond the level of anastomosis with the descending colon. Complications during the first year after operation are reduced when an end-to-side anastomosis is done between the distal rectum and a pouch formed from the distal descending colon. The resection should include the mesorectum and wide lateral margins and extension of the operation beyond the fascial planes.

Irradiation in the Management of Cancer of the Large Intestine

Irradiation has proved to be a valuable adjunct to managing cancer of the large intestine. Cancers of the anal canal have appeared more frequently in recent years among men, homosexuals, and those infected with acquired immune deficiency syndrome (AIDS), although they account for a small proportion of neoplasms found in the large bowel, and women continue to constitute the largest group with the disease. Other than biopsy, in the past operative management of necessity meant abdominoperineal resection with a permanent colostomy. More conservative management has been successful more recently and includes irradiation therapy. When irradiation was combined with chemotherapy as many as four-fifths of the patients have been treated successfully without recurrence. 5-Fluorouracil is the standard chemotherapeutic agent used in this regimen, combined with another agent such as cisplatin or mitomycin C. If biopsy is positive for cancer after 1 month following the termination of radiation and chemotherapy, an additional course of both is indicated. Positive biopsy subsequently must be followed by abdominoperineal resection and colostomy.

Both preoperative and postoperative irradiation have improved the management of patients with carcinoma of the rectum. The former has the disadvantage of delaying operation and being done at a time when the extent of the cancer is not known with the danger of inappropriate treatment. Postoperative irradiation has also been studied extensively. Both the rates of survival and recurrence are improved by irradiation and chemotherapy. Combined treatment gives better results than either given alone in the postoperative period for Dukes' B2 and C lesions. 5-Fluorouracil is the drug of choice for this type of ancillary treatment.

Chemotherapy for Cancer of the Large Intestine

5-Fluorouracil has consistently exhibited a response rate of 20 percent in patients with cancer of the colon. When used in combination with other compounds or biologic agents, the response is increased. Combinations of choice are 5-fluorouracil with either leucovorin or levamisole. Other agents reported to improve results are irinotecan and floxuridine, cisplatin, interferon-α, leucovorin, levamisole, and methotrexate. Some studies have suggested survival to be increased as well. Standard therapy for Dukes' C cancer is either 5-fluorouracil and levamisole or 5-fluorouracil and leucovorin. For advanced disease the combination of 5-fluorouracil and leucovorin yields 30 to 35 percent rates of response. Intrahepatic chemotherapy gives a higher rate of response for metastases to the liver but no difference in survival. The usefulness of chemotherapy is somewhat doubtful with either initial or late failure to respond to 5-fluorouracil.

ANUS

The proximal end of the anal canal is designated to begin at the anorectal ring. The distal limit used is either the dentate line or the anal verge. In any discussion the anatomic margins must be indicated to compare incidence and results of therapy accurately. The dentate line is used in this discussion as the lower limit of the anal canal and the proximal limit of the anal margin. Tumors originating in the anal margin usually have a better prognosis than those in the anal canal. Pruritis, pain, bleeding, and a change in bowel habits are typical symptoms of these tumors. At times inguinal lymphadenopathy is the indication of metastatic foci. Also leukoplakia and chronic fistulae may be present. Suggestive of a viral etiology for some of these tumors, is the isolation of human papilloma viral DNA from some of the patients with cancer of the anal canal. Computerized tomography and/or nuclear magnetic resonance imaging may help evaluate the degree of invasion and presence of metastatic disease. Endoscopy with biopsy is indicated before the initiation of therapy. At times the diagnosis is made for the first time when excised hemorrhoids are examined. In addition to epidermoid carcinoma, biopsy may reveal condyloma acuminata, lichen skin disease, leukoplakia, basal cell carcinoma, adenocarcinoma, melanoma, Paget's disease, and Bowen's disease.

Epidermoid carcinoma of the anal margin is treated by local excision making sure the margins are free. The 5-year survival is approximately 80 percent. When the resection is extensive, a skin graft may be necessary to close the defect, and an abdominoperineal resection is not mandatory unless there is deep invasion or recurrence. When abdominoperineal resection is necessary in the occasional case, the percentage of patients surviving 5 years is lower. Wide-beam external and interstitial irradiation usually are used only when resection fails after recurrence.

The management of epidermoid carcinoma of the anal canal is a more difficult problem to solve. Simple excision is not often applicable, although the 5-year survival is approximately 65 percent in those cases for which this approach is suitable, and it is advisable only for superficially invasive cancers less than 2 cm in diameter. In the past, abdominoperineal resection was done in many cases with a 5-year survival of approximately 50 percent. The irradiation used was not very effective and inferior to the megavoltage primary radiation used today which yields higher rates of survival. Colostomy has been necessary only when necrosis and scarring and obstruction have occurred as sequellae after irradiation. Currently neoadjuvant chemoradiation is being used whenever possible, consisting of initial mitomycin C followed or concomitant with fractionated radiation in tumor doses up to 50 cGy. Mitomycin C can be given alone or followed by 5-fluorouracil. Responses to cisplatin also have been reported. Complete responses have been obtained in more than two-thirds of patients treated. Complications that have occurred in some patients having this treatment are dermatitis, proctitis, diarrhea, thrombocytopenia, and leukopenia. An abdominoperineal resection is done in those showing no response. It is hoped that additional clinical trials combining chemotherapy, irradiation, and resection will improve the rates of survival for this most distressing type of cancer.

The results of treating neoplasms other than squamous carcinoma of the anus vary from satisfactory when basal cell carcinomas are resected to very discouraging when melanomas and adenocarcinomas require therapy. The rarely seen basal cell carcinomas must be excised widely with free deep and lateral margins. When this is done, cures are usually obtained and even recurrences can be resected without great difficulty. Also Bowen's disease can be excised satisfactorily without recurrence. Follow-up over a long period is advisable, however, since late recurrence may appear in the epithelium in which these lesions are found. Paget's disease of the anus presents the same pale crusted and scaling lesion seen in Paget's disease of the breast. Fortunately there is not an inevitable deeper neoplasm present, and removal with wide margins is frequently all that is required. When there is a deeper neoplasm present, a more extensive resection is required, but the prognosis is poor in this situation. Melanomas of the anus occur rarely and usually are pigmented. They have a poor prognosis with survival of about 6 percent. The presence of a mass and/or bleeding may call attention to the lesion. Most long-term survivors have had abdominoperineal resections. Prophylactic groin lymphadenectomy has been added in some cases without evidence that it affected survival, and chemoradiation trials show little evidence of response. Adenocarcinoma of the anal canal, also a rare neoplasm, has a similar poor prognosis and usually requires abdominoperineal resection for best results.

URINARY AND MALE GENITAL TRACTS

Cancer of the urinary and male genital tracts consists of neoplasms of the kidneys, renal pelvis, ureters, urinary bladder, prostate gland, urethra, testicles, and penis. Surgical therapy is the most effective way to achieve cures overall, but irradiation and chemotherapy can yield favorable responses in some cases. Chemotherapy is most successful for treating cancer of the testicle and least useful in attempts to cure renal cancer. Both irradiation and chemotherapy can be used in the management of metastatic disease and are administered frequently for metastases from prostate and kidney. Neoplasms of the testicle respond at times to biologic agents such as inteferon and interleukin. The management of neoplasms of each of these anatomic sites in the urinary and male genital tracts is reviewed separately.

Kidney

The two major types of tumors of the kidney are renal cell carcinomas of the parenchyma and urothelial tumors of the renal pelvis. The former are malignancies that are found in more than 26,000 patients and cause over 7000

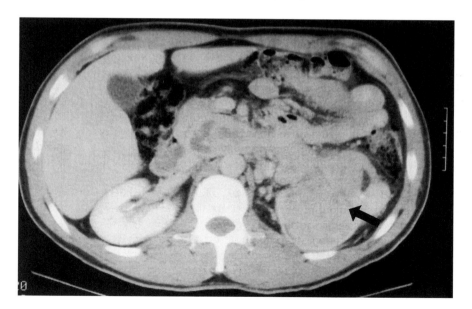

Figure 32 Computerized tomogram showing left renal cell carcinoma.

deaths annually in the United States. The incidence in men is twofold that in women, occurs most often in the sixth and seventh decades, and is seen more frequently in urban than in rural populations. The incidence is highest in Scandinavia and lowest in Japan and is increasing slowly in the United States. Renal cell cancer was known and treated more than 100 years ago. The appearance of the neoplasm when examined under the microscope at that time led to naming them hypernephromas because of some similarity to adrenal tissue. Although this term has persisted in the literature, the malignant cells in renal cell carcinomas originate in the parenchyma of the kidney and do not represent adrenal rests. Other terms that have been used and also are falling into disuse are nephroblastoma, clear-cell carcinoma, and Grawitz's tumor. Renal cell malignancies have been confused with oncocytomas as well.

Four out of five patients with renal cell carcinoma have one or more of the symptomatic triad of pain in the flank, palpable tumor, and hematuria, but the complete triad may not appear until quite late in the course of the disease. Additional signs and symptoms of the paraneoplastic syndrome characteristic of this tumor are pyrexia; night sweats; fatigue; hypochromic anemia; polycythemia; coagulopathies; amyloidosis; vasculitis; myopathies; neuropathies; loss of weight; varicoceles in men; elevated levels of alpha-fetoprotein, alkaline phosphatase, calcium (possibly because a factor originating in the tumor causes resorption of bone), plasma fibrinogen, erythropoietin, renin, parathormone, adrenocorticotropic hormone (ACTH), prolactin, glucagon, and gonadotropins; and hepatomegaly and hepatic failure not associated with metastases and subsiding with nephrectomy.

Increased risk for developing renal cell carcinoma is associated with smoking, obesity, exposure to cadmium, exposure to Thorotrast, working with coke ovens and petrochemicals probably including long exposure to gasoline, employment in leather and tanning production and shoe manufacturing, and contact with asbestos. It occurs both sporadically and as a familial disease. In von Hippel-Lindau disease approximately one-third of the patients develop renal cell carcinoma, which also is found often in patients with tuberous sclerosis and renal polycystic disease attributed to an autosomal dominant gene. Much molecular genetic and cytogenetic research has revealed that the sporadic and familial cases probably have similar genetic abnormalities. Reciprocal translocations between chromosome 8 and chromosome 3 were found in all cells of affected members in the families studied, and a somewhat similar abnormality was found only in the cells of the renal neoplasm in patients with sporadic disease. Susceptibility to the cancer appears to be related to deletion of a wild-type segment on chromosome 3 within the range of the *3p14*-26 region, and the location of the chromosomal abnormality associated with von Hippel-Lindau disease is within the same region of this chromosome. By using analysis of DNA polymorphism the altered gene carrier state can be detected in those with the familial disease and possibly may be useful for screening.

In addition to a medical history, physical examination, hematologic studies, blood chemistry, electrocardiogram, and urinalysis, most diagnostic studies are done to determine the location, size, and extent of the mass detected in the kidney. With the advent of computerized tomography and magnetic resonance imaging, more renal tumors now are detected incidentally in the course of examination for other clinical problems than formerly. Ultrasound surveys are very useful to distinguish cystic from solid masses, and both magnetic resonance imaging and computerized tomography are available with or without enhancement for a more complete assessment of the nature of the mass and its extent and nodal involvement. Urograms are often done and are very valuable to determine the status of the opposite kidney and whether the organ with the tumor is a solitary kidney. Renal cell carcinomas are often multiple and bilateral and may extend into the renal vein and vena cava. Arteriograms and venograms may be indicated. Enhanced tomographic venography and digital subtraction angiography are used at times to clarify any vascular involvement and extent of the tumor. Radiographic examination of the chest is indicated if not included in the field of the computerized tomograms or magnetic resonance imaging. Bone scintigrams are not done often preoperatively. Biopsies and aspiration of questionable cystic masses is sometimes done, but biopsy of solid tumors is seldom indicated before surgical exploration.

Three types of cells are found when biopsies are examined under the microscope: clear, granular, and spindle cells. Those with clear cells offer a somewhat better prognosis, and the spindle cells offer a somewhat less promising prognosis than the other two types. Also, the presence of abnormalities of the chromosomes, including aneuploidy, suggests a less encouraging prognosis than do tumors with diploid chromosomes. When estimating the outlook for patients with recurrent disease, favorable factors are previous resection, a lengthy interval between operation and the appearance of metastases, and the presence only of a solitary pulmonary metastasis.

The approaches to treating renal cell carcinoma include surgical, radiographic, chemotherapeutic, and biologic. Overall, resection has been the most successful means for achieving cures. The cancer can be exposed by means of an abdominal, flank, or thoracoabdominal incision depending on the habitus, the location of the neoplasm, and its extent. A flank incision limited to an extraperitoneal procedure is usually preferable whenever possible unless the size and extent of the neoplasm requires additional exposure. When the opposite organ is intact and functioning, nephrectomy is done frequently. The contents within the surrounding fascia along with the adrenal are removed. The resection may also include regional lymph nodes as well. Nephrectomy is permissible even when there is a solitary distal metastasis, since it may be possible to remove the metastatic focus, and cures are known when the kidney and the metastatic disease have been removed. When the stage of the disease indicates, nodal resection may extend from the diaphragm to the pelvic brim.

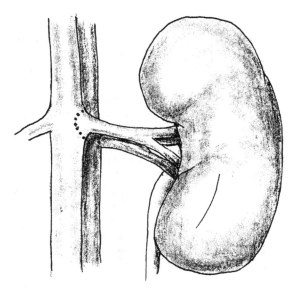

Figure 33 Renal transplant to iliac vessels.

In cases with a solitary kidney containing the neoplasm or when the disease is bilateral or the opposite kidney exhibits progressive benign disease, a partial or nephron-sparing resection can be successful in as many as 85 percent of these cases. Intraoperative ultrasonography is quite a useful adjunct in detecting additional occult tumors. When the opposite kidney is normal in appearance and function, a partial nephrectomy is usually not attempted unless the neoplasm is solitary, small, and preferably low grade. Complications after nephron-sparing resections include urinary fistulas and renal failure. The former usually heal satisfactorily with appropriate care, but the latter may require temporary or permanent dialysis in patients with a single kidney. An extracorporeal procedure makes partial resection much easier to accomplish but requires more time and is associated with more complications. When the neoplasm is very large, it may be neccessary to transplant the remaining segment with vascular anastomosis to iliac vessels and reanastomosis of the ureter lower in the abdomen. With the improvement of diagnostic techniques and diagnosis at earlier stages, extracorporeal procedures are done much less frequently.

Both preoperative and postoperative irradiation have been given in various studies. At the present time, preoperative irradiation is rarely given; postoperative therapy may be given when there is metastatic disease but usually is used as palliation for symptoms. The most common distal metastatic sites are bone, brain, and lung. When they are present, operative removal should be considered first, reserving radiation until later if the single or multiple foci are resected. If no operation is done, then radiotherapy may give symptomatic relief at least temporarily, although relief of pain is not invariably successful.

Chemotherapy has given disappointing results when tried for this type of cancer. For example, floxuridine (FUDR) has been given in various programs and dosages including timed sequences following circadian rhythm without much success. Biologic agents have given more encouraging responses. Best results have followed treatment with recombinant interferon-α with questionable responses with interferon-γ. Usage of interferon continues to be somewhat controversial, but occasional complete responses do occur along with lower responses in the usual course of events. Side effects including fever, fatigue, and an influenza-like syndrome are troublesome. Treatment is sometimes combined with cis-retinoic acid and vinblastine. Responses have also been obtained with interleukin-2, which activates the immune mechanism of the host. Some complete responses have been obtained, but the usual rate is low. Treatment is not combined with chemotherapy, and the combination of interferon and interleukin is not recommended at the present time. The latter is associated with toxicities that must be carefully controlled and is carried out best in a specialized center preferably in the context of a clinical trial. The toxic effects limit the number of clinical situations in which the treatment is appropriate. Hormonal therapy with medroxyprogesterone acetate, testosterone, and antiestrogen have been advocated and tried, much on the basis of good results of treating this type of tumor in the Syrian hamster. It is unfortunate that these clinical results have not duplicated those with the laboratory animals.

TNM classification and staging of renal cell carcinoma

TX	Primary tumor cannot be assessed
T0	No evidence of primary tumor
T1	Tumor <2.5 cm within kidney
T2	Tumor >2.5 cm within kidney
T3	Tumor invading major veins or adrenal but not beyond Gerota's fascia
T4	Tumor invading beyond Gerota's fascia
NX	Regional nodes cannot be assessed
N0	No metastases to renal nodes
N1	Metastasis to single node <2 cm
N2	Metastasis to single node >2 cm and <5 cm or multiple nodes none >5 cm
N3	Metastasis to node(s) >5 cm
MX	Distal metastasis cannot be assessed
M0	No distant metastasis
M1	Distant metastasis

(Continued)

GX	Differentiation cannot be assessed
G1	Well differentiated
G2	Moderately differentiated
G3	Poorly differentiated
G4	Undifferentiated
Stage I	T1, N0, M0
Stage II	T2, N0, M0
Stage III	T3, N1, M0
Stage IV	T4, Any N, M0
	Any T, Any N, M1

Staging of renal cell carcinoma (Robson)

Stage I	Limited to kidney
Stage II	Invasion to but not beyond Gerota's fascia
Stage III	Invasion into major veins and lymphatics
Stage IV	Invasion beyond Gerota's fascia or distal metastasis

Renal Pelvis and Ureter

Cancer of the renal pelvis is composed predominantly of transitional cell carcinomas, with squamous carcinomas and adenocarcinomas appearing less frequently. The cancer may be multifocal and may be found bilaterally in the pelvis and also in the ureter and bladder. Cancer of the renal pelvis is found more frequently in men, and kindreds having the neoplasm have been reported. Also familial Balkan neuropathy is associated with increased incidence of cancer of the renal pelvis, and it is found with increased frequency among patients with Li-Fraumeni syndrome. The mutant gene for this type of cancer may be on chromosome 9 with enhancement by mutation of suppressor genes on other chromosomes. Smoking is a prime etiologic agent, and abuse of analgesics containing phenacetin is a predisposing factor as well. Workers in industries producing analine dyes, plastics, rubber, and textiles are thought to be more susceptible. Ureteral carcinomas are encountered less frequently than those of the renal pelvis, but the histologic types are the same and the sex ratio and symptoms are similar. Solitary lesions are found in the lower third of the ureter with greatest frequency.

Symptomatology at both sites can include hematuria, palpable mass, and pain. Bleeding may be sufficient to result in an obstructing clot. Occlusion by either a clot or the bulk and extension of the neoplasm can be responsible for painful symptoms. Radiologic visualization with intravenous or retrograde contrast material is quite useful in refining the diagnosis, and the use of computerized tomography may be helpful additionally. Also angiography is useful when vascular obstruction or invasion has occurred. Prognosis is related to the type, grade, and stage of these neoplasms. Tissue diagnosis is made by endoscopic biopsy or brushing or study of the urine. The tables below give the designation for the stages of neoplasms of the renal pelvis and ureter.

Staging of carcinoma of the renal pelvis

Stage I	No invasion
Stage II	Invasion of lamina propria
Stage III	Invasion to muscularis and beyond if within kidney
Stage IV	Adjacent tissues involved and/or distant metastases

Staging of carcinoma of the ureter

Stage O	Mucosa only
Stage A	Superficial (lamina propria)
Stage B	Invasion to muscularis
Stage C	Through muscularis to adjacent structures
Stage D	Distant metastases

The best results of surgical management of cancer of the renal pelvis are obtained with radical nephrectomy including the surrounding fascia of Gerota, the ureter, and the cuff of the urinary bladder when a functional normal kidney and ureter are present on the opposite side. This is moderated of necessity when the affected organ is a solitary kidney, the disease is bilateral, or renal insufficiency is present. In those cases it may be possible to resect the tumor, including a rim of surrounding parenchyma, and preserve the remainder of the kidney with reimplantation of ureter below the former site of the neoplasm. When only the ureter is affected, then the cancer and adjacent section of ureter are removed and the kidney implanted below. Whether the use of endoscopic surgical techniques using laser and cautery will result in better results remains for the future to disclose.

Low-grade neoplasms are not usually treated with irradiation postoperatively, but high-grade advanced lesions are best treated with external beam radiographic therapy using multiple ports, cross-firing, and tumor dose of approximately 4500 cGy. If chemotherapy is to be administered as well, then the dose of irradiation should be reduced. Chemotherapy with combinations of drugs such as cisplatin and doxorubicin (Adriamycin) with cyclophosphamide or methotrexate and vincristine has elicited responses in both the renal pelvis and ureter which apparently have similar sensitivities to those in the urinary bladder.

Other Tumors of the Kidney

Nephroblastomas (Wilms' tumors) constitute approximately one-tenth of malignancies in childhood, with peak incidence between 2 and 4 years. Some patients with this neoplasm also have other congenital deformities. A genetic defect at the locus of a tumor suppressor gene on chromosome 11 is associated with the appearance of these tumors and was used in formulating the two-hit theory of carcinogenesis of Knudson. Symptoms and signs include pain, hematuria, mass in the flank, anorexia, fever, and nausea and vomiting. The tumors are found to be solid masses with ultrasound studies. Urograms, chest radiographs, venography and arteriography, computerized tomograms, and nuclear magnetic resonance studies are used to clarify the extent and location of these masses and whether there are bilateral cancers or a solitary kidney bearing the tumor, and to determine staging. Invasion and metastatic spread of these neoplasms is similar to that of renal cell carcinoma. Radical nephrectomy with thorough examination of the opposite kidney is usually possible through an anterior approach. Biopsy of node(s) may be done to complete accurate staging. When both kidneys are involved, treatment consists of unilateral radical nephrectomy and resection of as much of the neoplasm as possible from the less affected kidney. Responses have been obtained with agents such as cisplatin, ifosfamide, vincristine, and actinomycin D and doxorubicin combined with etoposide. Chemotherapy is sometimes used before tumor thrombectomy and frequently in combination with resection of pulmonary metastasis and after recurrence. Radiotherapy is not used in stage I and favorable stage II disease and in children younger than 2 years of age and only cautiously in older children. Responses are obtained with radiotherapy in stage III disease.

Sarcomas constitute about 1 percent of renal malignancies. Slightly more than half are leiomyosarcomas. They compress the renal parenchyma more than invading it but metastasize early and widely. Radical nephrectomy is indicated when these malignancies are encountered, and chemotherapy will extend survival at times.

Angiomyosarcoma is a hamartoma of the kidney about four-fifths of which occur in women, usually in the sixth and seventh decade. Most are associated with tuberous sclerosis. These tumors can be enucleated and may be followed if they are located peripherally and asymptomatic. Misdiagnosis can lead to an unnecessary radical nephrectomy. Pain, mass in the flank, and hematuria may call attention to the lesion or if a retroperitoneal hematoma occurs when the mass ruptures.

Oncocytomas are benign tumors originating in the distal tubules. They occur at approximately 60 years of age, affecting twice as many men as women. They must be distinguished from renal cell carcinomas. If small, peripheral, and asymptomatic, these tumors may be followed without therapy. When operation is indicated, a partial nephrectomy is all that is required.

Urinary Bladder

Cancer of the urinary bladder is composed of four types of neoplasms. Most are transitional cell lesions; the remaining 5 percent consist of adenocarcinomas, squamous carcinomas, and small cell cancers similar to those found in the lung. Occasionally the neoplasms may be mixed lesions. Many are multifocal, occurring not only in the bladder, but also elsewhere in the epithelium of the urinary tract. About three quarters of the lesions are superficial (in the mucosa, submucosa, and/or lamina propria), and the clinical objective is eradication and prevention of spread and recurrence. The remaining neoplasms are invasive of the deeper tissue of the wall including the muscles, and they may spread to distant sites as well. Management must be decisive with eradication of the primary site by single or combined therapy and discovery and appropriate treatment of metastases. These cancers occur more frequently in males than females, although it is slowly increasing in the group of females who smoke. The superficial tumors are found more frequently in the white than in the black groups in the population. The disease is encountered in the late decades of life. Factors associated with the appearance of these cancers are exposures sustained by workers in the aniline dye, rubber, paint, and organic chemical industries, smoking, positive family history, chronic urinary tract infections, bilharziasis, and abnormalities of chromosomes 9, 11, and 17.

Symptoms that may be encountered are frequency, hematuria, and pain. With more extensive lesions there may be vascular and lymphatic obstruction with edema and even rectal occlusion. In addition to thorough physical examination, useful diagnostic studies are cystoscopy, flow cytometry, cystograms and pyelograms, computerized tomograms, nuclear magnetic resonance imaging, and ultrasound studies at times. Radiographic studies of the chest, bone scan, and isotope studies can be helpful when there is some likelihood of metastatic disease. Localized biopsies at both suspected primary sites and distant locations are done at the time of cystoscopy. Also, cultures and cytologic studies of urinary sediment are helpful in planning treatment.

Both neoplastic changes and exposure to infection and injury are associated with hyperplasia and dysplasia of the cystic mucosa as well as that higher in the collecting system. Considerable skill on the part of the pathologist is often required to distinguish early malignant changes because of other epithelial abnormalities. The grading and staging of tumors of the bladder consist of microscopic evaluation of the depth of extension and spread beyond the wall obtained from biopsies and the clinical evaluation after diagnostic studies have been completed. Grading based on the microscopic appearance of these tumors is usually divided into four types, but quite often the last two are combined. The appearance ranges from papillomas with minimal invasion and low probability of metastases to cancer invading the muscle with great possibility of metastatic spread. The TNM system outlined below is used currently, although occasionally references to older classifications are encountered.

TNM classification of tumors of the bladder

T0	No detectable tumor
Tis	Superficial: Tumor in situ
Ta	Superficial: Confined to mucosa
T1	Superficial: Confined to stroma
T2	Infiltrating: Invading muscle
T3a	Infiltrating: Invading muscle and fascia
T3b	Infiltrating: Invading surrounding fat
T4	Invading: Adjacent structures
N+	Invading: Regional lymph nodes
M+	Metastatic: Organs and distant nodes

It is imperative that patients with tumors of the uroepithelium be followed carefully because of the tendency to occur at multiple sites, the possibility of recurrence, and difficulty of detecting metastases from small and early lesions. For example, carcinoma in situ is a potentially dangerous lesion with a history of rapid invasion after long quiescence. Recurrence and/or progression occurs in approximately one-third of the superficial tumors of the bladder after discovery and treatment.

Treatment of superficial tumors is transurethral resection or fulguration. In many cases this is followed by adjuvant intravesical chemotherapy. The agents most frequently utilized are bacillus Calmette-Guérin (BCG), doxorubicin, mitomycin C, and thiotepa. There may be myelosuppression because the chemotherapeutic agent is absorbed to varying degrees, but this is not a great problem. Also BCG management introduces the bacterium, which occasionally requires treatment. Some irritation of the bladder occurs, and patients receiving the therapy may experience some burning, frequency, and discomfort. The treatment can be given on an outpatient basis, and often no anesthetic is required. The sterile fluid carrier containing the agent is introduced into the bladder and retained by the patient usually for about 2 hours. The persistence of symptoms after a reasonable interval following treatment, especially when the diagnosis is Tis, often means that there has been recurrence requiring additional management.

Very small lesions invading muscle have been treated successfully with transurethral resection when it has been possible to eradicate all evidence of the tumor. A second visualization is always done to determine whether there is any evidence of recurrence. Partial cystectomy is indicated at times when muscle invasion has occurred, but it is not done when there are multiple superficial tumors. Best results are anticipated when the mucosa shows no evidence of dysplasia or hyperplastic lesions. The urethral mucosa is checked for suspicious changes, and preoperative external beam irradiation with a maximum tumor dose of 1200 cGy reduces the chance of seeding during the surgical procedure. The neoplasm must be located in the superior and at times the posterior wall, and biopsies of the margins of the segment resected must be free of malignant cells. Only about 1 in 10 patients is suitable as a candidate for this type of management. Unfortunately approximately half of those treated experience a recurrence.

Larger neoplasms with muscle invasion and/or distant metastases have been treated by more radical cystectomy and external beam irradiation through multiple ports alone and together. More recently chemotherapy has been added to the therapeutic armamentarium for managing these difficult problems. Many years of experience utilizing resection and irradiation have culminated in the current skill in using them. The most appropriate way to use chemotherapy is still being developed; but responses of the neoplasms, especially the most common type, transitional cell cancer, are encouraging. The numbers of patients tested and lack of controls when comparisons of different plans of treatment have been made in the past do not always permit conclusions about the best regimens for managing the different problems presented by cancer of the bladder with operation, irradiation, and chemotherapy alone or in various combinations. Many contemporary studies continue to explore these questions, and at times entering such a study is a wise choice for an individual patient.

The response to irradiation, especially when administered preoperatively, will indicate the sensitivity of the cancer being irradiated. Responses are often obtained when transitional cell cancers are irradiated, but the remaining types are often much more refractory. For example, a striking differential response is often evident when mixed neoplasms are irradiated. The degree of success has been found to be related to grade, stage, size, and extension of the tumor and general condition of the patient including level of hemoglobin. The objective of cure with irradiation depends on local control of the cancer. Unfortunately this is a difficult goal to achieve, and recurrence presents the surgeon with a formidable technical task when cystectomy is done in a field that has undergone prior irradiation. To extend the effectiveness of local control, brachytherapy using iridium 192, cesium 137, and radium needles has been used in highly selected cases. Also, open intraoperative external beam irradiation and MeV (megavolt) electron therapy have been tried in efforts to control the primary cancer. Currently, this approach has not gained general acceptance as having great promise for general use. However, the use of irradiation to prevent seeding and in various combinations with operative resection continues to be useful in managing the many problems presented by these neoplasms of the bladder.

Experience with chemotherapy indicates that both single agents and combinations of chemotherapeutic drugs induce responses and partial responses of transitional cell cancers of the bladder. Mixed tumors, adenocarcinomas, squamous cell cancers, and small cell cancers are less responsive. Agents used for adenocarcinomas are cisplatin, methotrexate, and vinblastine (CMV). Those used to treat squamous cell carcinoma are 5-fluorouracil and cisplatin. When various combinations of doxorubicin, vincristine, etoposide, cyclophosphamide, methotrexate, and lomustine have been used to treat small cell cancer, response has been short term when obtained. Among agents used for transitional cell cancer are methotrexate, vinblastine, doxorubicin (adriamycin), and cisplatin (MVAC) and similar combinations such as CMV.

Neoadjuvant chemotherapy, the term applied to chemotherapy given as the initial treatment, has two major objectives: to reduce the tumor load and to indicate the degree of sensitivity of the tumor cells, if any, to the agent or agents used. Adjuvant chemotherapy (that given concomitantly or after irradiation and/or resection) is given more empirically because it is not possible to monitor the response to chemotherapy accurately. Responses of cancer of the bladder have been obtained from administration of single agents such as carboplatin, cisplatin, cyclophosphamide, doxorubicin, 5-fluorouracil, gallium nitrate, methotrexate, mitomycin C, and vinblastine. Combinations of agents that have been used are cisplatin and methotrexate (CM); cisplatin, and methotrexate, and vinblastine (CMV); and methotrexate, vinblastine, doxorubicin, and cisplatin (MVAC). Epirubicin (Epidriamycin) can be substituted for doxorubicin in MVAC. Other combinations are cisplatin, cyclophosphamide, and doxorubicin and carboplatin, methotrexate, mitoxantrone, and vinblastine. In advanced disease the patient and family should decide on the objectives of chemotherapy, weighing palliation for relief of symptoms and prolongation of life against the undesirable side effects of treatment. Agents of choice for superficial malignancy are instillations of BCG, doxorubicin, mitomycin, or thiotepa. Recommended most often for systemic therapy are methotrexate, vinblastine, doxorubicin, and cisplatin (or carboplatin) (MVAC); gallium nitrate, gemcitabine, ifosfamide, and paclitaxel.

Resection is usually included when control of the primary cancer is thought possible; and, when the cancer is advanced, more extensive resection is done than the limited transurethral procedures described above. Computerized tomography of abdomen and pelvis now gives the surgeon better information preoperatively than was possible before computerized tomography became available. In advanced cancer, pelvic node dissection is usually advisable even when prior studies have failed to reveal metastatic nodal disease. In women resection includes removal of the bladder, the entire urethra, the anterior vaginal wall and uterus, and the ovaries in postmenopausal patients. In men impotence and incontinence are problems to be avoided if the extent of the neoplasm permits. The bladder, prostate and seminal vessels, and proximal urethra are removed. Care is taken to evaluate whether and where the urethra may be involved beforehand. A segment of ileum is proving to be the best portion of the bowel for constructing a substitute for the bladder. The small bowel substitute has less pressure than one constructed from the colon and therefore is less prone to be associated with problems of incontinence. Anastomosis is made with the urethra in the male, and the tubular configuration of the ileum is not retained. Before undertaking such a major procedure, the risk must be evaulated carefully. Not all patients are suitable, but this does not mean that irradiation and chemotherapy cannot be given, although renal and cardiac disease may alter the plan for administering chemotherapy as well as the effectiveness of the treatment. The treatment of cancer of the bladder wisely requires management that is specifically designed for the individual patient. There is a broad spectrum of clinical pictures which this type of cancer presents, and the usefulness of each mode of therapy varies widely from one set of circumstances to the next. Much can be accomplished when the appropriate measures are adopted, initiated, and altered when responses indicate a change in course.

Prostate

Cancer of the prostate ranks second in the causes of deaths from cancer among males in the United States. It occurs in older age groups, with the median age of 74 years for the clinical diagnosis. Approximately one-third of males are found to have carcinoma of the prostate at autopsy. The gland and malignancies within it require testosterone for proliferation; cancer of the prostate does not occur in eunuchs. The presence of such a carcinoma presents one of the most difficult problems in choosing and carrying out appropriate therapy, although it is known to respond to irradiation and endocrine therapy as well as resection. There is no reliable way to predict the future course and response of an individual cancer; as a result, management is somewhat controversial. The frequent finding of small localized neoplasms of the prostate at autopsy leads the clinician to be conservative in writing prescriptions for therapy. Black Americans have a higher incidence of the cancer than do whites. The prevalence in Western Europeans also is high, whereas Asians living in the East have fewer cancers of this type but exhibit increased incidence after moving to the West. There is this general indication of environmental influences on etiology, and the higher incidence of cancer of the prostate among close relatives of patients known to have the disease at an early age suggests genetic factors as well. The cancers arise both from epithelial and interstitial tissues. Approximately 97 percent are adenocarcinomas (acinar, comedo, cribriform, and papillary). The least prevalent are squamous carcinomas. Other types are adenocystic, mucinous, and small cell cancers. Also transitional cell, papillary, and ductal carcinomas are found but not very frequently. Rhabdomyosarcomas are known to occur in children. Free and total prostate-specific antigen (PSA) has become a valuable test of diagnosing cancer of the prostate and following the response to therapy. Elevation of prostatic acid phosphatase (PAP) is another useful adjunct to management but does not compare to the reliability of prostate-specific antigen.

The clinical workup of patients requires careful rectal examination, perineal transrectal biopsy with ultrasound visualization, computerized tomograms, liver function tests, magnetic resonance imaging, bone scans and lymphangiograms when indicated, flow cytometry for determining chromosomal abnormalities and DNA changes, and the usual studies of urine and blood and electrolyte levels. Spread of the cancer occurs through local, lymphatic, and hematogenous routes. Study of the microscopic appearance of the neoplastic tissue has been used for grading the cancers with the hope of predicting their future behavior. Several are in current use, including Gaeta, Gleason, Mayo, and Mostofi systems, all of which have about the same reliability. Departures from the normal diploid chromosome pairs to various aneuploid configurations have been found to increase the gravity of the prognosis. Also two other values have some prognostic significance, the volume of the neoplasm and the level of prostate-specific antigen. The staging of these tumors usually follows either the classification of the American Urological Association or that of the International Union against Cancer (UICC: Unio Internationale contre le Cancer).

Screening periodically for prostate cancer is carried out most effectively and practically by doing a rectal examination of the gland supplemented by determining the level of the prostate-specific antigen. When indicated, biopsy can be done transrectally without the necessity of an anesthetic after preparation with an enema and antibiotic. Ultrasound imaging is used to localize suspicious lesions and appropriate sites for needle biopsy. Computerized tomography has been useful in determining extracapsular and nodal extension but now is not used as frequently, having been partially supplanted by the use of the levels of prostate-specific antigen. Magnetic resonance imaging is more expensive but yields better images of prostate and nodes, although the accuracy of extracapsular extension is not as great as desirable. Metastatic disease of bones can be determined with considerable confidence by bone scans. The bones are rarely involved when the level of prostate-specific antigen is below 20 ng/mL. After the tissue diagnosis of cancer of the prostate and an evaluation of its extent is made, the options for management in general are observation, operation, radiotherapy, and hormonal management alone or in various combinations. Unfortunately chemotherapy does not offer the same success achieved with other types of cancer.

The difficulty in making the decision to observe the patient with careful follow-up examination and testing when the cancer is localized is the absence of any means for prognosticating accurately the natural course of an individual cancer. Observation is more reasonable in patients age 80 years or more, since the life expectancy is shorter and only therapy entailing minimal risk can be justified in the great majority of cases. For patients who have the diagnosis made at younger ages, the limitation of current data supporting observation alone should be made quite clear to the patient before embarking on such a course.

Operation for prostatic cancer is done under general or epidural anesthetic with antecedent enema, bowel preparation, and antibiotic prophylaxis immediately before operation. The surgical approach to treatment has changed over the years with improvement in the rate of complications and margins of the resection remaining free of cancer. The procedure most often advised is a revision of the retropubic approach with removal of the cancer, prostate gland, seminal vesicles, and bilateral resection of internal iliac and obturator lymph nodes. This radical prostatectomy is done with meticulous care, including preservation of the neurovascular bundles responsible for erection. As a result, the complications of impotence and urinary incontinence have been greatly reduced. The bladder and urethra are reunited with a vesicourethral anastomosis to complete the procedure and drains are left in place. Postoperative care is directed toward preventing the complications of venous thrombosis, pulmonary infections and atelectasis, stress incontinence, and abscess. Improving the technique of operation, which requires both skill and experience, has been the means of combating impotence, lack of margins free of cancer, strictures of bladder neck and urethra, lymphocele, and injuries of obturator nerves and ureters.

Irradiation is usually administered as external beam therapy with tumor dose up to 7000 cGy in divided doses. The use of photon, neutron beam, or brachytherapy with needles or applicators containing radioactive elements depends on the equipment available, the inclination of the therapist, and any unique quality of the neoplasm itself. Since multiple doses are given over varying lengths of time, it is imperative that the position of the patient in relation to the source of irradiation and the shielding is reproducible. Often casts are made to retain the patient's position during therapy. Scanning computerized tomograms can provide a three-dimensional contour of the anatomic target to be irradiated conforming to the individual gland and extent of the tumor involving it. This technique results in fewer undesirable side effects of therapy. High-energy photons in the range of 6 MeV or greater are used at times when the equipment is available. Neutrons may be focused accurately, and a mixture of neutron and photon therapy has been used with the presumed advantage of allowing greater dosage without increase in side effects. However, no clinical study has been completed with figures supporting this premise objectively.

Implantation of radioactive isotope sources has been used in the treatment of cancer of the prostate for many years. Sources such as gold 198, iodine 125, palladium, and iridium contained in needles or catheters have been implanted freehand, with use of a template constructed for equal distribution of dosage, and with the aid of ultrasound visualization for placement. Also phosphorus 32, strontium, samarium 53, and rhenium 186 localize in bone and have been used successfully to relieve pain resulting from osseous metastases. This brachytherapy has been used alone and in combination with external beam radiotherapy or operation. Frequently it has been preceded by lymphadenectomy. When used with resection of the prostate, the brachytherapy follows the operative procedure and the local sources of irradiation are placed in the tissue beyond the margins of resection. This means of treating prostatic cancer is thought to be useful for well differentiated cancer especially when localized and as adjunctive treatment in combination with other types of irradiation. The data currently available about the results of treatment unfortunately do not provide comparative results that withstand objective critical appraisal.

The removal of androgen yields a response by reducing the proliferation of prostatic cancer cells and is used frequently for treating metastatic disease. The production of approximately 95 percent of the circulating androgens is controlled by the pituitary gland and hypothalamus and the remainder is under the control of the adrenal glands. The level of androgen can be reduced at any place in the scheme of elaboration. Orchidectomy under local or general anesthesia is a relatively minor surgical procedure often used for this purpose. Plastic repair of the scrotum can be done, preserving the epididymus, or testicular prostheses can be included as a feature of the operation if desired by the patient. The value of complete androgen blockade is supported in part by clinical results showing prolongation of interval before progression and modest increase in length of survival. This can be brought about by means of an antiandrogen and either orchidectomy or gonadotropin hormone releasing hormone (GnRH) analogue (goserelin acetate or leuprolide). It should be kept in mind that an initial temporary flare period may increase the size of metastatic foci with danger of injury to the spinal cord or urinary obstruction. It can be controlled by antiandrogen in combination with GnRH antagonist. Also prednisone given to patients after orchidectomy can reduce dihydrotestosterone levels. Ketoconazole can reduce both adrenal and testicular testosterone very rapidly but has a number of side effects. Estramustine and diphosphonates and suramin are newer pharmaceuticals having some promise. Antiandrogens can be steroids such as megestrol acetate (Megace) or nonsteroidal such as flutamide, but undesirable side effects limit the usefulness of many of them. Additional hormonal treatment after initial failure may yield responses, but additional time for survival is not necessarily expected. Hydrocortisone alone and with glutethimide has been used successfully, as has flutamide. ketoconazole, octreotide acetate (Sandostatin), and somatulin may relieve pain, but side effects must be monitored carefully during their use.

The use of chemotherapy to combat carcinoma of the prostate has not been as promising as originally hoped. Since the advent of prostate-specific antigen levels and rates of increase as a means for objective evaluation of results, clinical trials are providing more precise evidence for conclusions. The success of hormonal therapy and the lack of any means to judge objectively the quality of life before and after treatment reduce the numer of patients suitable for entering case-control studies. This has impeded the rate of progress and made justification for chemotherapy somewhat equivocal up to the present time. Extension of survival has not been an obvious result of treatment with chemotherapeutic agents so far. Estramustine, etoposide, mitomycin C, suramin, vinblastine, and vindesine are examples of agents that have yielded results that are somewhat promising. Cyclophosphamide, 5-fluorouracil, and methotrexate are among those associated with more disappointing responses. The failure of hormonal therapy to continue symptomatic relief may lead the therapist to suggest enrollment of the patient in a clinical trial of chemotherapy. Angiogenesis inhibitors and other new agents aimed at controlling the spread of metastases are being investigated currently.

The choice of treatment at any given time usually depends on the stage of the prostatic cancer, the age and general condition of the patient. In stage A1 (American Urological Association classification) many clinicians prefer to follow levels of prostate-specific antigen and do periodic rectal examinations of the prostate. With an increase in prostate-specific antigen levels, then radical prostatectomy is considered for this stage of the disease and stages B1 and B2 in patients 70 years and younger. In those 70 to 80 years of age, external beam radiotherapy may be chosen. Hormonal therapy can be given to those over 80 years of age for progressive disease. The difficulty of successful resection following recurrence after irradiation is frequently the reason for choosing operation in the younger age groups rather than irradiation. Comparison of results obtained by irradiation and operative treatment shows approximately equal survival rates at the end of 10 years when localized well differentiated cancers of the prostate are treated. Complications appear after each. Deep vein thrombosis, pulmonary embolism, abscess, impotence, ureteral and obturator nerve injury, perforation of the bowel, incontinence, urinary obstruction, and bladder and urethral stricture can occur following operation. Complications that can follow irradiation are impotence, nausea, diarrhea, gastrointestinal bleeding, and obstruction and formation of fistulas, dysuria, urethral stricture, and proctitis. Recurrence or evidence for continued spread of cancer of the prostate following irradiation is an indication for salvage with operation. Absence of free margins after operation then can be treated with irradiation. In stage B3, radical prostatectomy is considered if the cancer is well differentiated with prostate-specific antigen levels <15 ng/mL. Otherwise external beam irradiation is usually chosen for definitive therapy. In stages C1 and C2 external beam irradiation is often the treatment of choice. For the D stages of metastatic disease, hormonal therapy is used for symptomatic disease, and bilateral orchidectomy is added in stage D3 with progression despite intensive hormonal therapy. Hormone therapy and chemotherapy have yielded encouraging palliation with leuprolide or goserelin with and without flutamide or bicalutamide. The level of response following therapy also supports the use of diethylstilbestrol; nilutamide; and combinations of aminoglutethimide or ketoconazole plus prednisone; estromustine and vinblastine or etoposide or paclitaxel; doxorubicin and ketoconazole; aminoglutethimede or ketoconazole plus prednisone; and mitoxantrone and prednisone.

Neoplasms of the prostate

Classification of the UICC (Unio Internationale contre le Cancer)

T: Primary tumor

Tx	Primary tumor not assessed
T0	No evidence of primary tumor
T1	Not evident by palpation or imaging
	T1a <5% of tissue resected
	T1b >5% of tissue resected
	T1c Identified only by needle biopsy
T2	Tumor confined to prostate +/− invasion of capsule
	T2a <1/2 lobe involved
	T2b >1/2 or one lobe involved
	T2c Both lobes involved
T3	Extends through prostatic capsule
	T3a Unilateral
	T3b Bilateral
	T3c Seminal vesicle invaded
T4	Neoplasm fixed or invades adjacent structures (other than seminal vesicles)
	T4a Neck of bladder, external sphincter, or rectum invaded
	T4b Invades levator ani and/or fixed to pelvic wall

N: Regional lymph nodes

Nx	Nodes cannot be assessed
N0	Regional lymph nodes not involved
N1	Single lymph node <2 cm
N2	Single lymph node >2 to <5 cm or multiple nodes <5 cm
N3	Lymph node >5 cm

M: Metastatic disease

Mx	Cannot be assessed
M0	No evidence for metastases
M1	Distant metastases
	M1a Nonregional lymph node(s)
	M1b Bone(s)
	M1c Other site(s)

Neoplasms of the prostate

Classification of the American Urological Association

Stage A

Unsuspected and found on examination of biopsy

A1	<4 foci well differentiated
A2	>3 foci well differentiated or any number of moderately or poorly differentiated foci

Stage B

Palpable but within prostatic capsule

B1	<2 cm one lobe

(Continued)

B2	>2 cm one lobe
B3	Both lobes

Stage C
Extension beyond prostatic capsule +/− seminal vesicle(s)

C1	Minor extension beyond capsule
C2	Major extension beyond capsule

Stage D
Metastases present

D0	Persistent elevation acid phosphatase only
D1	Pelvic lymph nodes invaded
D2	Lymph nodes above aortic bifurcation +/− distant metastases
D3	Progression of metastases despite intensive hormonal therapy

Male Urethra

Cancer of the urethra in the male is encountered rarely and less frequently than in the female. It may be confused with cancer originating in the bladder and prostate when it appears in the proximal portion of the male urethra. The presence of the tumor is called to the attention of the patient by urinary obstruction, hematuria, especially when bleeding occurs in the absence of trauma, the presence of a palpable mass within the penis, or lymphadenopathy, pain, abscess, and fistula. These tumors are not usually seen until middle age. Small and superficial carcinomas in situ and papillomas of the male urethra are treated more easily than the malignant tumors that occur in the prostatic, bulbomembranous, and distal (penile) uethra. Approximately three-fourths of the malignant lesions are squamous cell carcinomas with transitional cell neoplasms and adenocarcinomas appearing less frequently in descending order. More than half of these cancers are found in the bulbomembranous urethra. Tests for PSA (prostate-specific antigen) and acid phosphatase are not positive when a lesion is located in the prostatic urethra in the absence of prostatic cancer.

Examination of a male patient in whom cancer of the urethra is suspected should include careful inspection and palpation of the external genitalia and perineum, preferably bimanually under general anesthesia, cytologic study of the urinary sediment, determination of the presence of regional lymphatic enlargement, external needle biopsy or transurethral biopsy with urethroscopy, and computerized tomograms or magnetic resonance imaging of abdomen and pelvis to assess the status of draining lymphatics.

Treatment of urethral cancer is more successful for anterior than for posterior lesions. Small papillary lesions or cancers in situ can be treated by local endoscopic resection but must be followed carefully and frequently for recurrence and lymphatic involvement. When the distal penile urethra is the site of the cancer, partial penectomy can be done, but sufficient proximal tissue free of cancer, usually at least 2 cm or more, must be present for success. The presence of palpable inguinal lymph nodes almost always indicates the presence of metastases. When present, ilioinguinal lymphadenectomy is indicated. If the proximal urethra is involved with cancer, then amputation of the organ is mandatory. Orchiectomy is indicated when the scrotum is invaded. In rare cases it has been possible to remove the bulbomembranous segment of urethra when it is the site of cancer and perform an end-to-end anastomosis to repair the defect. Also small and early lesions can be removed endoscopically, but most of the time the invasion is sufficiently extensive to require radical excision with deep pelvic node dissection. The prostatic urethra is the rarest location for cancer. Although early cancer in situ can be treated endoscopically, by far most of the cancers are sufficiently invasive to require radical prostatectomy.

Radiation therapy of urethral neoplasms in the male has been used in dosages up to 6000 cGy of external beam therapy. Also, brachytherapy in the form of implants of radioactive sources has been done for advanced lesions that have recurred. Recurrences after radiation therapy take place with discouraging frequency.

Chemotherapy has been used more recently as supplementary treatment with some palliative success. For example, MVAC (methotrexate, vinblastine, doxorubicin, and cisplatin) therapy has effected responses of transitional cell neoplasms. Toxicities limiting dosages also limit the effectiveness of chemotherapy, but the advent of new regimens in the future may bring about a more optimistic outlook for treating urethral cancer.

Penis

Cancer of the penis occurs most frequently in uncircumcised males with attendant poor cleanliness and the presence of smegma. Smegma is the product of bacterial action on cells desquamated beneath the foreskin and is known to be carcinogenic in animal studies. The role it plays in human penile cancer is not entirely clear, however. This cancer is rarely seen in circumcised males or those not circumcised who are able to retract the foreskin and have good hygienic habits. It appears usually during the sixth decade and is the diagnosis in less than one percent of men with cancer. There is some suspicion that human papilloma virus is a causative agent, but the evidence so far is not conclusive. Benign but precancerous lesions of the penis are leukoplakia, Bowen's disease (erythroplasia of Queyrat), balanitis xerotica obliterans, and Buschke-Lowenstein verrucous tumors. All are known to have become malignant in some cases and fortunately are responsive to local excision and, in the case of the first two, 5-fluorouracil, and in the case of the third, local steroids.

Most cancers of the penis are squamous carcinomas. Various types of cancer such as basal cell cancer, Kaposi's sarcoma, and metastatic neoplasms occur much more infrequently. (Cancer of the male urethra is discussed under that title.) Jackson's classification of penile cancer is used more frequently than others. It consists of the following stages:

Stage I	(A) Tumors of glans and/or prepuce
Stage II	(B) Tumors involving the shaft of the penis
Stage III	(C) Tumors with operable inguinal metastases
Stage IV	(D) Tumors with adjacent spread or inoperable inguinal or distant metastases

Symptoms of the disease are the presence of a mass, ulceration, bleeding, and lymphadenopathy. The outlook for the patient depends very much on the extent of the disease, and diagnostic studies must include an analysis of possible involvement of draining lymphatics, which include the superficial and deep inguinal nodes, the femoral and iliac nodes, and those beyond. Drainage is bilateral, and treatment must take this into consideration. Either computerized tomography or magnetic resonance imaging are useful in addition to careful physical examination and clinical history to yield an accurate assessment of the extent of the disease. Enlargement of palpable lymph nodes does not necessarily indicate metastatic disease, since lymphadenitis gives the same clinical picture. At times antibiotic therapy may result in resolution of the problem. However, the importance of determining the extent of the disease is sometimes justification for biopsy of sentinal nodes. Metastatic cancer of the penis is also spread through hematogenous dissemination.

Superficial cancers can be excised widely and cured in early lesions. The location of the more invasive cancers determines the extent of resection in stage II disease. If distal, excision of the terminal portion of the organ can be done, leaving at least a proximal length of 2 cm or more free of cancer. More proximal cancers require complete resection and perineal urethrostomy. After the primary lesion has been controlled by excision, a rationale for the control of possible lymphatic invasion is not so easily reached. When the inguinal lymph nodes contain tumor, a bilateral inguinal node resection is indicated. In stage I, there is some rationale for deferring node dissection and following the course of the patient when there is no evidence of lymphatic invasion. In later stages, there are differences of opinion about prophylactic lymph node resection.

The justification often used for irradiation therapy is preservation of function. Techniques of treatment with this modality have steadily improved over the years. Up to one fifth of patients treated in the past have suffered relapse, and obstruction of the urethra also occurs at times after irradiation. When irradiation is the primary therapy and has failed, then operation is available as salvage management. Both external beam therapy and brachytherapy with iridium 196 and other radioactive sources have been used in total dosages up to 6000 cGy.

Chemotherapy is tailored to the histologic appearance of the cancer under the microscope. Both single agents alone, sequentially, and combined with others have been used with some palliative success. Currently methotrexate is used with some rewarding results; others used alone are bleomycin and cisplatin. Combination regimens of cisplatin and 5-fluorouracil and also bleomycin, cisplatin, and cyclophosphamide have been somewhat effective. Sequential therapy has included bleomycin and methotrexate, followed by irradiation. The problems of evaluating the relative advantages of different modalities of treatment are accentuated in penile carcinoma because of the scarcity of patients with the disease in places where this type of investigation is available. Undoubtedly, however, such studies will continue, and perhaps more cures will be obtained.

Testis

Cancer of the testis is the neoplasm found most frequently in males from the age of 15 to 35 years and also occurs with increased frequency in those aged 60 and above. The rate of cures is greater for cancer of the testis than for any other solid neoplasm. The use of multimodal therapy in recent years has led to cures in four-fifths of all cases and almost 100 percent of early lesions. The types of germinal cancer seen most often are sensitive to radiation and some chemotherapeutic agents, and frequently patients with the disease have few additional medical problems. More than 90 percent of testicular cancers arise from germ cells. The two types of these cells yielding markers in the serum are trophoblasts and yolk sac cells. The former produce beta-human chorionic gonadotropin and the latter produce alpha-fetoprotein detectable in the serum of patients with these types of cancer. Also the level of each in the serum indicates the amount of tumor present. Thus these convenient markers aid not only in the diagnosis but also in the follow-up evaluation of management. The lactic dehyrogenase level (LDH) in the serum can be elevated when the tumor load is quite large but is not considered a specific tumor marker. Up to 10 percent of patients with testicular cancer also have had a diagnosis of undescended testicle. The cancer may be contralateral to the location of the cryptorchidism.

Many times the presence of cancer of the testis is first discovered as a painless mass in the testicle by the patient. Cancer must be differentiated from epididymitis, torsion of the testis, hematoma, cystocele, and spermatocele. Physical examination of males must always include careful examination of the testes for masses. When a cancer is suspected, ultrasound examination will separate lesions within the testes from those external, will identify cystic lesions, and is helpful in identifying the location and nature of masses in the presence of a hydrocele. In addition to the presence of a lump in the testis, the patient may have lumbar discomfort, gastrointestinal and/or pulmonary symptoms, the presence of metastatic disease which may be discovered before the primary disease; a few patients with germ cell tumors have gynecomastia. Computerized tomograms are useful in detecting metastatic disease, and radiographic study of the chest may be helpful in staging the disease as well.

The initial treatment of germ cell tumors is surgical orchiectomy, removing the testis through an inguinal incision, first clamping, dividing, and ligating the spermatic cord at the inguinal ring to reduce the chance of proximal spread. The surgeon must be vigilant and not miss a second cancer on the opposite side. An accurate diagnosis of the type of neoplasm can be made on the basis of the microscopic appearance of sections of the tumor and subsequent therapy planned on the basis of the type and extent of the cancer. Biopsy should not be done, and a scrotal approach to resection is contraindicated.

Approximately 95 percent of the neoplasms of the testis originate in germinal cells. The remainder originate from Sertoli cells and Leydig cells. The principal types of cancer found in the testis are seminomas, spermatocytic tumors, teratomas, and yolk sac tumors (sometimes referred to as endodermal sinus tumors). Teratomas are divided into a first group of differentiated or mature tumors with some referred to as immature with malignant transformation and a second group of malignant teratomas, undifferentiated or trophoblastic. Sometimes those in the second group are referred to as embryonal carcinomas of the adult type or choriocarcinomas.

Neoplasms of the testis spread locally to cord and epididymis and adjacent structures, via the lymphatics upward to paraaortic nodes, and by hematogenous spread to lungs, liver, and brain. TNM staging includes T1 to T4 tumors depending on the extent of spread throughout the testis, N1 nodal extension denoting involvement of paraaortic nodes and N2 signifying extension to pelvic and/or mediastinal nodes, and M characterizing hematogenous spread to lung, liver, and/or brain. The Boden-Gibb staging is a simple classification into stages denoting the extent of the cancer as follows: A(I) testes, B(II) regional nodes, and C(III) beyond retroperitoneal nodes. The system of staging of the American Joint Commission for seminomas consists of the following designations: I(A) negative and II(B) positive. The designations of extent of involvement in stage II(B) are N1 microscopic involvement, N2 gross involvement with A(B1) having fewer than five nodes >2 cm and B(B2) having more than five nodes >2 cm, N3 resectable extension, and N4(B3) nonresectable or incompletely resected extension. Extragonadal germ cell tumors arise in midline structures and traditionally have a poorer prognosis. Before this diagnosis is accepted, every effort should be made to determine whether the cancer with this diagnosis is metastatic from an occult testicular primary.

After orchiectomy for nonsematomatous germ cell cancer, evaluation of the involvement of regional lymph nodes without retroperitoneal lymph node resection is not sufficiently accurate to diagnose those without lymphatic involvement in all cases. For that reason retroperitoneal lymphadenectomy is often carried out when clinical evaluation of the presence of lymphatic disease is negative. In the past, sterility ensued in many of these cases having the second operation. A recent alteration in the technique with thoracoabdominal approach and limitation of the inferior limit of the dissection on the side contralateral to the neoplasm has resulted in a gratifying reduction in postoperative problems with infertility. When no cancer is found after the operation, follow-up reveals spread of the malignancy later in about one-tenth of the cases. Chemotherapy is often successful in eradicating the metastatic disease in most of the cases. Bilateral retroperitoneal lymphadenectomy is carried out in all patients with grade II cancer. If some of the involved lymph nodes are large, supplemental chemotherapy is usually added to the regimen.

When the choice is made to follow a patient after orchiectomy instead of additional treatment, surveillance testing should be frequent and thorough including physical examination, x-ray studies, computerized tomograms, and levels of the marker compounds in the serum for 5 and preferably for 10 years. A decision to choose surveillance rather than immediate removal of regional lymph nodes is made less frequently in those patients with local and hematogenous invasion and a large component of embryonal carcinoma in the primary neoplasm because they are considered factors associated with higher risk for recurrent cancer. Greater success with chemotherapy in recent years has resulted in more patients entering surveillance programs. Some studies suggest that recurrence is at a more advanced stage in these patients without a second operation than the stage of the disease in those who have recurrence after lymphadenectomy. The wisdom of surveillance will become more apparent with the passage of time and the careful management of follow-up studies. Both types of management are yielding a gratifying number of cures.

The results of treating seminoma in stages I and IIA exemplify one of the more successful outcomes of continued clinical investigation of available therapy. The cancer is responsive to resection, irradiation, and chemotherapy, and almost all patients can be cured. After orchiectomy and the usual workup to discover metastatic disease, lymphangiograms can be helpful along with radiographic studies to detect spread above the diaphragm. Irradiation with total dosage of 3600 cGy fractionated is usually given with field(s) below the diaphragm and shielding of the remaining testicle. Prophylactic irradiation above the diaphragm is not usually done, and surveillance without treatment following orchiectomy is not currently in favor. The results of irradiation alone fall when the cancer is in stages IIB and III. Chemotherapy is very effective in raising the number of cures in this situation. It is useful in treating cases with disease above the diaphragm and when the resistant metastatic focus is localized. Also irradiation and resection can be used to treat localized disease.

Undoubtedly the most effective chemotherapeutic agent against cancer of the testis is cisplatin, a compound of platinum. Its discovery and use has increased the number of cures remarkably. It is used in various combinations with bleomycin, cyclophosphamide, dactinomycin, ifosfamide, vinblastine, and VP-16. The side effects of such treatment should be explained carefully to the patient before it is initiated. In cases with persistent disease autologous bone marrow transplantation can be used to extend the intensity of chemotherapy. The first-line regimen used most commonly is BEP (bleomycin, etoposide, cisplatin). Also paclitaxel and the combination of ifosfamide, mesna, cisplatin, etoposide or vinblastine yield encouraging responses. Chemotherapy does not cure the primary site and should not be used as a substitute for resection. Salvage of persistent disease after irradiation, chemotherapy, or both can be achieved by a surgical approach to the problem. Also an alternate regimen of chemotherapy can be used for salvage. The outlook for patients with cancer of the testis is usually optimistic, but problems increase with the extension and increase in tumor mass. The appropriate utilization of the effective triad of operation, irradiation, and chemotherapy continues to effect a remarkable number of cures even in advanced disease.

FEMALE GENITAL TRACT

Cervix

Cancer of the cervix is the most common female malignancy encountered globally, but it ranks eighth in frequency in the United States. This corresponds approximately to a 70 percent reduction, probably because so many women have Papanicolaou smears and probably would be even lower if more than the 15 percent of those who do not now have annual tests would comply. The current use of the automated provision of a monolayer of cells and scanning for identification of suspected malignancy for confirmation by the pathologist has improved the reliability of the cervical smears. This cancer is found in twice as many black women as in all other races combined in the United States. Also, the DNA of human papilloma virus is found in twice as many patients with the disease as is found in controls. Increased risk for cervical carcinoma is associated with sexual intercourse and its early onset, multiple sexual partners, poor pre- and postnatal care, the presence of herpesvirus type 2, genital herpes, condylomata acuminata, and low socioeconomic status. Women whose sexual partners are circumcised have a lower incidence of carcinoma of the cervix. These social and sexual aspects of the disease suggest it may be largely preventable.

Nine-tenths of invasive carcinomas of the cervix are squamous cell cancers, by far the majority of which consist of nonkeratinizing large cells. Adenocystic, adenosquamous, and small cell carcinomas usually have a poor prognosis. Verrucous and adenobasal cell cancer have a better history of successful management. A number of other types of neoplasms are found in the cervix, including malignant mixed müllerian tumors, carcinoids, embryomas, embryonal rhabdomyosarcomas, leiomyosarcomas, lymphomas, primary sarcomas, and melanomas, but they are relatively rare. Metastatic carcinomas are also encountered in the cervix from such organs as breast, colon, and uterus. The usual progression of the squamous cell cervical cancers is from dysplasia to preinvasion to invasion locally, progressing to lower uterus and upper vagina and spreading by extension through lymphatic and vascular channels to more distant sites. Lymphatic spread can extend to obturator and internal and external iliac nodes and then upward to paraaortic and supraclavicular nodes. Hematogenous spread to bones, liver, lungs, and mediastinum occurs in less than one-tenth of cases.

First symptoms of cervical cancer may be intermenstrual and/or postcoital bleeding. As the disease advances, it may be accompanied by pain. Cervical cancer can be indicated by a smear early in its course, but the diagnosis must always be confirmed by a biopsy studied microscopically. Diagnostic studies must be sufficiently accurate to result in valid staging of the disease including bimanual pelvic physical examination (sometimes requiring an anesthetic), ureterograms, cystoscopy, colposcopy and biopsy, radiographic studies, ultrasound studies, lymphangiograms, and, if indicated, tomograms.

Clinical management of carcinoma of the cervix depends on the stage of the disease being treated. In stage IA1 a cone biopsy including the cancer with sufficient margin or a simple hysterectomy may suffice. Similar management for stage IA2 disease leads to recurrence in about 5 percent of cases; this problem is not a feature when a radical hysterectomy including pelvic lymph node resection is included. In stages IB to IIA either radical hysterectomy or radical radiation therapy including whole pelvic external therapy and brachytherapy are used for both squamous and adenocarcinomas. (The latter lesion is somewhat more difficult to stage accurately at times). Disadvantages of surgical therapy are the possibilities of hemorrhage, thrombosis, and infections postoperatively and later the development of genitourinary fistula and atony of the bladder occuring in no more than 1 in 50 cases. Among advantages of operation are less expense, shorter duration, fewer long-term effects, ability to define precisely the extent of the disease, and preservation of the ovaries when indicated. Disadvantages of irradiation therapy are fibrosis of the vagina, chronic problems of bowel and bladder, inability to define specifically the extent of the tumor, failure to sterilize cancer in lymph nodes, and impaired sexual function. Radiation therapy alone is used in stages IIB to IVA with about one-fifth to one-half of patients surviving 5 years. Exenteration can be done when there are no distant metastases in stage IVA disease.

Chemotherapy has yielded responses lasting several months when single agents and combinations of agents have been used. Cisplatin elicits a response in approximately one-third of cases, and combinations of drugs give about the same response. The doses given are somewhat low since there is no dose response advantage. Other single drugs used have been bleomycin, carboplatin, 5-fluorouracil, ifosfamide, methotrexate, mitomycin C, vincristine, and VP-16. Combinations that have been tried are cisplatin, 5-fluorouracil, and hydroxyurea; doxorubicin, bleomycin, and cisplatin; and doxorubicin, cisplatin, and methotrexate. Bleomycin, ifosfamide, mesna, and cisplatin (BIP); ifosfamide and mesna; cisplatin; carboplatin, 5-fluorouracil; and paclitaxel are the best choices of single agents and combinations at the present time. More studies are desirable to determine accurately the value of both neoadjuvant and adjuvant chemotherapy. Percentage survival for 5 years with operation or irradiation or chemotherapy alone or combined approximates 98 for stage IA, 75 to 85 for stages IB to IIA, 55 for stage IIB, 10 to 50 for stage III, and 0 for stage IVB. Survival has not improved as much as palliation. However, the increasing number of early cases detected in the United States has been gratifying.

Prognostic factors for the results of treating cervical cancer are the histologic type of the cancer, its size, and the degree of invasion of stroma and parametrial tissues, lymph nodes, and blood vessels. In patients with cancer of the cervix, numerous comorbid conditions and complications present very difficult special problems such as the presence of AIDS, pregnancy, other tumors, and pelvic inflammatory disease. Sometimes cancer of the cervix is discovered during a routine hysterectomy for another cause. Comorbid conditions make improvement in survival figures even more difficult to achieve. The surgeon always retains the option of changing the plan for therapy if the findings at operation materially change the staging of the disease. In stage IIB and higher, the patient may wish to enter an experimental protocol for evaluating new methods of therapy. Recurrent cancer of the cervix presents a great therapeutic challenge which must be approached with caution. It is possible to resect some of these cancers, but the number is not great and every effort must be made so that a contraindication from past experience will not be missed.

Stages of cancer of the cervix
International Federation of Gynecology and Obstetrics

Stage 0	Intraepithelial carcinoma in situ
Stage I	Carcinoma of uterus
Stage IA	Microscopic preclinical invasion
Stage IA1	Minimal microscopic stromal invasion
Stage IA2	Invasion 5 mm deep × 7 mm wide or less
Stage IB	Tumor larger than stage IA2
Stage II	Invasion beyond uterus but not farther than lower third of vagina or to pelvic wall
Stage IIA	Withoug parametrial invasion
Stage IIB	With parametrial invasion

(Continued)

Stage III	Cancer extends to pelvic wall and/or lower third of vagina and/or causes dysfunction of kidney(s)
Stage IIIA	Cancer extends to lower third of vagina, not pelvic wall
Stage IIIB	Cancer extends to pelvic wall and causes dysfunction of kidney(s)
Stage IVA	Cancer extends beyond pelvis and/or invades bladder or rectum

Uterus

Uterine malignancies appear most frequently in the sixth decade. Endometrioid adenocarcinoma occurs most frequently with papillary serous, adenosquamous, and clear cell carcinomas constituting all but 10 percent of these neoplasms. The survival for 5 years is approximately 90 percent for endometrioid cancers, whereas that for papillary serous and clear cell cancer is about half that. Primary uterine and ovarian cancer can occur at the same time. Carcinosarcomas and sarcomas are the most common neoplasms of connective tissue, constituting about 5 percent of the total. Leiomyosarcomas are not found very often. Prognosis varies with the type and grade of the tumor, depth of myometrium invaded, cytology of peritoneal washings, DNA ploity and S-phase fraction, CA-125 marker, hormone receptor levels, and stage of the cancer determined by assessing all information acquired after a thorough workup. The unopposed effect of estrogen on the endometrium can lead to hyperplasia and premalignancy with intermenstrual and postmenopausal bleeding. Although administering progesterone with estrogen can lead to troublesome vaginal bleeding, this regimen protects against the effects of estrogen alone on the endometrium. Whether the addition of progesterone diminishes the effect of estrogen in preventing cardiovascular disease and cancer of the breast is not known.

Vaginal bleeding is an early sign of carcinoma and, if aberrant or postmenopausal, should always lead to diagnostic studies. The diagnosis can usually be made with adequate biopsy not requiring dilatation and curettage under anesthesia. Careful and thorough clinical examination of the patient and appropriate laboratory studies, evaluation of comorbid conditions, chest radiographic studies, and possibly cystoscopy and proctoscopy should be done. Decisions about staging also should depend on findings at operation with changes being made in staging and operative objectives if the results of exploration are unexpected. Sampling of lymph nodes and peritoneal washings are often quite helpful. After invasion of the myometrium, spread occurs by direct extension and by lymphatic and hematogenous extension. Metastatic disease in bone, brain, liver, and lung usually appears rather late.

The respective role operation, radiotherapy, and chemotherapy each play in treating uterine cancer depends on the stage of the disease. Operation is frequently the first therapeutic procedure, affording a clear diagnostic picture without the problem of radiation obscuring it, which sometimes occurs. The operation usually consists of total extrafascial hysterectomy and bilateral salpingo-oophorectomy and sampling of lymph nodes, peritoneal washings, intraoperative evaluation of the extent of the disease, and alteration of the plan of operation if the extent of the cancer shows invasion in the upper abdomen. Pelvic irradiation is the most frequent adjuvant therapy given. When it is given alone, the survival is less than after resection alone even in early disease. In stage I disease, postoperative irradiation is given when extension to the endocervix, vascular or lymphoid invasion, or deep myometrial invasion has occurred. When the cancer is extensive with extrauterine disease and malignant cells in peritoneal washings are found, the patient may wish to join a clinical trial testing a regimen for advanced disease. Progesterone may be of limited usefulness in combination with irradiation. Responses obtained with chemotherapy are characteristically of short duration. Those agents that have elicited some response when used alone or in various combinations are doxorubicin, cisplatin, cyclophosphamide (Cytoxan), ifosfamide, and VP-16. Cisplatin has given the most encouraging results. However, both hormonal treatment and chemotherapy are of limited usefulness for endometrial cancer. Papillary serous carcinomas, even when constituting a minor part of a larger cancer, behave very much like similar cancers of the ovary with the same refractory insensitivity to treatment. Sarcomas usually require total abdominal hysterectomy and bilateral salpingo-oophorectomy followed by adjuvant treatment. Currently probably the best treatments for endometrial carcinoma are megestrol or a similar progestin; doxorubicin and cisplatin with and without cyclophosphamide; carboplatin; altretamine; fluorouracil, paclitaxel, and tamoxifen.

Stages of uterine malignancy
International Federation of Gynecology and Obstetrics

Stage IA	Tumor limited to endometrium
Stage IB	Invasion <1/2 of myometrium
Stage IC	Invation >1/2 of myometrium
Stage IIA	Only endocervical glands invaded
Stage IIB	Stroma of cervix invaded
Stage IIIA	Invasion of serosa and/or adnexa and/or positive peritoneal cytology
Stage IIIB	Cancer metastatic to vagina
Stage IIIC	Cancer metastatic to pelvic and/or paraaortic lymph nodes
Stage IVA	Invasion of mucosa of bowel and/or bladder
Stage IVB	Distant metastases including abdominal and/or inguinal lymph nodes

Choriocarcinoma

Choriocarcinomas arise in the placenta as a result of abnormal proliferation of the chorionic villi following normal and abnormal uterine pregnancies, abortions, and ectopic pregnancies. Benign tumors occur on this basis as well and are labeled hydatidiform moles; moles also can be invasive (chorioadenoma destruens). Patients with the problem may have irregular uterine bleeding with passage of villiform fragments of tissue, fetal heart sounds may be absent when expected, the uterus may be abnormally large, a positive pregnancy test may be present after abortion, the radioimmunoassay for beta-human chorionic gonadotropin (HCG) may be elevated or fail to return to normal levels following termination of pregnancy, and pelvic examination and x-ray examination of the chest may reveal metastases to vagina and lungs. Both choriocarcinomas and invasive moles require treatment, and careful and detailed studies must be done to determine the extent of the disease and its location, including scans of liver and brain, examination of cerebrospinal fluid for cells and HCG, hepatic and renal function tests, and pelvic ultrasound. Choriocarcinoma and chorioadenomas with poor prognosis are treated with combination of chemotherapeutic agents along with irradiation to sites of metastases. Methotrexate, actinomycin D, and chlorambucil (MAC) and doxorubicin, hydroxyurea, leucovorin, melphalan, methotrexate, and vincristine are two combinations that have yielded responses. Patients with lower risk such as those with no metastases or no more than to vagina or lungs can be cured in almost all cases, often with single chemotherapeutic agents. The treatments having the best chance of response are methotrexate with and without leucovorin; dactinomyxcin; cisplatin; methotrexate, etoposide, dactinomycin, cyclophosphamide, and vincristine (EMA-CO); and methotrexate, dactinomycin, and cyclophosphamide (MAC).

Fallopian Tubes

Primary cancer of the fallopian tubes is found less frequently than any other neoplasm of the female genital organs; metastatic lesions to the tubes from other portions of the urogenital system appear more frequently. For the origin of the cancer to be localized in the fallopian tubes, either no cancer must be present in either ovary or uterus or the type of cancer in either must not be identical with the fallopian neoplasm. The types of malignancies found in the tubes are adenocarcinomas (alveolar, papillary, and medullary), both homologous and heterologous mixed adenocarcinoma-sarcomas, leiomyosarcomas, chondrosarcomas, choriocarcinomas associated with pregnancy, and lymphomas. The adenocarcinomas are by far the most common. The behavior and appearance of these neoplasms and those of the ovary are somewhat similar, but those arising in the fallopian tubes tend to be more advanced with poorer prognosis.

The diagnosis is made preoperatively quite infrequently. Vaginal smears for Papanicolaou's staining are not positive very often, and the triad of profuse vaginal discharge, adnexal mass, and abdominal pain is not found in many cases. Cancer of the fallopian tube is difficult to distinguish on clinical examination from hydrosalpinx and tubovarian abscess. Both tubes are involved in about half the cases. The cancer spreads by direct mural extension through the wall, through the lumen, and by lymphatic or, less frequently, hematogenous dissemination. Pelvic and aortic nodes can become involved; less frequently the inguinal nodes contain cancer.

Operation is usually the first procedure of choice in stage I lesions, and conservative resection is not the recommended approach. Shedding of neoplastic cells into the lumen of the tubes is one unfortunate characteristic that increases the likelihood of dissemination of the disease when first seen. Operation consists of complete abdominal hysterectomy, salpingo-oophorectomy, omentectomy, peritonal biopsies including biopsies of the diaphragm and peritoneal washings, resection of all visible malignant tissue possible, sampling of pelvic and aortic nodes, and thorough exploration of the upper abdomen as well as the pelvis. Adjuvant therapy, especially in stages II through IV, is usually indicated. Hormonal therapy has not been effective, but radiotherapy and chemotherapy both have elicited additional responses in the later stages of the disease. External beam irradiation to pelvis with a tumor dose of 5000 cGy is known to extend life expectancy. The fields are expanded to upper abdomen in stages III and IV. Intraperitoneal ^{198}Au and ^{32}P can be effective for treatment of thin layers of peritoneal malignant cells. Chemotherapy with both single agents and combinations of agents have been used with some success as adjuvant therapy. Those eliciting some response are alkylating agents (chlorambucil, cyclophosphamide, melphalan, and thiotepa), cisplatin, and doxorubicin. A combination that has been used is cyclophosphamide, doxorubicin, and cisplatin (CAP). Chlorambucil combined with irradiation therapy elicits some response, but the contribution of the chemotherapy, if any, is not clear. More extensive cooperative clinical trials to evaluate adjuvant therapy with irradiation and/or chemotherapy are needed. The problem is the difficulty of accumulating enough entries into a trial because the cancer occurs so infrequently.

Adapted staging of cancer of the fallopian tubes

International Federation of Gynecology and Obstetrics

Stage I	Cancer of fallopian tubes
Stage IA	Cancer one fallopian tube, no ascites
Stage IB	Cancer both fallopian tubes, no ascites
Stage IC	Cancer one or both fallopian tubes, ascites cancer cells
Stage II	Growth limited to true pelvis
Stage IIA	Spread to uterus or ovary
Stage IIB	Spread to other tissue in pelvis

(Continued)

Stage III	Cancer one or both ovaries, peritoneal metastases
Stage IV	Cancer one or both fallopian tubes, distant metastases beyond peritoneal cavity

Source: Dodson et al.

Ovary

Cancer of the ovary is the leading cause of death from neoplasms of the reproductive system, accounting for almost half of the total number. This figure has not changed appreciably in the last quarter century except for the pronounced improvement in the survival of patients with germ-cell tumors. The primary problem is the difficulty in reaching an early diagnosis. At least half of patients are seen because of symptoms or signs of advanced disease such as ascites and extensive spread throughout the abdomen. Early disease is associated with minor or negligible symptoms, and at times the neoplasm is discovered unexpectedly during an operation performed for another condition. Ovarian neoplasms occur more often after the age of 45 than at earlier ages, although they do occur in younger patients before the menarche. Ovarian tumors detected before the menarche are less likely to be malignant.

Ovarian cancer is seen more often in single women, those who became pregnant at a more advanced age, and those with problems of infertility. The use of contraceptives seems to reduce the risk of developing this type of neoplasm. The breast cancer susceptibility gene *BRCA1* location 17g, accounts for most multiple familial early onset cases of both breast cancer and ovarian cancer. Higher socioeconomic status and descent from residents in North America and Northern Europe are associated with the disease. Those having had cancer of the breast are at increased risk for cancer of the ovary and vice versa. Familial histories of cancer of the ovary also have been reported to be related to autosomal dominant genes with incomplete penetrance. Site-specific ovarian cancer syndrome and the hereditary nonpolyposis colorectal cancer (Lynch II) syndrome account for very little risk of ovarian cancer in the general population. Genetic disorders such as Peutz-Jeghers syndrome, basal cell nevus syndrome, and Turner's syndrome are associated with tumors of the ovary, most of which are benign. Except possibly for asbestosis, no evidence for a role attributable to carcinogens in the etiology of ovarian cancer has been discovered.

Screening tests that are available are bimanual rectovaginal pelvic examination, CA-125 serum tumor marker detected by radioimmunoassay, and transvaginal ultrasonography including color Doppler imaging of ovarian vessels. Pelvic examination has not yielded the desired percentage of early diagnoses, and the remaining tests have less accuracy than desired. Currently, annual physical examination including rectovaginal examination, ultrasonography, and CA-125 tests are indicated. Entrance into a clinical screening trial is wise as well. In those with a familial history of ovarian cancer, a thorough study is suggested to evaluate the nature of the risk. Ovariectomy after the age of childbearing is an alternative advocated by some physicians for those with higher risk because of inherent genetic factors. However, noncompliance with estrogen replacement therapy reduces life expectancy because of osteoporosis and cardiovascular disease in premenopausal women who undergo bilateral oophorectomy. This should be made known to any patient contemplating the procedure before the menarche. Other factors that possibly are protective are the use of oral contraceptives, breast-feeding, and more than one completed pregnancy.

World Health Organization classification of ovarian cancer

Epithelial malignancies
  Serous malignancy
  Mucinous malignancy
  Endometrioid neoplasm
  Clear cell malignancy
  Brenner malignancy
  Mixed epithelioma
  Undifferentiated carcinoma

Gonadal stromal neoplasms
  Granulosa stroma cell neoplasm
  Androblastoma; Sertoli Leydig cell neoplasm
  Gynandroblastoma
  Unclassified

Germ cell malignancies
  Dysgerminoma
  Endodermal sinus neoplasm
  Embryonal carcinoma
  Polyembryoma
  Choriocarcinoma
  Teratoma
  Mixed tumor
  Gonadoblastoma

Staging for carcinoma of the ovary
International Federation of Gynecology and Obstetrics

Stage I	Growth limited to ovaries
Stage IA	Limited to one ovary; no ascites
Stage IB	Limited to both ovaries; no ascites
Stage IC	Stage IA or IB with ascites or positive peritoneal washings

(Continued)

Stage II	Growth limited to ovaries with pelvic extension
Stage IIA	Extension and/or metastases to uterus and/or tubes
Stage IIB	Extension to additional pelvic structures
Stage IIC	Stage IIA or IIB with ascites or positive peritoneal washings
Stage III	Growth involving one or both ovaries with implants in abdominal organs and peritoneum and spread to lymph nodes
Stage IIIA	Gross neoplasm in true pelvis; seeding in abdominal peritoneum
Stage IIIB	Nodes negative; peritoneal implants ≤2 cm
Stage IIIC	Implants >2 cm and/or positive inguinal or retroperitoneal nodes
Stage IV	Metastases to hepatic parenchyma and/or growth involving one or both ovaries with distant metastases (cytologic confirmation required for pleural effusion to be labeled malignant)

Tumors of the ovary are classified in three principal categories: epithelial, gonadal stromal, and germinal cell origin. By far the tumors most frequently encountered are the epithelial lesions most of which are malignant. Each of the remaining types account for less than 5 to 10 percent of the total number of ovarian neoplasms. Epithelial adenocarcinomas are subclassified as serous, mucinous, endometrioid, clear cell, and undifferentiated. A summary of the World Health Organization classification is contained in the accompanying table. Epithelial neoplasms spread by shedding of cells from the surface of the ovary even when no detectable rupture of the capsule is apparent, through the lymphatics, and by hematogenous dissemination. Extension can occur to uterus, bladder, tubes, and opposite ovary. All too often peritoneal seeding has occurred before the presence of the cancer is detected. The lymphatic flow carries metastases upward from the under surface of the diaphragm and may extent into mediastinal lymphatics. Obstruction of these lymphatic channels leads to ascites, and the islands of malignant cells invade the omentum and surface of the bowel. Involvement of the paraaortic, hypogastric, external iliac, and less frequently the inguinal nodes occurs with the passage of time. Hepatic, pulmonary, renal, osseous, adrenal, and splenic metastases have been reported. Because of this pattern of dissemination, operation for ovarian cancer must include meticulous and thorough examination of the entire abdomen including the undersurfaces of the diaphragm, especially on the right side. If metastatic foci are discovered, then it is mandatory to remove as much of the tumor mass as possible, including the omentum and reproductive organs when indicated.

Granulosa cell tumors are the type of stromal cell neoplasm seen most frequently. These tumors give symptoms similar to those of epithelial neoplasms but tend to be detected earlier and have a more benign course. They usually occur during the fifth to the seventh decade and may be associated with endometrial carcinoma. They are usually unilateral, tend to be localized

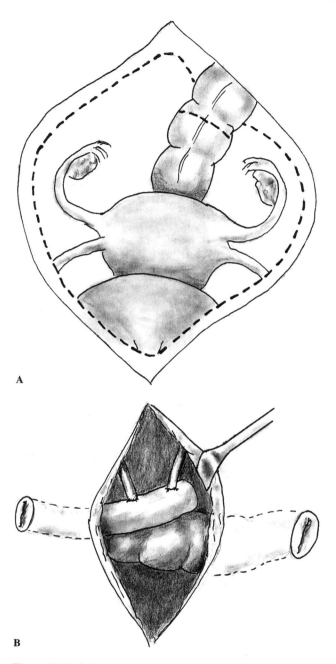

A

B

Figure 34 Pelvic exenteration for cancer. A. Limits of resection. B. Position of ureters, ileal conduit and ileostomy, and colostomy before complete closure of the wound.

when discovered, and can usually be treated successfully with salpingo-oophorectomy and total hysterectomy but can recur many years later. Response to irradiation has been disappointing, but treatment with dactinomycin D, cyclophosphamide, and 5-fluorouracil has been useful. A variant is the gynandroblastoma, which also may contain Leydig cells and tubules. All types of ovarian neoplasms exhibit various degrees of differentiation, and this is of prognostic significance in predicting future behavior. Because of the relatively small number of stromal cell tumors encountered, the data on responses to various types of therapy are not very extensive. Germ cell tumors are usually found in patients younger than 30 years of age and may be unilateral. Those encountered most frequently are dysgerminomas, embryonal carcinomas, and endodermal sinus tumors. Although some are highly malignant, considerable success has been obtained by using a combination of surgical resection with chemotherapy such as vincristine, dactinomycin, and cyclophosphamide.

Accurate staging is an important aspect of management of ovarian cancer. The accompanying table contains a summary of the classification of the International Federation of Gynecology and Obstetrics. This standardization is useful because the results of management reported from various studies can be applied accurately to an individual case of the disease. Also it provides reliable controls for evaluation of new modalities of treatment.

Ovarian and adnexal masses may be cystic and benign or malignant tumors of the ovary. Other conditions that must be differentiated are abscesses, endometriosis, polycystic ovarian disease, pregnancy, diverticula, urinary calculi, fibroid or other tumors of the uterus, enlarged lymph nodes, or neoplasms of other organs. Ultrasound is useful in determining the size and location of cystic features and in guiding an aspirating needle. Such aspirations may not distinguish a benign from a malignant tumor, however. It is important always to determine whether the premenopausal patient affected is pregnant and, if so, not to remove a corpus luteum cyst before the 12th week of pregnancy. It is possible to remove a large benign cyst and preserve the ovary. If a cancer cannot be ruled out, then the pregnant patient should be operated on during the second trimester and a salpingo-oophorectomy performed if an ovarian cancer confined to the ovary is found. If it has spread beyond, then a full exploration and debulking procedure is indicated. The uterus is not removed and the pregnancy terminated unless appropriate cytoreduction requires it. Since the usual chemotherapy does not affect the fetus, it can be instituted when indicated.

Characteristically there are few symptoms related to the presence of ovarian cancer early in the course of the disease. Later symptoms can be nausea, flatulence, dyspepsia, bowel dysfunction, anorexia, loss of weight, vaginal bleeding, pelvic pressure and discomfort, menstrual irregularity and postmenopausal bleeding, or abdominal pain; the patient can become aware of an abdominal mass and ascites, but usually symptoms and signs are not sufficiently prominent to arouse suspicion. Also Papanicolaou smears are not positive for adenocarcinoma cells very often. The presence of an ovarian mass 5 to 8 cm in diameter in peri- or postmenopausal patients always should be regarded as possibly malignant and should be treated as such. In younger patients small masses may not be malignant but nevertheless should be followed carefully. Ovarian tumors are nodular, cystic, and when malignant may present as a complex mass on ultrasound. The use of laparoscopy for diagnosis currently is controversial. Vaginal probe ultrasound with color Doppler imaging is preferred by some doctors. The omission of a pelvic examination during physical examination can result in missing the presence of an ovarian tumor. Computerized tomograms are helpful in delineating the extent of metastases, and lymphangiograms can indicate the presence and location of lymphatic extension.

When a positive diagnosis of ovarian cancer is made, an exploratory abdominal operation by an experienced surgeon should follow promptly. The abdominal cavity should be entered through a longitudinal incision to obtain the best exposure. In young women the decision to conserve reproductive capacity and only do unilateral oophorectomy should be reached after careful microscopic diagnosis and accurate staging from information obtained during the abdominal exploration. Malignant germ cell tumors occur around the age of 30 years, and ovarian tumors of borderline malignancy tend to occur in patients younger than 45 years of age. When the extent and malignancy of the neoplasm indicates, not only should the primary cancer be removed along with the uterus and tubes, but also the volume of the tumor should be reduced as much as possible by resecting the omentum, involved lymph nodes, and portions of other organs affected, if possible. Undoubtedly cytoreductive surgery is beneficial in terms of reducing the problem addressed by subsequent chemotherapy and irradiation. A second-look procedure to determine whether a cure has been obtained and the extent of any residual disease can be justified if multiple courses of chemotherapy have been given and a secondary group of agents is available for extended therapy.

Patients with stage I disease, having no malignant cells in the peritoneal fluid, are usually treated by bilateral salpingo-oophorectomy, abdominal hysterectomy, and omentectomy without the addition of adjuvant therapy. When malignant cells are present in the ascitic fluid (stage II disease), the same operation is performed, and adjuvant therapy is usually instituted. This additional therapy which can be offered includes various trials with chemotherapy and intraperitoneal isotope treatment (usually with ^{32}P). How or whether these various adjuvant modalities affect survival is not entirely clear at the present time. Because the cancer is confined to the peritonial cavity for long periods of time in so many cases, chemotherapy by intraperitoneal lavage is being used in therapeutic trials at times but only when there is minimal residual disease and adhesions do not block adequate distribution of fluid in the peritoneal cavity.

External irradiation has been used to treat cancer of the ovary for many decades and is indicated after maximal cytoreductive operative treatment when the cancer is inoperable, when a second look operation indicates recurrence, for localized treatment of distant metastases, and at times for alleviation of symptoms. When the therapy is delivered in divided doses by open field technique, the tumor dose is approximately 4500 cGy to the pelvic ports and 2500 cGy to upper abdominal ports. Because it is less complicated, is shorter in duration, has less late toxicity, and has equivalent results, this technique is used more frequently than the moving strip technique. The response of ovarian neoplasms to irradiation varies with their histologic appearance, and treatment is more effective when cytoreduction of the tumor mass is optimal. Complications of irradiation include nausea and vomiting, epidermitis, diarrhea, loss of weight, basilar pneumonitis and fibrosis, and renal and bone marrow damage. Usually most of these problems regress promptly and disappear. The liver and spleen must be shielded, reducing the dosage and effectiveness of irradiation in those parts of the abdomen. The size and position of ports, number of fractionated doses, shielding, and amount of irradiation are adjusted to minimize complications.

Chemotherapy has increased the median survival of patients treated for ovarian cancer from approximately 1 year to approximately 1.5 years. Survival may even be longer with the current most effective combination, taxol and cisplatin. The most effective agents found so far are platinum compounds, and platinum-based combinations with other agents yield even better rates of response and complete responses with increased likelihood of complete remission in advanced disease. Cisplatin and carboplatin are two of the best agents for treating ovarian carcinoma. Also effective are alkylating agents, such as AZQ (azirididynbenzoquinone), chlorambucil, cyclophosphamide, ifosfamide, mechlorethamine, melphalan, and thiotepa, which have been used extensively. Taxol, a plant alkaloid, is very useful; other such compounds are vinblastine and VP-16. The antibiotics, doxorubicin (Adriamycin) and mitomycin C, and antimetabolites, 5-fluorouracil and methotrexate, have also been used successfully. Dianhydrogalacticol, hexamethylmelamine, and peptichemio are included among useful agents as well. Some combinations of agents that have been used successfully are cyclophosphamide and doxorubicin; cisplatin, cyclophosphamide, doxorubicin, and hexamethylmelamine; cisplatin, cyclophosphamide, and doxorubicin; cisplatin and cyclophosphamide; and cyclophosphamide and hexamethylmelamine with and without 5-fluorouracil. Best results of treating epithelial neoplasms currently are obtained with cisplatin or carboplatin plus paclitaxel; and germ cell tumors respond best to bleomycin, etoposide, and cisplatin (BEP).

Toxicities and acquired drug resistance are two major problems which must be recognized and combated in treating patients with chemotherapy. Toxicities of some agents can include nausea and vomiting, suppression of bone marrow, alopecia, hypersensitivities, ototoxicity, nephrotoxicity, arthralgia, and peripheral neuropathy. The development of leukemia is a late complication which, fortunately, is not encountered very frequently. The external and implantable tubes and pumps for the delivery systems of these agents are being improved constantly, making treatment less trying for the patient and increasing the proportion that can be given as an outpatient procedure.

Receptors for estrogen and progesterone are present in approximately half of ovarian cancers. Antiestrogens, antiandrogens, and gonadotropin-releasing analogues have been used extensively as treatment for these neoplasms in many trials. Unfortunately the responses to hormonal therapy have been quite disappointing. Also the use of monoclonal antibodies and interleukin-2 have not led to successful alterations in therapy for ovarian cancer.

Vagina

Metastatic cancer from sites such as colon, endometrium, and breast are found more frequently in the vagina than primary cancer, which constitutes no more than 2 percent of neoplasms of the female genital tract. Approximately 90 percent of these primary lesions are squamous carcinomas similar to those appearing in the cervix; the median time of appearance is early in the fifth decade. Verrucous carcinoma with exophytic cauliflower appearance is more easily cured than the squamous neoplasms. Exposure to diethylstilbestrol in utero may lead to adenosis and clear cell carcinomas appearing most frequently around the age of 19. Primary melanomas are found very rarely in the vagina, but they do occur in this location along with melanomas elsewhere and are one of the most common primary lesions other than squamous carcinoma. Neoplasms of connective tissue include leiomyosarcomas, stromal sarcomas, and lymphosarcomas. Rhabdomyosarcoma botryoides of the vagina is seen in childhood. Risk factors for vaginal cancer that have been reported are prior positive Papanicolaou's smear, early hysterectomy, prior cancer of the cervix, low socioeconomic status, previous radiation therapy, and the exposure to diethylstilbestrol in utero mentioned above.

Carcinoma of the vagina spreads by direct extension and through the lymphatics. It is difficult to treat successfully when it is detected late in the course of the disease and because so many other organs are only a few millimeters away. Actually early superficial cancers will respond and can be cured by topical 5-fluorouracil. Carcinoma in situ can be treated by excision, 5-fluorouracil, and supplemental intracavitary or interstitial irradiation. In stage I when the upper portion of the vagina is involved, treatment consisting of radical hysterectomy, partial vaginectomy, and pelvic lymphadenectomy can be used successfully. Exenteration may be required when the lower portion of the vagina is involved. Also external beam and intracavitary radiotherapy is sometimes used. At times a 6500-cGy tumor dose directed to lymph nodes and paravaginal tissue is required. Stage II disease is treated with external beam and brachytherapy. In stages III and IV external irradiation to the pelvis and ports arranged with distant metastatic targets in brain, bone, and elsewhere is used. Either radical resection or radiotherapy are used to combat clear cell carcinoma grade I. Radiation is the primary treatment for other stages. Radiotherapy frequently includes vaginal cylinders and interstitial therapy utilizing ^{226}Ra, ^{137}Cs, and ^{192}Ir as well as external beam irradiation.

Only doxorubicin has been found to have significant antitumor effect on most neoplasms of the vagina, and very disappointing results have been obtained in treating melanoma. Endodermal sinus tumors respond to combination therapy and conservative resection. The agents that have been used are PEB (cisplatin, etoposide, bleomycin), PVP (cisplatin, vinblastine, bleomycin), and VAC (vincristine, doxorubicin, cyclophosphamide). VAC is also used in addition to operation and radiation for treating childhood embronal rhabdomyosarcoma.

Stages of cancer of the vagina
International Federation of Gynecology and Obstatrics

Stage 0	Intraepithelial carcinoma in situ
Stage I	Cancer limited to vaginal wall
Stage II	Cancer in subvaginal tissue but not pelvic wall
Stage III	Cancer extending to pelvic wall
Stage IVA	Cancer spread to adjacent organ(s)
Stage IVB	Cancer spread to distant organs

Female Urethra

Studies, including biopsy, similar to those described for the male urethra are indicated to establish the diagnosis in the female as well. Cancer of the female urethra occurs in patients in older age groups, it is more frequently seen in white women, and most of the neoplasms are squamous carcinomas. Transitional cell and adenocarcinomas also occur, but the treatment is usually the same for all types of the disease. Distal urethrectomy can be used for treating cancer in that location, but at times a more radical procedure including total urethrectomy, cystectomy, and pelvic and sometimes inguinal node resection may be necessary in the treatment of more extensive lesions. Interstitial radioactive implants can be used as treatment of superficial meatal cancer. External beam radiotherapy is used for more extensive disease with invasion of labia, vagina, and urinary bladder, or anterior exenteration may be the best choice of treatment in these cases. Needles can be used for brachytherapy with iridium 192 or other radioactive source in combination with resective and external beam therapy. It is possible to use a total divided dose or irradiation up to 7000 cGy when external beam irradiation and brachytherapy are used concomitantly. One plan that is advocated is preoperative irradiation with radical cystourethrectomy or concomitant 5-fluorouracil and mitomycin C chemotherapy. Complications with these more extensive treatment regimens often occur and require careful surveillance and appropriate management. Clearly the usefulness of new chemotherapeutic agents and continued assessment of new approaches to combination therapy must be continued.

Vulva

Carcinoma of the vulva constitutes approximately 5 percent of cancers of the female genital tract in the United States. Most are squamous carcinomas, and patients with this diagnosis are more prone to develop cancer of the cervix. These carcinomas may appear in areas of chronic hyperplasia or atrophy as multicentric and confluent white, pink, or brown lesions that are sometimes elevated. They can develop in vulvar condylomata, and herpesvirus type II and human papilloma virus have been implicated in their origin. The cancers also can be preceded by leukoplakia of the vulva, and more appear on the labia majora than elsewhere. Growth is usually by slow microinvasion with ultimate extension to adjacent organs, regional lymph nodes, and distant sites.

These cancers are seen in older women from the fifth decade to later ages. It is found more frequently in lower economic groups and possibly in those in laundry and cleaning occupations. Approximately one-fifth of the patients are asymptomatic; others complain of pain, a mass, pruritis, and bleeding. The International Federation of Gynecology and Obstetrics classification of the disease appears in the accompanying table. The proper staging of the disease is essential for optimum results of treatment. Survival for 5 years ranges from almost 100 percent in stage I to approximately 85, 75, and 30 percent, respectively, in stages II, III, and IV. Clinical workup for patients with the diagnosis of cancer of the vulva requires bimanual pelvic examination, Papanicolaou's smear, radiographic study of the chest, possibly a computerized tomogram, and investigation of additional medical problems especially in elderly women.

The treatment of cancer of the vulva utilizes resection, radiotherapy, and chemotherapy but whether each is used and how it is used depends on the stage of the disease. Carcinoma in situ is usually excised widely, and at times a graft is used to cover the defect. Laser treatment can be used to vaporize extremely small superficial lesions; a disadvantage is that there is no specimen to examine at the close of the procedure. A modified vulvectomy or even hemivulvectomy is sometimes justified in stage I lesions with limited invasion. Whether a dissection of inguinal nodes should be carried out or a sample for microscopic diagnosis taken is a decision resting on preliminary diagnostic studies and physical examination. A margin of 1.0 cm free of cancer should be removed with the tissue excised. A radical vulvectomy is usually done for stage II disease, removing vulvar subcutaneous tissue to the pubic ramus, adjacent muscle, and inguinal lymph nodes. Great care in operative technique and postoperative care must be exercised to avoid problems of wound healing, stricture, lymphedema, and function. This approach is modified at times with less extensive vulvectomy but including inguinal and femoral lymphadenectomy followed by irradiation with a tumor dose of approximately 5000 cGy. Unilateral operations are never done for midline lesions. The use of radiation alone is somewhat controversial. Stage III lesions rarely require exenteration, and treatment usually consists of radical vulvectomy with resection of distal vagina, urethra, and/or anal canal if involved and postoperative irradiation if excised lymph nodes are found to be invaded. Stage IV disease requires radical vulvectomy with resection of regional nodes. An anterior exenteration may be necessary if the rectum and/or vagina, bladder, and other organs are involved. Stage IVB disease with fixation of the cancer and/or involvement of bone is treated with irradiation and chemotherapy. The tumor dose of radiation may be extended to 7000 cGy for large inoperable neoplasms with lymph nodes included in the fields as well. Recurrent carcinoma of the vulva is usually treated first with radiation, the remaining management depending on the response.

Superficial squamous lesions respond to 5-fluorouracil; also systemic administration of bleomycin or doxorubicin have elicited responses. Administration of cisplatin results in little response. Combinations that have been used for vulvar carcinoma are bleomycin, lomustine (CCNU), and methotrexate as well as bleomycin, cisplatin, mitomycin C, and vincristine. Radiation along with a combination of 5-fluorouracil and mitomycin C has also been used for advanced cancer of the vulva.

In addition to the squamous lesions, adenocarcinomas, Bartholin's gland carcinomas, basal cell carcinomas, and melanomas occur. Sarcomas and verrucous carcinomas are seen infrequently. Basal cell and verrucous carcinomas can usually be cured by local excision alone. Adenoid cystic carcinoma of Bartholin's gland also is usually treated by resection, the extent and whether lymphadenectomy is included depending on the degree of invasion. The same is true for melanomas. Metastatic cancer of the vulva is excised, with additional management depending on the original primary site and extent.

Staging of cancer of the vulva
International Federation of Gynecology and Obstetrics

Stage 0	Intraepithelial, preinvasive carcinoma in situ
Stage I	Tumor ≤2 cm in diameter confined to vulva Nodes not clinically suspicious
Stage II	Tumor >2 cm in diameter confined to vulva Nodes not clinically suspicious
Stage III	Tumor of any size with spread to urethra and/or anus, perineum, and vagina Metastases in unilateral or bilateral regional lymph nodes
Stage IVA	Tumor of any size infiltrating any of the following structures: bilateral regional lymph nodes, bladder, pelvic bone, rectum, and upper urethra
Stage IVB	Distant metastases

LEUKEMIAS AND LYMPHOMAS

The types of leukemia include the following:

Acute lymphocytic (lymphoblastic) leukemia (ALL)
Acute nonlymphocytic (myelocytic) leukemia (ANL, AML)
Chronic lymphocytic leukemia (CLL)
Chronic myeloid (myelogenous, granulocytic) leukemia (CML)

The acute lymphocytic leukemias occur more frequently in children, whereas the acute nonlymphocytic (myeloid) and chronic leukemias present problems more frequently in adults. One causative agent is irradiation occurring from wartime exposure and industrial accidents and in the course of therapy for various diseases. Also some chemotherapeutic chemicals such as alkylating agents, benzene, chloramphenicol, nitrosourea, phenylcarbazone, and procarbazine have been implicated as well. Chromosomal abnormalities have been detected in both acute lymphocytic and acute myeloid leukemia, and studies on the role of oncogenes in the origin and characteristics of the leukemias continue. A complete response to therapy consists of the return of peripheral blood and marrow to normal and the disappearance of lymphadenopathy and hepatosplenomegaly. A partial response yields little benefit in acute leukemia but may alleviate clinical problems in chronic leukemia.

ACUTE LYMPHOCYTIC LEUKEMIA

Most of the cells constituting acute "lymphocytic" leukemia are lymphoblasts, and the disease is often referred to as acute lymphoblastic leukemia.

Three major types of cells are distinguishable on the basis of their appearance:

L1 cells with high nuclear cytoplasmic ratio and none or one small nucleolus seen most often in children with the disease

L2 cells consisting of a mixture of small and large types with larger nucleoli seen most often in adults

L3 cells of uniform large size with B-cell markers representing the type seen most infrequently.

The classification of the acute leukemias is based on study of the bone marrow including morphology of blast cells, their antigenic characteristics, enzymes, histochemistry, and chromosomal pattern. The disease arises in a stem cell, and the subsequent clones lead to failure of the bone marrow. Several translocations have been identified in some patients with acute lymphocytic leukemia, and the c-*myc* protooncogene and Philadelphia chromosmal abnormality have also been noted. Clinical symptoms and signs are the result of reduction in numbers of erythrocytes, leukocytes, and platelets and extramedullary extension of the disease from the bone marrow to organs and periosteum. Common findings are fever, purpura, infections, lymphadenopathy, splenomegaly, hepatomegaly, and bone pain or refusal of children to walk. Central nervous system involvement is usually apparent after the diagnosis is made. In children symptoms may not differentiate the problem as acute leukemia, and careful history, physical examination, and laboratory studies may be necessary before ruling out other diseases including tumors such as neuroblastoma, non-Hodgkin's lymphoma, retinoblastoma, and rhabdomyosarcoma.

The response to therapy is more favorable in those with a hyperdiploid chromosome count, but the outcome is less favorable in adults older than 45 years and children younger than 2 years and older than 9 years, adults and children with chromosomal translocations, the presence of T or B markers, high leukocyte count, hypodiploidy, and extramedullary extension to organs including the meninges. Also there is a poorer prognosis in the black than in the white race. The plan of therapy consists of induction, prophylaxis of extension to central nervous system, and management during remission. The response to acute lymphocytic leukemia in most children is one of the bright pictures achieved with therapy; that for adults is much less encouraging.

Before induction therapy is initiated, the patient must be started on treatment with allopurinol to prevent hyperuricemia and consequent renal damage. Also concurrent physical problems must be treated vigorously to provide the best condition of the patient before treatment begins. Electrolyte and fluid imbalance, infections, cardiac failure, uncontrolled diabetes, and renal disease are examples of this kind of problem. Also menses should be suppressed, since menorrhagia can ensue with the thrombocytopenia accompanying therapy. Finally a multiluminal catheter must be installed for vascular access.

In children at low risk with acute lymphatic leukemia the induction treatment aimed at remission may consist of the following:

L-Asparaginase IM or IV
Prednisone (or dexamethasone) PO
Vincristine IV

When L-asparaginase is administered, preparation for possible anaphylaxis or other complication must be initiated beforehand. If complete remission has not been obtained based on study of the bone marrow, additional therapy can be given such as substitution of 6-mercaptopurine PO for L-asparaginase. During the induction or consolidation phase, prophylaxis for involvement of the central nervous system consists of cranial irradiation in divided dosage and either spinal irradiation or intrathecal methotrexate. When there is enlargement or evidence of infiltration of testicles on the evidence from biopsy, irradiation of the testicles is given in low divided doses. Headache, bone marrow suppression, parotitis, stomatitis, dental caries, and in children and even young adults alteration in growth pattern and ability to learn as well as leukoencephalopathy have occurred after irradiation of the cranium. When irradiation of the spine is carried out or when intrathecal chemotherapy is used, hydrocortisone is given after a suitable response occurs in order to alleviate arachnoiditis or neuritis. Many patients are placed on experimental protocols, especially adults with acute lymphocytic leukemia (ALL).

Maintenance therapy is begun when platelet count is above 100,000 and absolute neutrophil count (ANC) is greater than 1000. One regimen used consists of the following agents:

6-Mercaptopurine PO
Methotrexate PO
Prednisone PO
Vincristine IV

Patients, chiefly children, classified as intermediate risks are managed using the following scheme. The risk is based on platelet and leukocyte count, age, and sex. The regimen for induction utilizes the same drugs as for patients at low risk, L-asparaginase, prednisone, and vincristine. Irradiation management for central nervous system and testicular involvement is the same, and methotrexate intrathecally may be given as well. 6-Mercaptopurine, prednisone, and vincristine are used for consolidation therapy, the first agent not being used unless the platelet count is more than 100,000 and the ANC is more than 1000. Maintenance treatment is continued for as long as 3 years, depending on the sex of the patient and the response to medication. Many therapists continue the methotrexate as well.

Patients classified as being at high risk, chiefly adults, have induction therapy such as daunorubicin, vincristine, prednisone, and L-asparaginase. Also cytarabine as well as methotrexate may be used intrathecally. Consolidation therapy usually begins the first part of the second month of therapy and includes cyclophosphamide IV, prednisone PO, 6-mercaptopurine, and cytarabine IV or SQ. Methotrexate may be given intrathecally. Prophylactic irradiation of the central nervous system is given as described above. Interim maintenance therapy such as oral 6-mercaptopurine and methotrexate then may be succeeded with delayed intensification treatment consisting of reinduction of dexamethasone PO, doxorubicin IV, L-asparaginase IM, and vincristine IV and reconsolidation with cyclophosphamide IV, cytarabine IV or SQ, dexamethasone PO, and thioguanine PO. Also maintenance therapy may consist of 6-mercaptopurine PO, methotrexate PO, and vincristine IV for as long as 3 years. Intrathecal (IT) therapy with methotrexate may be indicated in addition to other therapy.

When relapse occurs in low-risk patients, particularly those in whom it occurs a year or more after induction, therapy is still quite useful in prolonging survival. Intravenous cytarabine and vindesine have been used for this problem with good results. In other patients the outlook is not as promising. When the central nervous system and testicle are the sites of recurrence, local irradiation or IT chemotherapy is usually initiated before systemic chemotherapy. Because of the very good prognosis with chemotherapy, transplantation of bone marrow is usually not considered appropriate during the first remission for patients in the low-risk category, whereas those at higher risk with acute lymphocytic leukemia as well as those with B-cell acute leukemia and acute lymphoblastic leukemia-lymphoma should be considered for transplantation of bone marrow earlier.

Acute lymphocytic leukemia in adults can be treated first with vincristine IV, prednisone PO, and daunorubicin IV (often referred to as VPD therapy) or variations featuring other agents such as DATVP (cytarabine IV, daunorubicin IV, thioguanine PO, vincristine IV, and prednisone PO), intravenous cytarabine, and daunorubicin in a schedule referred to as "7 plus 3" plus vincristine IV and prednisone PO, and MOAD (methotrexate IV, vincristine IV, L-asparaginase IV, and dexamethasone PO). In adults prophylactic irradiation of the cranium in fractional dosages and intrathecal methotrexate are used in the same way as this approach in younger patients. Maintenance therapy of methotrexate PO and 6-mercaptopurine PO may be combined with vincristine IV and prednisone PO. Treatment of relapse is usually not as successful in adults as in children. Treatment used may be VM-26 (teniposide IV) and cytarabine IV). Transplantation of allogeneic bone marrow should be considered at least by the second remission and may be considered earlier in young patients. The management of hybrid and stem cell acute leukemia usually includes therapy usually used for both acute lymphocytic and non-lymphoid leukemia such as vincristine and prednisone in combination with the 7 plus 3 regimen. The prognosis in these cases is always guarded. Prophylactic treatment for central nervous system spread is always included in the plan for therapy.

ACUTE NONLYMPHOCYTIC LEUKEMIA

Acute nonlymphoid or myelocytic leukemia has been divided into several groups based on morphologic appearance of the predominant type of cell. Groups M1, M2, and M3 are granulocytic, groups M4 and M5 monocytic, group M6 erythrocytic, and group M7 megakaryocytic. Patients classified as having group M3 disease have a tendency to develop cerebral hemorrhage and intravascular coagulation. Those with M6 disease often have a clinical syndrome consisting of hyperplasia of the gums, infiltration of the skin, low serum potassium, lymphadenopathy, and usually a poor prognosis.

Before beginning definitive therapy directed toward complete remission, treatment with allopurinol must be initiated and continued along with chemotherapy until response of the bone marrow is adequate. Although some physicians favor the use of antibiotic therapy, many others prefer to depend on environmental asepsis to reduce the risk of infection. The two regimens often adopted in various combinations are the use of intravenous cytarabine and daunorubicin in the 7 plus 3 dosage scheme and DAT consisting of thioguanine PO, cytarabine IV, and daunorubicin IV, doxorubicin, idarubicin, and mitoxantrone have all been substituted for daunorubicin with some success, but all anthrocyclines including mitoxantrone are cardiotoxic and cannot be used when the patient has comorbid cardiovascular problems. Postinduction therapy is often given, provided the patient has not developed one or more prohibitive complications. Intensification, consolidation, and maintenance approaches usually utilize high degrees of cytarabine (ara-C).

Decisions about the continuation of chemotherapy require careful review of current condition of the patient and previous response. Those patients developing the disease de novo usually respond much better than those in whom the appearance is secondary to some other exposure or illness. Reduction of dosages in the elderly with acute myelogenous leukemia requires objective evaluation of specific conditions which may justify such an alteration. Patients developing the signs justifying the diagnosis of leukemia after having a dysplastic syndrome have a less favorable prognosis along with those developing the disease after induction by irradiation or therapeutic medication. Birth control should be considered by those women with myelogenous leukemia who are able to become pregnant. Treatment during pregnancy constitutes risks of fetal death and premature labor, but possible long-term dangers are not entirely clear. Relapse after the approaches to therapy described above is a clear indication for consideration of allogeneic bone marrow transplantation. Problems that are exceptionally difficult to manage are myelogenous leukemia of the central nervous system, disseminated intravascular coagulation (DIC) associated with acute promyelocytic leukemia, and leukostasis leading to vascular obstruction and necrosis with bleeding associated with hyperleukocytosis, and hyperviscosity which suggests conservative use of transfusions. Leukapheresis is useful in the management of leukostasis, and the judicious use of appropriate fractions of the blood are used in the treatment of DIC, which may also be ameliorated by the use of heparin, although its value remains somewhat controversial. Bone marow transplantation (BMT) is advocated by some therapists during the first or the second remission.

CHRONIC LYMPHOCYTIC LEUKEMIA

Chronic lymphocytic leukemia is the type of leukemia found most frequently, with approximately two-thirds of the cases occurring in males and one-third in females. It is a monoclonal derangement predominantly of B cells with only about 5 percent of T-cell origin. The clinical picture results from proliferation of these cells with enlargement of lymph nodes and spleen and infiltration and reduction in function of the bone marrow. Chlorambucil has been effective in obtaining responses alone and in combination with other agents such as prednisone. Higher doses of chlorambucil have increased the survival in some trials, but unfortunately the median survival from the disease is approximately 6 years or less. The use of prednisone for treating anemia and thrombocytopenia is somewhat limited by the increased danger of infections. Although chlorambucil and prednisone have been the standard treatment for many years, other combinations of agents are known to induce responses and remissions. They include cyclophosphamide, doxorubicin, prednisone; cyclophosphamide, melphalan, prednisone; cyclophosphamide, doxorubicin, prednisone, vincristine; cyclophosphamide, vincristine, prednisone, melphalan, carmustine (BCNU); and nucleoside analogues such as 2-chlorodeoxyadenosine and fludarabine. The therapy used most frequently currently is cyclophosphamide, vincristine, and prednisone. Bone marrow transplantation has been useful in some cases with remission when it is necessary following intensive chemotherapy.

Chronic T-cell lymphocytic leukemia tends to occur in young patients in whom the lymphocytosis may be overwhelming with lymphadenopathy, bone marrow infiltration, and dermal involvement at times. Responses to chemotherapy effective for other types of chronic lymphatic leukemia often are not found when there is T-cell monoclonal lineage. Treatment with corticosteroids, 2-chlorodeoxyadenosine, and splenectomy are somewhat effective, and cortisone and splenectomy may be useful in combating neutropenia.

Hairy cell leukemia derives its name from the appearance of the cells under the scanning electron microscope. Lymphadenopathy usually is not a prominent feature of the clinical picture. Treatment may include therapy with interferon-α, 2-deoxycoformycin, and 2-chlorodeoxyadenosine. Splenectomy is not used as frequently now as in the past. Pronounced splenomegaly and high circulating leukocyte count are prominent features of prolymphocytic leukemia. It also is associated with various chromosomal abnormalities. Responses do occur at times with cyclophosphamide, doxorubicin, vincristine, and prednisone; fludarabine; and splenectomy. The median period for survival is less than 3 years.

CHRONIC MYELOGENOUS LEUKEMIA

Chronic myelogenous leukemia in childhood occurs in two forms, adult and juvenile. The juvenile form is a disease of infancy, whereas the adult form occurs in adolescence. The former disease is quite unlike the latter. Apparently it is a form of myelomonocytic leukemia in which no Philadelphia chromosome is found, thrombocytopenia and associated hemorrhagic manifestations occur, immunoglobulin abnormalities are found, there may be a facial rash, and lymphadenopathy can be suppurative. The course of the disease grows progressively worse, with median survival less than 1 year. Chemotherapy, including busulfan, has not been very useful; bone marrow transplantation should be considered, since favorable results have been reported.

Chronic myelogenous leukemia in adolescents and adults begins with the occurrence of a translocation between chromosomes 9 and 22 resulting in the characteristic appearance of the Philadelphia chromosomal abnormality detectable by several means. These new cells replace normal diploid cells with mature myeloid cells which do not respond to extracellular growth factors acting to suppress abnormal increases in the mass of myeloid cells. If unchecked, this leads to a prodigious increase in the leukemic cells at the expense of normal leukocytes, successive infiltration of organs, and ultimately death from infection, thrombosis, and/or hemorrhage. Treatment in the past consisted of administration of radioactive phosphorus and splenectomy. With the advent of chemotherapy for this disease, these measures have been either abandoned or reserved for special situations and responses. Both busulfan and hydroxyurea have been found effective in inducing partial remissions without eliminating the Ph chromosome. The latter brings about a more rapid response in reducing splenomegaly, the leukocyte count, and symptoms, but one which is of shorter duration. Busulfan at times is responsible for more serious complications than hydroxyurea, however. Now splenectomy is reserved for patients not responding adequately to chemotherapy. Patients who are both nonresponsive and not candidates for operative intervention can be treated with cytarabine. Usually this disease is managed easily during the chronic phase which may last as long as several years, but response is reduced after it enters the accelerated or blast phase.

Interferons consist of a group of peptides produced by normal cells responding to several types of stimuli. Their action consists of antiviral effects, promotion of differentiation, antiproliferative responses, and modulation of immune phenomena. When interferons have been tried as therapy for chronic myeloid leukemia, patients at low risk responded most favorably with reduction in the numbers of cells exhibiting the Philadelphia chromosome. Undesirable side effects ensue at higher dosages, limiting usefulness of this therapy. Both interferon alfa-2 and the γ-interferon have been tried, the latter in combination with interferon alfa-2 and chemotherapy. Side effects of interferon alfa-2 include respiratory, gastrointestinal, renal, neurologic, and hematologic problems. These consist of a syndrome similar to influenza, diarrhea, nausea, abnormal memory and cognitive functions, parkinsonism, psychoses, depression, rare thrombocytopenia and hemolysis, and late autoimmune problems and hypothyroidism. To reduce the appearance of these complications, a different approach to therapy has been used consisting of induction of remission with busulfan or intensive therapy with a combination of cytarabine, daunorubicin, prednisone, and vincristine to induce remission followed by maintenance therapy with interferon alfa-2. Allogeneic or syngeneic bone marrow transplantation is indicated at times in the management of chronic myelogenous leukemia, usually in young patients. The approach is to give intensive chemotherapy and/or irradiation to destroy all cells from the leukemic clone, then to use the transplant to replace the marrow with normal cells to restore hemopoiesis. Specific means to do this are high-dose cyclophosphamide and irradiation or high-dose cyclophosphamide and busulfan. Bone marrow transplantation in patients in the accelerated phase of the disease or with a blast crisis is associated with a poor prognosis. Better results have been obtained in patients in the chronic phase of the leukemia. It should be kept in mind that the risk of developing the acute phase of the disease following bone marrow transplantation has been reported as high as 25 percent. With the continuing development of safe vectors for transport of missing and needed genes into human cells, genetic and molecular methods of treatment should lead to improvement in the therapy of leukemias in the future.

MALIGNANT (NON-HODGKIN'S) LYMPHOMA

The clinical course of the various types of non-Hodgkin's lymphomas is quite divergent, and a classification based on response to treatment, although somewhat unsatisfactory, is usually employed in dealing with the management of these neoplasms. In most of them the malignant cell is derived from the B cell, but the malignant cell is derived from the T-cell lymphocyte in others.

Classification is usually simplified into three grades of lesions: high, intermediate, and low. Some low-grade lesions appear to be somewhat localized when first encountered, but many low-grade lymphomas are widely disseminated at times including spread to the bone marrow. They may respond even to minimal therapy and live for an extended period. Higher-grade tumors are most likely to be disseminated on presentation and require intensive therapy to avoid a fatal outcome, but cures can be obtained with combination chemotherapy. Cures are obtained much less frequently in cases of low-grade tumors which may be fatal within a decade; Unlike Hodgkin's disease, stage I and II disease is seldom found and may respond to local treatment with radiotherapy.

Classification of malignant lymphomas

Low grade
  Small lymphocyte
  Small cleaved cell
    (follicular)
  Small and large cleaved cell mixed
    (follicular)

Intermediate grade
  Large cell predominant
    (follicular)
  Small cleaved cell diffuse
  Mixed small and large cell diffuse
  Large cell, cleaved cell, noncleaved cell diffuse

High grade
  Immunoblastic large cell
    (plasmacytoid, clear, polymorphous, epithelioid)
  Lymphoblastic
    (convoluted, nonconvoluted)
  Small noncleaved cell
    (Burkitt's, follicular)

Others

Staging for intermediate- and high-grade lymphomas*

I   Localized nodal or extranodal disease

II   Greater than one nodal or one or two extranodal sites with draining nodes but without symptoms, performance <70, mass >10 cm lactic dehydrogenase >500

III   Greater unfavorable prognostic findings than in stage II

*The staging for Hodgkin's disease is often preferred for malignant lymphomas as well.

The classification and staging of malignant lymphomas is somewhat more difficult than is the case for many other neoplasms. A careful record of symptoms and signs and physical examination must be obtained, including a history of weakness, loss of weight, sweating, presence of masses, skin lesions. Examination of the blood should include a complete count, sedimentation rate, hematocrit, tests for hepatic and renal function, and biopsies of bone marrow and masses such as enlarged axillary, cervical, epitrochlear, inquinal, femoral, and popliteal nodes are required. Examination for possible involvement of Waldeyer's ring involves indirect laryngoscopy. Radiographic studies to be considered are x-ray studies and computerized tomography of chest, abdomen, head, and spine, and magnetic resonance imaging of bone when these examinations are indicated. Ultrasound studies of the abdomen can be helpful, but lymphangiograms are seldom required when computerized scans have been done. At times, exploratory abdominal operation is indicated for certain types of management; this may or may not include splenectomy.

After the clinical studies and examinations have been completed, classification and staging of the disease can be determined. The classification summarized in the table is the one most frequently used by clinicians. This working formulation not only includes a description of the appearance of the various types of malignant lymphomas but also is useful in determining the outlook for success in the management of the disease. The use of the word *follicular* indicates that the lymphoma forms clusters of cells resembling germinal centers that appear in normal tissue. The choice of treatment is dependent on the classification, which simplifies this most important decision. The classification illustrated above is based on the histologic appearance of the tumor. The stage is of lesser importance in these intermediate and high-grade neoplasms because of the initial extent of the disease when treatment begins. This type of malignancy occurs in a wide range of ages, some patients being sufficiently elderly to have diseases of heart, lung, liver, and kidney. When such problems exist, then alteration in the type of chemotherapy may be justified as well as when they are present at any age. Bone marrow sensitivity to irradiation can be greater in the elderly as well. However, age alone should not lead to lowering the dose of chemotherapy to palliative level when the usual dosage can possibly be curative. Choosing an alternative regimen not containing a drug known to be very dangerous in an immunodeficient patient is wiser than continuing the same combination therapy with the drug in question at lower dosage.

The staging given for Hodgkin's disease is satisfactory for low-grade lymphomas but not for the remainder of the lymphomas. A more satisfactory way for staging intermediate- and high-grade lymphomas appears in the table. The usefulness of irradiation and chemotherapy is not always easy to determine even after careful classification and staging of the disease, and additional clinical trials with various combinations of available chemotherapeutic agents with and without irradiation will be required for clarification. Several factors are taken into consideration in deciding on the approach to treating a patient with malignant lymphoma. The principal characteristics to be considered are the histologic type of tumor determined by microscopic diagnosis of biopsy material, the stage of the disease, and the physical condition of the patient.

Irradiation for Malignant Lymphomas

The best results reported for irradiation of lymphomas has been achieved in treating low-grade lymphomas in the early stage of the disease. There is an encouraging potential for cure in those patients younger than 45 years of age with small volume disease. Some uncertainty remains about the relationship between the extent of the field irradiated and success and when irradiation and chemotherapy should be combined. Although irradiation has a less prominent role in treating intermediate- and high-grade malignant lymphomas than in managing Hodgkin's disease, there remains a more limited usefulness despite the fact that the lymphomas are located beyond the margins of the field for irradiation when discovered. Doses of 2500 to 4500 cGy are capable of controlling most nodular lymphomas. Irradiation is quite effective locally for treating large lesions. Rates for curing large-cell lymphomas in stage I rises to 90% when chemotherapy with or without irradiation is used. Irradiation is sometimes used for large-cell lymphomas that have become refractory to prior chemotherapy.

Chemotherapy for Low-Grade Malignant Lymphomas

Breakdown of tumor tissue often occurs with chemotherapy. Sometimes, before starting treatment, a course of allopurinol is begun to prevent the development of hyperuricemia that may accompany the destruction of the malignant cells. Treatment of low-grade lymphomas varies from observation to combination chemotherapy, since the treatment is regarded as palliative. However, almost a decade may elapse before the patient's condition becomes critical, and symptoms may not require combination chemotherapy for many years. Even spontaneous remissions are not unknown. It is always desirable to avoid the distressing toxic effects of the type of chemotherapy useful in this disease, but unfortunately the disease is usually widespread when first diagnosed and the time comes for treating the patient when elevated temperature, sweating, falling blood count, involvement of internal organs and bone marrow occur. Complete remission may be achieved by various combinations of therapeutic drugs, although recurrence occurs later. Sometimes the interval is prolonged. Under the circumstances presented by this type of malignant lymphoma it is necessary for the chemotherapist to exercise careful judgment about fitting treatment to the characteristics of the clinical picture presented by the individual being treated. Eventually the disease may become refractory to various chemotherapeutic agents alone or in combination, and this may be accompanied by changes in the tissue itself. When this transpires, any type of effective treatment is most difficult to achieve. When symptoms and lymphadenopathy are not great, oral cyclophosphamide or chlorambucil can be useful. At times it is administered with prednisone. With the advancement of symptoms and extent of the disease, combination therapy such as COPP, CHOP, or CVP (defined in the table) can be useful. When low-grade lymphomas become refractory, the regimens used for intermediate and advanced grades of the disease as primary treatment can be used but with much less success than when used for the higher grades of the disease.

Chemotherapy for Intermediate- and High-Grade Malignant Lymphomas

The management of intermediate- and high-grade malignant lymphomas is continually changing as new agents, new combinations, and better understanding of the response of the various types of cells constituting the tumors become available. The chemotherapist must keep in mind the natural history of the disease and do everything to avoid losing the opportunity for promoting cure or remission and reversing symptoms. Although toxic effects are an undesirable feature of many effective regimens, they are the price for the chance for cure or at least palliation. The patient and doctor must arrive at an approach to therapy that takes into consideration the patient's objectives and understanding of the treatments possible and proposed. When experience does not indicate a clear choice between regimens, at times the opportunity to enter as a patient included in a clinical trial may be acceptable.

Since these tumors are usually extensive when diagnosed, initial treatment is less apt to be delayed and will consist of some of the more effective combination regimens. CHOP has been used extensively, and other regimens have given encouraging results as well. Even in the case of aggressive lymphomas in an advanced stage, some of the newer combinations of drugs have been administered. Examples are COP-BLAM III, F-MACOP, LNH, MACOP-B, MegaCOMLA, ProMACE-CytaBOM, and VACOP-B (defined in the table). However, some investigations have not demonstrated pronounced superiority of CHOP. Lymphomas of B-cell origin are more numerous than those of T-cell origin and usually respond more favorably to treatment. Patients with AIDS have a very high incidence of malignant lymphomas. They usually are of B-cell origin, and the neoplasm frequently extends into the brain with concomitant deterioration of the prognosis. Treatment usually follows that given to members of the population at large; the difficulty is the necessity for decreasing dosages, which is necessary when any patient is immunosuppressed. This diminishes the effectiveness of the therapy and shortens life expectancy. The regimen chosen for managing each type of intermediate- and advanced-grade lymphoma and the stage in which it is found is based on experience gained in numerous and extended clinical trials, some of which are ongoing. It requires information that is current and extensive and past experience with this type of neoplasm for a wise choice. It can be given only by physicians who bear these qualifications.

Regimens for chemotherapy of non-Hodgkin's lymphomas

BACOP
  Bleomycin IV
  Cyclophosphamide IV
  Doxorubicin (Adriamycin) IV
  Prednisone PO
  Vincristine (Oncovin) IV

CAP-BOP
  Bleomycin IV
  Cyclophosphamide IV
  Doxorubicin IV
  Prednisone PO
  Vincristine IV

CHOP
  Cyclophosphamide IV
  Doxorubicin (Adriamycin) IV
  Prednisone PO
  Vincristine (Oncovin) IV

COMLA
  Cyclophosphamide IV
  Cytarabine IV
  Leucovorin PO
  Methotrexate IV

COP-BLAM
  Bleomycin IV
  Cyclophosphamide IV
  Doxorubicin IV
  Prednisone PO
  Procarbazine PO
  Vincristine (Oncovin) IV

COPP
  Cyclophosphamide IV
  Prednisone PO
  Procarbazine PO
  Vincristine (Oncovin) IV

CVP
  Cyclophosphamide IV
  Prednisone PO
  Vincristine (Oncovin) IV

F-MACHOP
  Doxorubicin (Adriamycin) IV
  Cyclophosphamide IV
  Cytosine arabinoside IV
  5-Fluorouracil IV
  Methotrexate IV
  Prednisone PO
  Vincristine IV

LNH-84
  Induction
    Doxorubicin (Adriamycin) IV
    Bleomycin IV
    Cyclophosphamide IV
    Methotrexate IV
    Prednisone PO
    Vindesine IV
  Consolidation
    Cytarabine IV
    Etoposide IV
    Ifosfamide IV
    L-Asparaginase IV
    Methotrexate IV

MACOP-B
  Bleomycin IV
  Cyclophosphamide IV
  Doxorubicin (Adriamycin) IV
  Leucovorin PO
  Methorexate IV
  Prednisone PO
  Trimethoprim-sulfa PO
  Vincristine (Oncovin) IV

m-BACOD
  Bleomycin IV
  Cyclophosphamide IV
  Dexamethasone PO
  Doxorubicin (Adriamycin) IV
  Leucovorin PO
  Methotrexate IV
  Vincristine (Oncovin)

(Continued)

ProMACE-CytaBOM	ProMACE-MOPP
Bleomycin IV	Then
Cotrimoxazole PO	Mechlorethamine IV
Cyclophosphamide IV	Prednisone PO
Cytarabine IV	Procarbazine PO
Doxorubicin IV	Vincristine (Oncovin) IV
Etoposide IV	
Methotrexate IV	VACOP-B
Prednisone PO	Bleomycin IV
Vincristine IV	Cimetidine PO
ProMACE-MOPP	Cotrimoxazole PO
First	Cyclophosphamide IV
Cyclophosphamide IV	Doxorubicin IV
Doxorubicin (Adriamycin) IV	Etoposide IV
Etoposide IV	Ketoconazole PO
Leucovorin IV	Prednisone PO
Methotrexate IV	Vincristine IV
Prednisone PO	

HODGKIN'S DISEASE

The treatment of Hodgkin's disease is one of the successes in the treatment of malignant disease. All cases are potentially curable, even when the stage of the disease is advanced. It is one of the disorders affecting the lymphatic system which constitutes approximately 1 percent of all malignancies in the United States with a bimodal incidence and peaks occurring around ages 25 and 55, which is not the case in most undeveloped countries. Cases of Hodgkin's disease were first described by Thomas Hodgkin, a London physician, in 1832. In most patients, involvement of the lymph nodes and sometimes the spleen is the initial pattern that is detected. The disease characteristically spreads in contiguous fashion from node to node. Invasion of adjacent organs does occur later in the disease, and more disease may be found in the left upper chest and neck than in the right probably because of the location of the thoracic duct which is the thoroughfare for drainage of the lymph into the left subclavian vein. The microscopic appearance of this cancer exhibits large cells that contain two or more nuclei with one nucleolus called Reed-Sternberg cells after two of the men who described these giant cells in 1898 and 1902. Although these cells are striking in appearance, most of the bulk of the tumor consists of cells usually found in the normal lymph node: stroma, lymphocytes, and plasma cells. The microscopic appearance of the neoplasm has been divided into four types. The most frequently encountered is one showing nodular sclerosis. Mixed cellularity is found in the one less often seen, and the ones seen most infrequently are those with lymphocyte predominance and depletion of lymphocytes, respectively.

The stage of this disease is the most important feature for prognosticating its behavior and scheduling the appropriate treatment. Most therapists use the following scheme or a variation of it for staging:

Stage I   Involvement of a single lymph node or structure
               such as spleen, thymus, or Waldeyer's ring
Stage II   Involvement of two or more lymph-node regions on
               the same side of the diaphragm
Stage III   Involvement of lymph node regions or structures on
               both sides of the diaphragm
               1 Hilar, splenic, portal, or celiac lymph nodes
               2 Mesenteric, paraaortic, or iliac lymph nodes
Stage IV   Involvement of extranodal site(s)
               A No symptoms
               B Loss of weight, sweats, fever
               E Involvement of single extranodal site
               X Extensive disease.

Since the response of Hodgkin's disease to various combinations and dosages of irradiation and chemotherapy depends on the stage of the disease, it is very important to determine the location and extent of the disease as accurately as possible before a definitive course of therapy is initiated, even if this requires an abdominal operation.

A detailed history, careful physical examination, and appropriate laboratory and radiographic studies must always be carried out before treatment is initiated. A history of loss of weight, pruritus, profuse sweating without the apparent usual causes, fever, and enlargement of lymph nodes is frequently elicited. The physical examination should include special attention to the regions containing lymph nodes and the abdomen for the presence of enlarged nodes, masses, and abnormalities of liver and spleen. Examination of the blood should include a complete blood count, determination of alkaline phosphatase, and sedimentation rate. Both anterioposterior and lateral x-ray views of the chest are always obtained and supplemented with computerized tomograms if the former is abnormal. Tomograms of the abdomen may also be indicated at times along with lymphangiograms of the lower extremities and abdomen. X-ray studies of the bones should be carried out in any areas that are tender. Bone marrow biopsies are omitted sometimes for stages I and II. A positive biopsy of the suspected tissue is always required before the definitive diagnosis of Hodgkin's disease can be established. In some cases a diagnostic laparoscopy or celiotomy may be required. When done, it usually includes examination of the entire abdominal cavity, biopsies of splenic, celiac, paraaortic, mesenteric, portal, and iliac lymph nodes, splenectomy, and small wedge resection of left lobe and needle biopsies of both right and left lobes of the liver. The information obtained from the studies outlined can be used to determine with assurance the stage of the disease, and then appropriate treatment can be planned and started immediately.

Irradiation therapy is quite an effective feature of the successful treatment of Hodgkin's disease. The dose-response curves of these tumors to irradiation are well known and used in calculating appropriate dosages. Supervoltage is used for treatment. Cobalt machines have been and are used for this purpose, although linear accelerators offer the radiologist some advantages in reaching his goals. The dosage for local tumor masses is in the range 4000 to 4400 cGy. Care must be taken in drawing up a scheme of treatment that includes pulmonary and cardiac fields. The whole heart is not irradiated, and the amount of the lung included in the field depends on the extent of the tumor. Masses in the mediastinum offer special problems for obtaining effective dosages. The three principal areas for irradiation are mantle (neck, axilla, mediastinum, preauricular, and occipital regions), paraaortic, and pelvic regions. Complications occur chiefly in the mantle field and include radiation pneumonitis, alteration in pulmonary function, pericarditis, and pericardial effusion. Great care must be taken to prevent overlapping ports (especially in the mantle and paraaortic fields) from increasing dosage sufficiently to cause damage to the spinal cord. Radiation fibrosis of the brachial plexus is a danger when dosage is great, and thyroid problems can be one of the sequellae of mantle irradiation. Leukopenia and thrombocytopenia can occur after pelvic irradiation. Care not to include the ovaries by shielding or moving them at the time of celiotomy is also important.

Treatment can consist of irradiation or chemotherapy alone or in combination, depending on the stage of the disease at the time of therapy. To give a brief overview of this general approach, it is useful to summarize the type of management most frequently used for the various stages. Mantle irradiation alone is often sufficient for cure in stages I and II. Chemotherapy may be added in the presence of a large mediastinal mass in stage II. The field of irradiation may be extended or combined with chemotherapy in stages I and II. Total nodal irradiation or combination management may be adopted for stage III. Chemotherapy using various combinations of chemotherapeutic agents yields remarkable results in stages III, IVA, and IVB disease. Even if a control is not achieved after the approaches described, it may be possible to salvage a cure, particularly if the recurrence is nodal.

Regimens for chemotherapy usually consist of administration of a combination of several different chemotherapeutic drugs, with a schedule set in advance. Before starting chemotherapy, allopurinol is given to avoid the hyperuricemia that often occurs concomitant with lysis of the tumor by the medications used for treatment. This is usually necessary only with the first course of the combined drug therapy. Various combinations of the following drugs, listed in alphabetical order by the letter used to designate each acronym, have been used to label programs designed for the management of therapeutic problems encountered in the care of patients with Hodgkin's disease. Some of the combinations used are listed below as acronyms adopted from the names of the agents used.

Chemotherapy regimens for Hodgkin's disease

A	Doxorubicin (Adriamycin)
B	Bleomycin
C	Lomustine (CCNU), chlorambucil, cisplatin, cyclophosphamide, cytarabine
D	Dacarbazine, dexamethasone, doxorubicin (Adriamycin)
E	Etoposide
I	Ifosfamide, prednisone
L	Lomustine (CCNU)
M	Mechlorethamine, melphalan, methotrexate, MethylGAG
O	Vincristine (Oncovin)
P	Prednimustine, prednisone, procarbazine
V	Vinblastine, vincristine (Oncovin), vindesine
N	Nitrogen mustard

MOPP
   Mechlorethamine IV
   Vincristine (Oncovin) IV
   Procarbazine PO
   Prednisone PO

ABVD
   Doxorubicin (Adriamycin) IV
   Bleomycin IV
   Vinblastine IV
   Dacacarbazine IV

ABV
   ABVD without dacacarbazine

MOPP/ABV

ABDIC
   Doxorubicin (Adriamycin) IV
   Bleomycin IV or IM
   Dacacarbazine IV
   Lomustine (CCNU) PO
   Prednisone PO

BCAVe
   Bleomycin IV or IM
   Lomustine (CCNU) PO

(Continued)

BCAVe
  Doxorubicin (Adriamycin) IV
  Vinblastine IV
CEP
  CCNU PO
  Etoposide PO
  Prednimustine PO

The dose of each compound, interval between courses, length of each course, and number of courses varies, depending on clinical response to therapy. When failure to respond to the MOPP regimen occurs, trial with CEP, ABVD, and combination chemotherapy similar to ABVD can be successful. In children, radiotherapy must be limited and chemotherapy designed more conservatively.

Complications have been encountered during the late follow-up of patients treated for Hodgkin's disease, including solid tumors, non-Hodgkin's lymphoma, leukemia, pneumococcal sepsis, pneumonitis, varicella, dental caries, retardation of growth in children, avascular necrosis, cardiomyopathy, acute and chronic pericarditis, dyspareunia, and infertility. The likelihood of developing these problems is diminished by foresight in the careful management of therapy, and appropriate corrective measures are available to alleviate and eradicate them. For example, solid tumors and leukemias require specific measures to which they respond, vaccines and antibacterial drugs are available for infections, hormonal treatment is available for thyroid deficiency, and radiation therapy in childhood must be managed very conservatively.

MALIGNANCIES OF PLASMA CELLS

Neoplasms of plasma cells are a group of monoclonal malignancies, each of which arises from a single plasma cell. These originate from B-cell lymphocytes (a type of white blood cell) which have the characteristic of secreting antibodies. The products synthesized by these cells can be measured and are useful in following the course of the disease and its response to treatment. The monoclonal M protein appears in cases of multiple myeloma, macroglobinemia, amyloidosis, heavy chain disease, and monoclonal gammopathy (of undetermined significance).

Multiple Myeloma

When multiple myeloma occurs, malignant plasma cells may be found in many locations, but the characteristic refractory response to treatment and

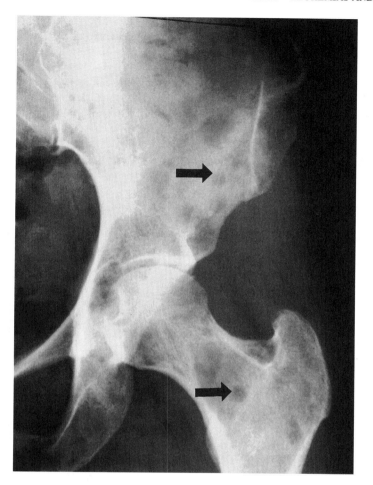

Figure 35 Roentgen image of multiple myeloma in left ilium and femur.

symptomatology are primarily the result of infiltration of the bone and bone marrow, the effect of the cellular secretory products, and suppression of the immune response of the normal cells remaining. Usually the patient with multiple myeloma seeks relief from bone pain which is then found to be accompanied by diffuse infiltration of the marrow with malignant plasmacytes characteristically numbering more than 10 percent of the plasma cells. Bence Jones protein (antibody light chains) is found in the urine, and the level of monoclonal immunoglobulin in the serum is elevated. (Monoclonal gammopathy occurs occasionally in patients without the clinical findings characteristic of multiple myeloma. Under these circumstances it is designated as monoclonal gammopathy of undetermined significance.) In cases of multiple myeloma, x-ray studies reveal striking lytic lesions of the bone and, occasionally, osteoporosis. At times renal insufficiency accompanied by elevated uric acid and calcium in the serum is encountered and many patients develop amyloidosis, but enlargement of the liver and spleen is not found very frequently. Impaired immune response makes the patient susceptible to infections that may increase renal damage. Compression of spinal cord and nerves and the development of anemia are additional problems. Fortunately, chemotherapy can extend life expectancy, and treatment is always a prime consideration in management. The acute nonlymphocytic leukemia that develops in the occasional patient is thought to be the result of chemotherapy with alkylating agents, but this risk is far outweighed by the benefits that treatment offers.

Staging of multiple myeloma is based on calculations of the tumor burden judged by the level of hemoglobin, immunoglobulins, calcium, light chain fragments, and osseous lesions. Response to therapy appears to be inversely proportional to tumor burden. Stages I and III have specific levels to be satisfied, and stage II is assigned to patients whose status satisfies the criteria for neither stage I nor stage III.

Clinical stages of multiple myeloma

Stage I (all items listed below)
   Hemoglobin >10 g
   None or single osseous lesion only
   Myeloma protein
     IgA <3 g
     IgG <5 g
   Urinary light chains <4 g in 24 h
   Serum calcium 12 mg or less

Stage III (at least one item listed below)
   Hemoglobin <8.5 g
   Multiple osseous lesions
   Myeloma protein
     IgA >5 g
     IgB >7 g
   Urinary light chains >12 g in 24 h
   Serum calcium >12 mg

Stage II
   Values for items fit neither stage I nor stage III

Subclasses
   Subclass A
     Serum creatinine <2 mg
   Subclass B
     Serum creatinine ≥2 mg

Radiation therapy When multiple myeloma is present only at a localized site, then radiotherapy is quite effective and may delay progression of the disease until the time chemotherapy is indicated, which may not occur until an extended period has elapsed. Irradiation is also useful for palliation when the disease is present at extraskeletal sites, there is spinal cord compression, and fractures seem imminent. The amount of irradiation must be controlled carefully to prevent consequent restriction of the effect of chemotherapy and damage to the normal marrow. Fractionation of a tumor dose of 2000 to 3000 cGy is usually sufficient for relief when the source of pain and structural damage can be included in the field of irradiation, since the lesions are quite sensitive to radiotherapy. It is very important not to increase the dose of irradiation in such a chronic disease and to be aware of what systemic chemotherapy has to offer. Unusual indications for irradiation are lesions of orbital bones and sphenoids associated with proptosis, of mandible and maxilla associated with facial distortions, and of skull associated with various central nervous system problems. When multiple myeloma is in stage III, hemibody irradiation (usually below the umbilicus) in a fractionated total tumor dose of no more than 850 cGy has been administered with some success. Hemibody irradiation above the umbilicus carries a great risk of attendant pneumonitis and usually requires the dosage to be diminished.

Chemotherapy   When the disease is indolent with minimal symptoms and signs of clinical disease, some physicians prefer to delay the onset of therapy. If this option is selected, the course of the disease must be followed very carefully for signs of progression and treatment initiated when they appear. Before the initiation of chemotherapy, it is always advisable to correct complications that are present, such as infections, hypercalcemia, or renal failure, insofar as possible. Also allopurinol often must be given during the first weeks of therapy to avoid the problems attendant on the elevation of serum uric acid that usually occurs during the first portion of treatment.

Most patients, including those at high risk related to age, symptoms, laboratory studies, or poor performance level, often have initial chemotherapy with oral MP (melphalan and prednisone). The dosage of prednisone is adapted to the characteristics of the individual patient's condition and disease. A difficult decision is when to stop therapy in responsive patients during what is sometimes called the plateau stage, since previous symptoms sometimes recur promptly when treatment is discontinued. Patients in stages I and II are known to have remissions as long as 2 years; those in stage III remain in unmaintained remission for no longer than 8 months in the usual course of events. Unfortunately, the disease recurs and eventually becomes refractory to treatment, no matter how well it responded to treatment initially. When treatment has not been given for a long period of time, the regimen bringing about a response originally may be effective again and should be tried. Therapy that may be tried when the disease becomes refractory includes those regimens appearing in the table below as listed or as alternating and intermittent treatment. Unfortunately some combinations such as VBMCP have toxicities interfering with their effectiveness. Complications occurring as the disease progresses, including hyperviscosity, amyloidosis, electrolyte imbalance, anemia, coagulopathies, neurologic problems, renal failure, hypercalcemia, and acute leukemia, require the greatest exercise of skill on the part of the physician treating the patient with multiple myeloma. In children, when very high doses are indicated for either chemotherapy or radiotherapy, a bone marrow transplant may be the most promising alternative. Clinical responses have been reported after the use of interferon alfa-2 alone and in combination, but it is not widely used as a part of routine therapy in current practice. Undoubtedly chemotherapy and radiotherapy may prolong an active and enjoyable life in this disease, and continuing efforts to improve the treatment are amply justified.

Chemotherapeutic agents for multiple myeloma alone and combined

BCP
  Carmustine (BCNU), cyclophosphamide, prednisone

C
  Cyclophosphamide

MCBP
  Melphalan, cyclophosphamide, BCNU, prednisone

MCBPA
  Melphalan, cyclophosphamide, BCNU, prednisone, doxorubicin

MeCCMVP
  Methyl-CCNU, cyclophosphamide, melphalan, vincristine, prednisone

MOCCA
  Melphalan, vincristine, CCNU, cyclophosphamide, doxorubicin

MP
  Melphalan, prednisone (most frequently used first-line therapy)

VAD
  Vincristine, doxorubicin, dexamethasone (most frequently used second-line therapy)

VBAD
  Vincristine, BCNU, doxorubicin (Adriamycin), dexamethasone

VBAP
  Vincristine, BCNU, Adriamycin, prednisone

VBCMP (M-2)
  Vincristine, carmustine (BCNU), melphalan, cyclophosphamide, prednisone

VCAP
  Vincristine, cyclophosphamide, Adriamycin, prednisone

VMCP
  Vincristine, melphalan, cyclophosphamide, prednisone

VMCP/VCAP
  See above

(Continued)

VMCP/VBAP
  See above

VMP
  Vincristine, melphalan, prednisone

Alternating
  VMCP + VBAP or VCAP (see above)

ABCM
  Adriamycin, BCNU, cyclophosphamide melphalan

Intermittent
  Cyclophosphamide, melphalan, carmustine, lomustin

High dose
  Dexamethasone

Macroglobulinemia (of Waldenström)

A number of diseases are characterized by the presence of monoclonal anti-bodies of the IgM class or macroglobulins. Plasmacytoid lymphocytes proliferate and are responsible for the macroglobulinemia in the variant designated Waldenström's macroglobulinemia. It occurs in older individuals and is characterized by mucocutaneous bleeding; anemia; fatigue; vascular abnormalities of the retina; enlargement of liver, spleen, and lymph nodes; polyneuropathy associated with hyperviscosity and peripheral neuritis; and pancytopenia at times. Although an infiltrate of plasmacytoid lymphocytes, plasma cells, and small lymphocytes invade the bone marrow and organs that are enlarged, the lytic destruction of bone with attendant problems and hypercalcemia characteristic of multiple myeloma do not occur very often. Infection, hyperviscosity syndrome, the presence of additional types of tumors, and bleeding are the serious complications that are encountered. This indolent disease usually progresses slowly, and a decision about interventional therapy is frequently delayed until the diagnosis seems quite certain. The management of anemia must be conducted very carefully in order not to induce problems with hyperviscosity. Alkylating agents can alleviate symptoms and possibly extend survival. Oral chlorambucil in low daily dosage continuously or intermittently in high dosage with prednisone is one regimen sometimes used. Also, cyclophosphamide orally in daily dosage with or without the addition of prednisone on a separate schedule is also used. When indicated, VBMCP (M-2) can be effective in the presence of resistance to antecedent drugs. In addition, VBAP, fludarabine, pentoistatin, and interferon-α have yielded remissions in refractory cases. When high levels of IgM monoclonal proteins accompany lymphoma or chronic lymphocytic leukemia, the treatment should correspond to that advocated for those diseases. Also when the clinical picture in macroglobulinemia closely approximates the bone destruction seen in multiple myeloma, the therapy for the latter disease should be given. Plasmapheresis may be necessary in the initial stages of treating hyperviscosity. Also, repeated plasmapheresis over a long period may be effective management in some cases refractory to alkylating agents.

Heavy Chain Disease

Heavy chain diseases consist of a very rare group of plasma cell abnormalities consisting of clones of plasma cells or B lymphocytes that secrete abnormal polypeptides with segments missing from alpha, gamma, and mu heavy chains of immunoglobulins (antibodies) resulting in a wide range of clinical symptoms. The respective treatment of gamma and mu disease is similar to that for non-Hodgkin's lymphoma and chronic lymphatic leukemia. Therapy for alpha disease includes both antibiotic treatment and chemotherapy.

TUMORS OF BONE

Up to approximately 8000 bone tumors are diagnosed in the United States annually with a ratio of benign to malignant lesions of 4:1. With the exception of giant cell tumors, they occur predominantly in men. Benign tumors, osteogenic sarcomas, and Ewing's tumors appear most commonly from the ages of 10 to 25 years. Usually the remainder are found in later life. Benign tumors include osteomas, chondromas, osteocartilaginous exostoses, angiomas, lipomas, giant cell tumors, fibromas, bone cysts, subperiosteal desmoids, and histiocytosis. Malignancies of bone include various types of osteogenic sarcomas and chondrosarcoma as well as adamantinomas, Ewing's sarcoma, chordomas, and others found less frequently. Initially a decision must be made about whether the tumor is benign or malignant, of osseous or marrow origin, or is metastatic. Pain, tenderness, tumefaction, or even heat, redness, fever, and chills (occasionally confused with infection) are symptoms and signs encountered at times.

Diagnostic studies other than the usual physical examination and blood count should include radiographic examination of bone and chest, nuclear magnetic resonance imaging (or computerized tomograms) when indicated, alkaline phosphatase, lactic dehydrogenase, calcium and phosphorus levels, and consideration of radionuclide bone scans and angiograms. Biopsy should be reserved as the final procedure of the diagnostic workup, since it could interfere with the evaluation of other studies. Needle biopsy is sometimes adequate and desirable but may not yield sufficient tissue for comprehensive diagnostic studies. An open biopsy requires considerable skill in selecting the site and approach and carrying out the operation. An immediate assessment of the adequacy of the specimen should follow. Also every effort to limit hemorrhage is mandatory and may require the use of bone cement (polymethylmethacrylate) to close the osseous defect. Any subsequent resection should include removal of the biopsy site.

Benign lesions of bone may require no treatment, biopsy, curettage, resection, or observation for signs of malignancy and metastases. Those seen most frequently in children are nonossifying fibromas and fibrous cortical defects in the metaphyses of bones in lower and upper extremities. No treatment is required when the diagnosis from radiographs is assured and pathologic fractures are not threatened. Biopsy and curettage and even bone grafting are necessary in cases offering the possibility of fractures. Osteoid osteomas present with a characteristic nidus which may be obscured by surrounding reaction in adjacent tissue. Removal of the lesion is curative but may be quite difficult when the spine is involved. Severe pain is often a characteristic feature of the problem.

Benign enostotic and exostotic chondromas may be difficult to distinguish from malignant lesions, although the latter usually appear beyond the age of 30. Solitary enchondromas rarely require curettage with packing. Multiple lesions at times present in a familial pattern and require observation for development of malignancy. They may necessitate prevention and management of deformity with intramedullary nailing and osteotomies. Solitary osteocartilaginous exostoses rarely become malignant and can be excised with little chance of recurrence. A dominant autosomal gene is responsible for multiple exostoses that require careful management including complete removal of the cartilaginous cap in childhood and subsequent observation for the development of malignancy.

Fibrous dysplasia occurs as monostotic and polyostotic disease and Albright's syndrome. The latter is associated with endocrine manifestations such as Cushing's syndrome, hyperthyroidism, hyperparathyroidism, rickets, acromegaly, and precocious puberty along with epithelial pigmentation. Prevention and treatment of deformities frequently present in fibrous dysplasias require continued management which is often very challenging. Most interesting bone cysts are the aneurysmal cysts. They may be difficult to distinguish from malignant tumors and giant cell tumors. Treatment consists of curettage, resection, and grafting as indicated. Simple cysts may require instillation of methyl prednisolone, curettage, resection, or grafting, depending on the extent of the problem, the presence of a fracture, and failure to respond to steroid therapy.

Giant cell tumors occur most frequently in the metaphyseal and epiphyseal regions of long bones in the second through fourth decades. They are found more frequently in females than males and metastasize in no more than 5 percent of the cases. The lesions are exceptionally destructive locally, may threaten joint integrity, and present even greater challenges when present in the axial skeleton. Treatments required range from simple resection and curettage and use of bone chips and methyl methacrylate to more extensive procedures such as extensive resection with allografting and use of metal implants. Embolization and irradiation have been used, but the latter can induce sarcoma and result in necrosis. Pulmonary metastases can be resected successfully.

Metastases to bone are approximately twice as frequently found as primary neoplasms. Metastases from Ewing's tumors and leukemia can occur at early ages in children, and almost all malignancies of bone after the sixth decade are metastatic in origin. The most frequent sources are prostate, breast, and lung, with cancer of the gastrointestinal tract and kidneys accounting for a large number of cases as well. Treatment varies according to the site of metastases, their number, their size, and the behavior of the type of cancer found. The use of estrogen for prostatic lesions and antiestrogens for mammary carcinoma is sometimes useful. Occasionally surgical resection is the treatment of choice for solitary lesions or those in favorable locations. Surgical techniques, including the use of rods and bone cement in long bones and spine, can be used when there is a threat of pathologic fracture and danger of damage to adjacent vital structures. Decompression of the cord is necessary when the growth, pressure, and location of metastases indicate the procedure. Even multiple metastases to the lung can be removed successfully. In a wide variety of malignant foci, irradiation can be indicated for the relief of pain and when resective therapy is not suitable. The type of chemotherapy suitable for responses depends on the type of malignancy. Therefore, it is necessary to establish the diagnosis with accuracy, which may be very difficult for lesions such as small round cell tumors but worth whatever analyses are required.

It is fortunate that primary malignancies of bone are relatively rare neoplasms. They may arise in any location, the diagnosis is often difficult to establish with certainty, and their behavior varies widely. Effective treatment has improved with the addition of adjuvant chemotherapy, and the number of amputations has decreased as well, but the outcome in many cases is much less than desirable with many aggressive lesions beyond cure when discovered. In advanced disease, intensive chemotherapy with bone marrow transplantation is being investigated. Currently the chemotherapy usually chosen initially for osteosarcoma consists of high dosages of methotrexate plus doxorubicin and cisplatin. Other combinations giving responses are bleomycin, cyclophosphamide, and doxorubicin; cisplatin, doxorubicin, and methotrexate with and without ifosfamide with mesna; etoposide, ifosfamide, and mesna; and ifosfamide with mesna, cisplatin, and etoposide (ICE). Myelomas involving the entire bone marrow and plasmacytomas consisting of solitary foci are monoclonal gammopathies increasing the levels of serum gamma globulin and constitute the malignant bone tumor most frequently diagnosed. Recommended chemotherapy for multiple myeloma is melphalan; cyclophosphamide and prednisone; or vincristine, doxorubicin, and dexamethasone (VAD). Also, responses occur after treatment with dexamethasone in high dosage; interferon alfa; and the combination of carmustine, cyclophosphamide, melphalan, prednisone, and vincristine. Bone marrow transplantation or stem-cell infusion may be required with chemotherapy in high dosage.

TNM classification and staging of osseous tumors

Histologic grade
G1	Well differentiated
G2	Moderately well differentiated
G3	Poorly differentiated (anaplastic)

Primary tumor
T0	No evidence for primary tumor
T1	Tumor within cortex
T2	Tumor beyond cortex

Regional lymph nodes
N0	No nodal metastases
N1	Regional nodal metastases

Distant metastases
M0	No distant metastases
M1	Distant metastases

Stage groups
IA	G1, G2	T1	N0	M0
IB	G1, G2	T2	N0	M0
IIA	G3	T1	N0	M0
IIB	G3	T2	N0	M0
IIIA	Any G	Any T	N1	M0
IIIB	Any G	Any T	Any N	M1

SARCOMAS

Soft tissue sarcomas are derived from the mesoderm and arise in extraskeletal tissues such as muscles, tendons, vascular endothelium, and mesothelium of the viscera. They have a pseudocapsule and metastasize via blood vessels much more frequently than through lymphatic channels. They account for approximately 0.1 percent of all cancers, but in children about 6 percent of tumors are soft tissue sarcomas. Benign tumors of soft tissue can be both aggressive and nonaggressive. The former include desmoid tumors, dematofibrosarcoma protuberans, atypical fibrous histiocytomas, and atypical lipomas. They do not metastasize, but tend to recur if resected without wide margins and sometimes are locally destructive. At times postoperative irradiation is used with the objective of preventing recurrence. Benign nonaggressive soft tissue tumors such as lipomas, sclerosing hemangiomas, neurofibromas, ganglions, nodular fasciitis, leiomyomas, and hemangiomas are treated by simple removal. Patients with benign tumors of soft tissue are more than 100 times more numerous than those with soft tissue sarcomas.

Lipomas and angiolipomas are known to appear in a familial setting of multiple tumors. Soft tissue sarcomas occur with greater frequency in several hereditary syndromes such as Gardner's syndrome, hereditary basal cell nevus syndrome, tuberous sclerosis, and von Recklinghausen's disease than in the general population. Prior exposure to irradiation is probably an etiologic factor in some sarcomas, and lymphedema predisposes to lymphangiosarcoma. Exposure to polyvinyl chloride, thorium dioxide, and asbestos have been reported to be associated with these tumors, and the incidence and extent of Kaposi's sarcoma is very high in patients with AIDS.

The sarcomas most frequently encountered are fibrosarcomas, liposarcomas, rhabdomyosarcomas, neurofibrosarcomas, synoviosarcomas. and leiomyosarcomas. With the passage of time the classification of fibrosarcomas has changed sufficiently to exclude some tumors previously classified as fibrosarcoma and to confine the diagnosis only to those arising from fibrocytes. Liposarcomas are classified as differentiated, myxoid, pleomorphic, fibroblastic, and round cell (lipoblastic). Rhabdomyosarcomas are classified as embryonal and alveolar, which appear most frequently in children, and pleomorphic, which appear most frequently in adults. Neurofibrosarcomas are derived from the neural sheath and are sometimes labeled neurigenic sarcomas, neurilemmomas, or schwannomas. Synoviosarcomas are derived from tendosynovial tissue and are classified as monophasic having sheets of spindle cells or biphasic having clefts lined with epithelium.

The first sign leading to the clinical diagnosis of these tumors is almost always the presence of a palpable mass. Other symptoms do not usually occur until later, after metastases are present. In addition to physical examination and laboratory studies, computerized tomography of the primary site and lungs is essential. Also nuclear magnetic resonance imaging and angiography may be helpful at times. Since the grade of a sarcoma is predictive in terms of the outcome of treatment, the initial biopsy and how it is procured is of major importance. Needle biopsies have the disadvantage of sometimes depositing neoplastic cells along the needle tract and bringing forth a specimen that is too small for the pathologist's needs. Much of the time an incisional biopsy is the procedure of first choice. When the tumor is deep, a general anesthetic may be necessary. Excisional biopsy is usually limited to tumors less than 3 cm in greatest diameter with excised margins no less than 2 cm. Enucleation is not a useful way to biopsy sarcomas since there is a psudocapsule with extension of the neoplasm well beyond capsular limits, and the rate of recurrence following enucleation is exceedingly high.

After a diagnosis is firmly established by histologic criteria, clinicians have three modalities of therapy at their disposal: operation, irradiation, and chemotherapy. When radiation therapy has been tried alone, very few malignancies have been controlled, even with tumor doses as high as 8000 cGy, with recurrence rate following resection more than 50 percent. When a much more radical approach to operative intervention was adopted, including more amputations of extremities including hindquarter and disarticulation procedures, the recurrence rate was reduced to 20 percent or less, but many of the patients were disabled and more were unhappy with the extent of therapy.

A combination of preoperative and/or postoperative irradiation and limited resection has changed the outcome of treatment with recurrences of less than 13 percent and concomitant superior functional and cosmetic results.

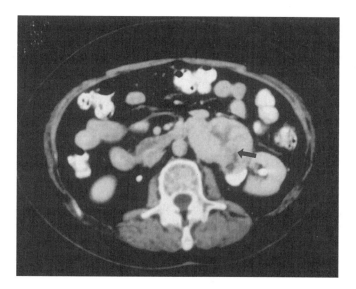

A

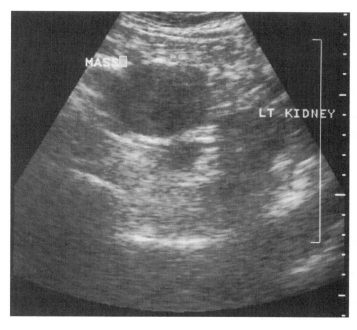

B

Figure 36 Retroperitoneal leiomyosarcoma. A. Computerized tomogram showing neoplasm and adjacent kidney. B. Ultrasound study of the partially necrotic tumor.

Preoperative irradiation has the advantage of immediate initiation, reduction in size of the lesion at times changing an inoperable to an operable mass. Delay in starting initial resection, complications of wound healing, edema, and increased susceptibility to traumatic fractures and infections are disadvantages. After irradiation high-grade tumors still have a poorer prognosis, but the primary lesion can be removed with a less radical procedure and a better chance for cure. Limited resection includes all the gross tumor with narrow margins beyond the visible limits, and then radiation is capable of eradicating the smaller microscopic extension around the central mass. (Irradiation therapy given to microscopic foci is much more efficient than treatment of gross disease.) The defect remaining can be managed by repositioning tendons, muscles, and skin flaps for better function, appearance, and obliteration of dead space. Closure of the wound without tension can avoid distressing complications as well. When the operation involves an extremity, the leg or arm should be immobilized and all drains left in place for the length of time required for sufficient healing of the wound and cessation of drainage. In some cases of large proximal sarcomas, extensive resections are indicated including hemipelvectomy, internal pelvectomy, and forequarter resection. Modifications are possible when the blood and nerve supply to the distal limb can be salvaged, preserving varying lengths of the extremity and avoiding undesirable deformities. These procedures are possible only by experienced surgical teams having adequate resources for prosthetic and plastic repairs. Debulking of retroperitoneal sarcomas does not usually improve the management of these tumors.

Both external beam therapy and brachytherapy with photons, electron beams, and protons have been used to control neoplastic cells beyond the limits of resection. Intraoperative therapy has the advantage of sparing adjacent organs within the abdominal cavity. The administration of brachytherapy utilizing afterloading with 192 I wires is sometimes useful in conjunction with resection. Preoperative irradiation usually does not exceed a tumor dose of 5000 cGy, but booster doses later can extend this as high as 7000 cGy. The value of radiosensitizers has been investigated, but their use is still in the realm of inquiry.

Many clinical trials using chemotherapy for soft tissue sarcomas have been reported. Evaluation of results of chemotherapy requires separation of results by type and grade of sarcoma and location (extremities, head and neck, or trunk). The responses are related to dosage, and the highest dosage possible is indicated. Aids for increasing permissible dosages have been the use of hematopoietic growth factors and bone marrow transplants. Doxorubicin is a most effective single agent, but toxicity limits dosage and effectiveness. Also remissions have been reported after the use in various ways of a large number of chemotherapeutic agents such as azotomycin, bleomycin, carboplatin, carminomycin, cisplatin, cycloleucine, cyclophosphamide, dacarbazine (DTIC), dactinomycin, epirubicin, etoposide, 5-fluorouracil, ifosfamide, melphalan, methotrexate, semustine (Methyl-CCNU), vindesine, and vincristine. Because sarcomas do not appear with great frequency, progress in improving the results of chemotherapy has been slower than desired. Numerous combinations of agents have been found to induce remissions with additions to doxorubicin, dactinomycin, epirubicin, ifosfamide, and methotrexate. For example those with doxorubicin include doxorubicin with dacarbazine; with dacarbazine and cyclophosphamide; with dacarbazine and ifosfamide; with dacarbazine and dactinomycin; and with dacarbazine, cyclophosphamide and vincristine. The highest rates of response have been with the combination of doxorubicin, ifosfamide, mesna, and dacarbazine (MAID). Recommended chemotherapy for rhabdomyosarcoma is etoposide, ifosfamide, mesna, vincristine or dactino-mycin and vincristine with either cyclophosphamide or ifosfamide and mesna.

Chemotherapy has been useful as adjuvant therapy for resectable sarco-mas and also for the treatment of advanced local tumors and those with extensive metastases. Isolated limb perfusion for chemotherapy of sarcomas and other tumors was used frequently in the past, but more recently difficulty in obtaining suitable agents and improvement in other means of treatment has resulted in a decided decline in this mode of therapy. Both chemotherapy and irradiation are effective in permitting more limited operations to control the primary lesions. A comparison of the relative efficiency of irradiation and chemotherapy in achieving this result is not available at the present time. On the basis of the presence of estrogen and progesterone receptors, hormonal therapy has been advocated and tried with disappointing results so far. Also interferon-α, interferon-β, and interleukin-2 have not been promising addi-tions to the management of these sarcomas.

The most frequent location of distant metastases is in the lung. It is worthwhile to consider resection of these foci if careful investigation reveals no other metastatic lesions or local recurrence. Success is dependent some-what on whether a long time has elapsed before the pulmonary lesion(s) appeared after treatment of the primary neoplasm, the presence of only a small number of metastases, and a slow doubling time. After metastases have been removed, a second thoracotomy is sometimes successful when more lesions appear in the lungs subsequently. All patients who have been treated without metastases being found should be followed with periodic radiographic studies of the chest for several years to detect any metastatic disease as soon as it appears. An aggressive surgical response to local recurrence is also justified, especially when there is no evidence for metastatic lesions. Sarcomas of the extremities are less prone to recur locally than those originating in other sites.

The results of changing clinical management of soft tissue sarcomas have steadily improved over the past 50 years. The number of cures and responses has increased, and the patients have a more acceptable type of disability during and following therapy. When there are reasonable alternatives to the types, combinations, and extent of treatment, patients should be made aware of the choices and respective complications and their wishes respected.

TNM classification of soft tissue sarcomas

Histologic grade	G1	Well differentiated (low grade)
	G2	Moderately well differentiated (moderate grade)
	G3	Poorly differentiated (high grade)
Primary tumor	T0	No tumor found
	T1	Greatest diameter: 5 cm or less
	T2	Greatest diameter: >5 cm
	T3	Invasion bone, artery, or nerve
Regional nodes	N0	No invasion verified
	N1	Invasion verified histologically
Distant metastases	M0	No distant metastases
	M1	Distant metastases

Staging of soft tissue sarcomas

Stage IA	G1	T1	N0	M0
Stage IB	G1	T2	N0	M0
Stage IIA	G2	T1	N0	M0
Stage IIB	G2	T2	N0	M0
Stage IIIA	G3	T1	N0	M0
Stage IIIB	G3	T2	N0	M0
Stage IIIC	Any G	T1-2	N1	M0
Stage IVA	Any G	T3	Any N	M0
Stage IVB	Any G	Any T	Any N	M1

ELEVEN

SOLID TUMORS OF CHILDHOOD

WILMS' TUMOR

Wilms' tumor (nephroblastoma) is a malignancy of childhood appearing most often as an abdominal mass before the age of 5 years. The clinical picture may include gastrointestinal symptoms of pain, nausea, vomiting, and bloating as well as hematuria, anemia, hypertension, and failure to thrive. Also an ipsilateral hydrocele is found occasionally. A few cases are bilateral, and the disease occurs in boys and girls in approximately equal numbers. The tumors are composed of epithelial cells, stromal cells, and blastema cells in various proportions and stages of differentiation. Anaplasia with rhabdoid or clear cell sarcomatous changes suggests a poor prognosis with tendencies for metastasis to brain or bone, respectively. Clinical conditions that can be associated with Wilms' tumors are renal abnormalities, cryptorchidism, gonadal dysgenesis, hypospadias, aniridia, hemihypertrophy, and retarded mental development. Also the presence of chromosomal abnormalities, neurofibromatosis, and Drash, Perlman, and Beckwith-Wiedemann syndromes are coincident at times. Familial inheritance of Wilms' tumor, which has been detected in a relatively small number of cases, suggests an autosomal dominant gene with variable penetrance. The significance of changes in chromosome 13 found in patients with aniridia and the exact genetic basis, genes, and chromosomes involved lack complete clarification.

These tumors must be differentiated from hydronephrosis and polycystic kidney, and associated thrombi in the vena cava, contralateral tumor, and pulmonary and abdominal metastases should be kept in mind as possibilities in the diagnostic workup. Ultrasound and magnetic resonance imaging are two of the most useful means for study, and angiography may be indicated to determine the presence of thrombi and guide the surgeon in operative management of the vena cava.

Staging of Wilms' tumors used in the National Wilms' Tumor Study is a useful standardization for comparison of results of clinical management of the disease.

Staging of Wilms' tumors
(National Wilms' Tumor Study)

Stage I	Tumor localized in kidney and removed completely
Stage II	Tumor beyond kidney and removed completely
Stage III	Tumor within abdomen with incomplete removal, spread to lymph nodes, and peritoneal implants
Stage IV	Hematogenous metastases
Stage V	Bilateral primary renal tumors

Before operating, the surgeon must decide whether a biopsy is indicated and whether a needle biopsy or open biopsy is appropriate. Preoperative chemotherapy with an agent such as vincristine will often reduce the size of large neoplasms sufficiently to curtail the technical difficulties and risks of resection. Also, in the case of large hemorrhagic tumors, preoperative embolization may be advisable. Surgical exploration for diagnosis of the extent of the neoplasm and resection, if possible, is usually done through a transverse abdominal or abdominothoracic incision. The renal venous and arterial blood supplies are controlled first before excision of the tumor. Also the vena cava is ligated temporarily when thrombi must be removed, and afterward the vessel is repaired. Involved lymph nodes are resected with the tumor and at least one node is biopsied even if nodal spread is not evident from gross inspection. When bilateral tumors are present, it may be possible partially to preserve at least one kidney. Even if bilateral resection is necessary, salvage is possible by starting dialysis immediately and doing renal transplantation later when there is no evidence of recurrence. Resection of pulmonary, hepatic, and cerebral metastases should always be considered, since their removal has been accomplished successfully in many cases. Neonatal mesoblastic nephromas are not classified as Wilms' tumors, usually require only surgical resection, and have an excellent prognosis for cure.

Late sequellae of retarded growth, development of another malignancy in later life, nephritis, and damage to heart, lungs, and liver following radiation have been reported and suggest conservative use of this modality for treatment. Preoperative chemotherapy with vincristine and dactinomycin has replaced preoperative irradiation in the practice of most radiologists and oncologists. Radiation is useful as an adjuvant in controlling metastases and abdominal dissemination of tumor cells at the time of operation. When and how it is used depends very much on the stage of the disease and results of operation.

Wilms' tumors do respond to chemotherapy, and its usage varies with the stage of the neoplasm being treated. Chemotherapeutic agents useful in treating Wilms' tumors are cisplatin, cyclophosphamide, dactinomycin, doxorubicin, and vincristine. The combinations usually recommended are dactinomycin and vincristine with or without doxorubicin with or without cyclophosphamide. Other useful agents are carboplatin; cisplatin; etoposide; and ifosfamide and mesna. Bone marrow and stem cell infusion are often required with chemotherapy in high dosage. As in chemotherapy for other tumors, the treatment must be altered appropriately when toxicity, leukopenia, and organopathy ensue. The results of an increasing number of case-control studies are helpful to avoid these complications.

NEUROBLASTOMA

Neuroblastomas are malignant tumors arising from the neural crest and composed of small cells arranged in rosettes containing secretory granules and neurofibrils. The mature ganglioneuromas are benign. Most neuroblastomas appear before the age of 8 years, and fully half of them are found by the age of 2. Some exhibit a familial pattern and others occur in association with Kippel-Feil, Beckworth-Wiedemann, and other syndromes as well as Hirschprung's disease. Half of these tumors are found in the adrenal medulla and the remainder along the sympathetic chain in the neck, thoracic cavity, paraspinal ganglia, and pelvis. Symptoms depend on the site of origin, location of metastases, and presence of neurosecretions. They include anorexia, nausea, vomiting, abdominal pain, Horner's syndrome, hypertension related to catecholamines, fever, loss of weight, and encephalopathy. Frequently the presence of an abdominal mass is the first clinical sign of the disease.

The diagnostic workup may profitably include levels of neuron-specific enolase in the serum and catecholamines in the urine which are elevated in the presence of neuroblastoma. Ultrasound studies and radiologic investigation with nuclear magnetic imaging, chest and skeletal studies, uropyelograms, and scans with (^{131}I) *m*-iodobenzyl guanidine (MIBG) are all useful in establishing the diagnosis and extent of the disease.

Staging of neuroblastomas frequently used is that proposed by the Children's Cancer Study Group. Stage I disease should be treated by resection and does not require the addition of radiotherapy and/or chemotherapy. The latter are added in stage II disease and given preoperatively to shrink the tumor in stage III disease with initially unresectable tumor. When responses are obtained with combination chemotherapy in stage IV disease, resection may be possible in some cases. In stage IVs radiotherapy may be indicated for relief of symptoms resulting from an enlarging liver.

Staging of neuroblastoma
(Children's Cancer Study Group)

Stage I	Tumor confined to primary site
Stage II	Tumor beyond origin but ipsilateral and with or without ipsilateral nodal involvement
Stage III	Tumor beyond midline
Stage IV	Distant metastases
Stage IVs	Small resectable primary tumor with metastases to liver, skin, and/or bone marrow (not cortex)

Responses to chemotherapy and radiotherapy for neuroblastoma have been disappointing especially in stage III and stage IV disease. Treatment has been extended to total body irradiation, localized radiation with ^{131}I-labeled MIBG, high-dose chemotherapy, and additional combinations of agents initiating a response. Recommended chemotherapy is currently cyclophosphamide, cisplatin, and doxorubicin with either teniposide or etoposide; cisplatin and cyclophosphamide, and cyclophosphamide and doxorubicin. Other agents that effect responses are carboplatin, etoposide, topotecan, and vincristine. Therapy at times must include bone marrow transplantation.

RETINOBLASTOMA

Retinoblastomas, the most common tumors of the eye in childhood, occur chiefly in children under the age of 5 years and rarely in adults. They arise in the nuclear layer of the retina and may invade the optic nerve and extend intracranially to meninges and beyond. Metastases are found at distant sites in bone and bone marrow and to a lesser extent in lungs and lymph nodes. The tumors consist of small cells with a rim of cytoplasm arranged in rosettes reminiscent of the microscopic appearance of medulloblastomas and neuroblastomas. The calcification that can be present in these tumors is a helpful diagnostic sign. Symptoms consist of blindness, leukocoria, strabismus, proptosis, pain, and ocular inflammation. The lesions may be unilateral or bilateral, rare regressions have been reported, and some of them (retinomas) are benign. They occur sporadically and also may exhibit an autosomal dominant familial pattern. A great many studies have been carried out to elucidate the chromosomal and genic abnormality responsible for the tumors. A retinoblastoma locus (RB1) has been identified on chromosome 13. The loss of both alleles apparently leads to the appearance of the neoplasm. The presence of retinoblastomas may include other tumors as well, including Ewing's tumor, fibrosarcoma, osteosarcoma, and Wilms' tumor. The presence of hereditary retinoblastoma in a family requires parental genetic counseling and extended follow-up of the patient.

Extensive diagnostic studies should be done before a plan of therapy is adopted. It should include physical examination, ophthaloscopy, bone marrow biopsy, cytologic examination of the cerebrospinal fluid, bone scan, computerized tomograms or magnetic resonance imaging of skull and contents, lactic acid dehydrogenase (LDH) determination, and radiographic study of the chest.

Staging of retinoblastomas useful in planning and evaluating treatment has been devised in several ways. The following table is adapted from the St. Jude's Research Hospital system.

Staging of retinoblastoma
(St. Jude's Research Hospital)

Stage I	Unifocal or multifocal tumor confined to retina
	A. One quadrant or less
	B. Two quadrants or less
	C. More than one-half of retinal surface
Stage II	Unifocal or multifocal tumor confined to globe
	A. Vitreous seeding
	B. Extending to head of optic nerve
	C. Extending to choroid
	D. Extending to choroid and head of optic nerve
	E. Extending to emissaries
Stage III	Regional extraocular extension
	A. Extending beyond cut end optic nerve including subarachnoid
	B. Extending through sclera into orbital contents
	C. Extending through choroid beyond cut end optic nerve including subarachnoid
	D. Extending through sclera into orbital contents beyond cut end optic nerve including subarachnoid
Stage IV	Distant metastases
	A. Extending through optic nerve to brain
	B. Hematogenous metastases to bone and soft tissues
	C. Metastases to bone marrow

Treatment of retinoblastomas usually requires anesthesia in children with fixation of the head and globe for precise localization of ports when irradiation is used. The tumor dose administered may be as high as 5400 cGy. Small primary or recurrent lesions can be treated by cryotherapy or photocoagulation. In localized unilateral disease either surgical or radiation therapy can be used. Enucleation is avoided in cases with bilateral disease by using irradiation.

Most cases are more advanced, and enucleation is necessary, resecting the optic nerve beyond the extension of the tumor and giving postoperative radiotherapy. When tumors are bilateral and the optic nerve is not involved, both eyes are irradiated. When there is loss of vision and/or involvement of the optic nerve in one eye, it is enucleated and the remaining eye is given radiotherapy. When both eyes have extensive disease and some vision persists, bilateral radiation is used. Both neoadjuvant and adjuvant chemotherapy have been used for treating this neoplasm, but responses have not been encouraging. Among the agents in use alone or in combination are cisplatin, cyclophosphamide, dactinomycin, doxorubicin, ifosfamide, methotrexate, nitrogen mustard, triethanolamine, and vincristine. Chemotherapy is used more often in far advanced disease. The preferred chemotherapy for retinoblastoma is cyclophosphamide and doxorubicin with or without cisplatin, with or without etoposide, and with or without vincristine; also intrathecal methotrexate with or without cytarabine or with or without hydrocortisone. Other effective drugs are carboplatin, etoposide, and ifosfamide with mesna.

RHABDOMYOSARCOMA

Rhabdomyosarcomas arise in embryonic mesenchymal tissue that differentiates into striated muscle. They are the soft tissue tumors found most frequently in children and are distributed widely throughout the body at any site containing striated muscle or its predecessor. The types of these tumors in descending order of incidence are embryonal, alveolar, undifferentiated, botryoid, and pleomorphic. When tumors have mixtures of these types, the name adopted is that of the major component. The tumors have a pseudocapsule and spread by direct invasion and by both lymphatic and hematogenous routes. The appearance of rhabdomyosarcomas is sometimes associated with the presence of neurogenic tumors, other sarcomas, familial carcinoma of the breast, and other familial neoplasms such as those in Li-Fraumeni syndrome, as well as tumors of the brain and adrenal gland in siblings, Gorlin's basal cell nevus syndrome, and fetal alcohol syndrome. Usually the tumors appear before 15 years of age, with the highest incidences during the first and last part of this time. Embryonal tumors, those in the head and neck, and those in the distal genitourinary tract tend to occur in the younger patients, and those that are paratesticular and found in the trunk appear more often in those who are older. Embryonal tumors have the most unfavorable prognosis and botryoid tumors the best. Sites with the most unfavorable results are the trunk, mucosa, and extremities; those with the best results are the orbit and distal urinary tract. In addition to rhabdomyosarcoma, a number of other sarcomas of soft tissues occur in childhood. Among them are Ewing's sarcoma in soft tissues, synovial sarcoma, fibrosarcoma, liposarcoma, neurofibrosarcoma, malignant fibrous histiocytoma, leiomyosarcoma, and hemangiopericytoma. Treatment in general follows the same approaches followed for rhabdomyosarcoma.

Symptoms of rhabdomyosarcoma are related to the site of the primary tumor; examples are tumors of the head and neck creating neurologic problems (such as increased intracranial pressure, cranial nerve deficiencies, and meningeal symptoms), epistaxis, sinusitis, pain in the ear, and otitis media and those located in the thorax and abdomen giving rise to dysphagia, an abdominal mass, gastrointestinal symptoms, and urinary obstruction and hematuria. The planning of treatment is dependent on the diagnosis following microscopic study of tissue removed at operation or biopsy. Additional investigation with ultrasound and computerized tomography or nuclear magnetic resonance imaging is usually done before treatment begins. Other studies often indicated are bone scans, bone marrow biopsies, cerebrospinal fluid examination, and lymphangiograms.

Staging of rhabdomyosarcomas used in the Intergroup Rhabdomysarcoma Study has been widely adopted as a useful adjunct to evaluation of management of these tumors. An adaptation appears below.

Staging of rhabdomyosarcomas
(Intergroup Rhabdomyosarcoma Study)

Stage I	Localized disease; no nodes involved; completely resected
	   A. Confined to site of origin
	   B. Contiguous infiltration outside site of origin

Stage II	Regional disease
	   A. Gross tumor resected; microscopic residual; nodes negative
	   B. Tumor and involved regional nodes completely resected; no microscopic residual
	   C. Tumor and involved nodes resected; microscopic residual

Stage III	Incomplete resection; gross residual
Stage IV	Metastatic disease initially

Resection is frequently the first step in treatment, but neochemotherapy may be given especially when it may be possible to convert an inoperable to operable tumor after the chemotherapy. In recent years resection of these tumors has become more conservative and limited with advances in radiotherapy and chemotherapy, although some tumors such as paratesticular neoplasms require decisive and extended operation and at times transplantation of the contralateral testis into the thigh when radical orchiectomy, node dissection, and postoperative radiation are necessary. Functional disabilities and anticipated undesirable deformities limit the surgical approach in many cases, and the only operation indicated is biopsy of primary tumor and suspected lymph nodes. In appropriate cases, resection is indicated when gross or microscopic tumor remains after the first procedure. Tumors of the extremities tend to recur following resection especially when they are the alveolar type. Also they frequently have metastases to the lymph nodes.

Irradiation is often used to treat residual tumor and involved nodes. Parameningeal rhabdomyosarcoma requires high doses of radiation with extended ports. Also radiation with wide margins is necessary along with chemotherapy for other rhabdomyosarcomas of the head and neck. In genitourinary disease lymph nodes are biopsied frequently and, if positive, irradiation is administered including paraaortic nodes if necessary. Prior to radiotherapy, chemotherapy may be given to reduce the size of the tumor, and then limited resection is carried out followed by irradiation. Brachytherapy and intracavitary therapy are useful in appropriate cases.

These tumors respond to a number of chemotherapeutic agents such as doxorubicin (Adriamycin), actinomycin D, cisplatin, cyclophosphamide, ditriazoimidazole carboximide, ifosfamide, and vincristine alone or in various combinations. Combinations used frequently include cyclophosphamide, doxorubicin, and vincristine; and dactinomycin with vincristine may be the only combination required in stage II tumors with microscopic residual. The survival from rhabdomyosarcomas has been improved impressively by the addition of chemotherapy to surgical and radiation therapy. Future improvement will depend in part on accession of new effective agents and objective clinical evaluation of the results of treatment with them. For example, melphalan was added to the armamentarium by using human rhabdomyosarcoma cell lines xenotransplanted into immunocompromised mice to screen possible new agents. Currently chemotherapy is administered frequently in those patients with micrometastases and residual tumor sites, and neoadjuvant chemotherapy without subsequent radiation may be given before resection of stage I tumors without residual disease. Also adjuvant chemotherapy with agents such as dactinomycin and vincristine is useful in managing orbital neoplasms. The chemotherapy of choice for rhabdomyosarcoma is etoposide, ifosfamide, mesna, and vincristine or dactinomycin with either cyclophosphamide or ifosfamide and mesna.

EWING'S SARCOMA

Ewing's sarcoma is comprised of small round cells in bones chiefly in the pelvis and lower extremities. It is often confused with primitive neuroectodermal tumors, and many pathologists classify both as the same tumor. It occurs more in adolescent males than in females. The radiographic picture shows both proliferative and destructive changes in the bone affected and is accompanied by a soft tissue mass almost without exception.

These tumors produce a clinical picture consisting of a mass, pain, elevated sedimentation rate and leukocyte count, elevated serum lactic dehydrogenase level, and intermittent fever. They must be differentiated from infections and other primary and metastatic lesions of bone. Before therapy is started the workup should include computerized tomograms or magnetic resonance scans, complete blood count, lactic acid dehydrogenase level, and sedimentation rate.

Both surgical resection and irradiation are used to treat the primary site, and the use of combined chemotherapeutic agents including doxorubicin as adjuvant treatment may also improve the results of management. Autologous bone marrow transplantation has been advocated for more advanced disease. Late secondary malignancies, fractures, retardation of growth in children, and necrosis following radiotherapy have led some clinicians to favor surgical resection as the primary approach to treatment with supplementary radiotherapy.

GERM CELL TUMORS

Germ cell tumors originate from primitive germ cells and appear in the reproductive system or elsewhere by migration. They consist of three types, benign teratomas appearing most often at birth, yolk sac tumors within the first 5 years, and dysgerminomas and malignant teratomas in adolescence. The clinical symptoms and signs may include pain, masses, elevated levels of alpha-fetoprotein in tumors of yolk sac origin, elevated human chorionic gonadotropin levels in tumors of trophoblastic origin, and masculinization and precocious secondary sexual features in dysgerminomas.

Surgical resection is the primary approach to treating these tumors. Radical orchiectomy after high ligation of the spermatic cord followed by removal of retroperitoneal lymph nodes when indicated is the treatment used most frequently for testicular neoplasms. Unilateral salpingo-oophorectomy is the usual treatment for ovarian tumors. Adjuvant radiotherapy is required infrequently. Responses are obtained with chemotherapy. Actinomycin, cyclophosphamide, and vincristine are used quite often. In addition, bleomycin and VP-16 are active as well, and methotrexate elicits responses in trophoblastic tumors.

PRIMARY MALIGNANT HEPATIC TUMORS

Although found infrequently, both hepatoblastomas and hepatocellular carcinomas occur in childhood. Hepatoblastomas are present most commonly in infancy and early childhood. They may be well differentiated with a better prognosis than undifferentiated malignancies. Hepatocellular lesions occur most frequently around the age of 4 years and in early adolescence, and up to half the cases have cirrhosis associated with galactosemia. An abdominal mass and/or hepatomegaly usually call attention to these tumors. Diagnostic workup should include unltrasound studies, computerized tomography, and levels of alpha-fetoprotein and human chorionic gonadotropin.

The principal treatment of these tumors is surgical resection. The liver has remarkable powers of regeneration, and up to 80 percent can be removed with the expectation of restoration with four-fifths of the patients surviving for 2 years after complete resection of the neoplasms. Radiotherapy is used only selectively. Responses to adjuvant chemotherapy occur with the use of agents such as doxorubicin, cyclophosphamide, 5-fluorouracil, and vincristine.

LYMPHOMAS AND HISTIOCYTOSES

Hodgkin's disease, usually the nodular sclerosing type, occurs most frequently in early adolescence and features enlarged lymph nodes. Non-Hodgkin's lymphomas in children are widely disseminated with primary sites in abdomen, mediastinum, and periphery, including the head and neck region. Symptoms also may suggest appendicitis, Meckel's diverticulitis, intussusception, and intestinal obstruction.

Biopsy is necessary to establish the diagnosis. A staging celiotomy in older children may be useful; when this is done, a subsequent change in staging is adopted in approximately half the cases. When splenectomy is contemplated in a child, prophylactic antibiotic therapy and pneumococcal vaccination should be considered because of the risk of devastating sepsis, especially in children with Hodgkin's disease. The survival for 10 years after the usual treatment of lymphoma in childhood ranges from 70 to 90 percent with the best results obtained in cases of Hodgkin's disease.

Histiocytoses originate from stem cells in the bone marrow whose ordinary function is erythrophagocytosis resulting in the formation of granulating lesions. There are three classes of these abnormalities. Class I, or histiocytosis X, is composed principally of Langerhan's cells responding to immunologic stimulation. The three conditions included are Hand-Schuller-Christian syndrome, Letterer-Siwe disease, and eosinophilic granulomas. Class II lesions include all other nonmalignant histiocytoses with chief component of mononuclear phagocytes that are not Langerhans' cells. Class III lesions are malignant and consist of acute monocytic leukemias. Malignant histiocytoses are often rapidly fatal with features of pain, fever, subcutaneous infiltration, enlarged lymph nodes, hemolytic anemia, pancytopenia, and enlargement of spleen and/or liver. These malignant lesions are treated with various combinations of bleomycin, cyclophosphamide, cytosine arabinoside, doxorubicin, etoposide, semustine (Methyl-CCNU), prednisone, and vincristine.

OTHER NEOPLASMS

Melanoma is the malignancy of the skin appearing most frequently, but squamous and basal cell carcinomas also occur. Protective measures and avoiding exposure to the sun is as important in childhood as later in life. Tumors of the breast that occur most frequently are fibroadenomas. Cystosarcoma phylloides can be exceedingly large. Carcinomas of the breast appear much less frequently than in adults and have been reported in both boys and girls. Treatment is similar to that for adults affected.

Included among malignancies of the head and neck in childhood are nasopharyngeal carcinomas, adamantinomas, oropharyngeal cancer, and neoplasms of the larynx and thyroid. In general the frequency with which these malignancies are encountered is much less often than in adults. Nasopharyngeal cancer is treated by irradiation of up to 6500 cGy and chemotherapy including bleomycin, cisplatin, 5-fluorouracil, and methotrexate. Mandibular, maxillary, and other ameloblastomas are treated with resection and irradiation. The use of tobacco in adolescence is probably a major factor in the increasing appearance of cancer of the oral cavity, which is treated in a similar fashion to therapy for adults. Juvenile papillomatosis, carcinoma which is rare, and rhabdomyosarcoma are the tumors of the larynx found in children and require the same management as in adults. Carcinomas of the thyroid are usually papillary or follicular and are treated by resection with radiation therapy for any postoperative residue.

Thoracic neoplasms found in childhood include thymomas, metastatic neoplasms, and tumors of the lung. Neoplastic epithelial cells must be present for a tumor to be diagnosed as a thymoma. Carcinomas of the lung are rather rare, but bronchial adenomas, bronchogenic undifferentiated cancers and adenocarcinomas, and pulmonary blastomas do occur. Approaches to treatment used for similar tumors in adults are adopted for these neoplasms.

Gastrointestinal cancer of the stomach, gallbladder, pancreas, and colon as well as renal cell carcinomas are rare in children. When they do occur, the same principles of management apply as for similar lesions in adults. Adrenal carcinomas and the MEN syndrome (multiple endocrine neoplasms) are known to appear in childhood with the same problems and therapeutic management as in adults.

TWELVE

TUMORS OF THE NERVOUS SYSTEM

Intracranial neoplasms include both intracerebral and extracerebral malignancies. The former consist of metastatic tumors which are found most frequently and gliomas (astrocytomas, ependymomas, medulloblastomas, oligodendrogliomas), primary lymphomas of the brain, and tumors of the choroid plexus and pineal gland. Extracerebral tumors include meningiomas, neuromas including acoustic neuromas, tumors of the pituitary, craniopharyngiomas, chordomas and metastatic tumors to bone, and hemangioblastomas. They must be distinguished from other lesions occupying space such as abscesses, vascular abnormalities, granulomas, and cysts. Tumors of the brain are the type of solid neoplasm most frequently found in children. More than 14,000 intracranial neoplasms are discovered annually in the United States, and more than 10,000 patients succumb to the disease each year. There is an increase in the incidence between the ages of infancy and 4 years, a decrease from the age of 15 for about a decade, and then a gradual increase to the age of 65 when the peak incidence is reached and sustained.

Although there has been no lack of speculation about the causes of intracranial neoplasms, definitive proof about proposed etiologic relationships between these tumors and antecedent trauma, viral infection, and exposure to chemicals other than vinyl chloride has been lacking. The appearance of intracranial tumors has followed chemotherapy and irradiation occasionally, and primary cerebrospinal lymphoma occurs in patients treated for AIDS and those with transplanted organs. A few hereditary syndromes such as Hippel-Lindau and Li-Fraumeni syndromes, tuberous sclerosis, and neurofibromatosis are associated with the appearance of a miscellaneous group of tumors in those affected. As genetic studies have progressed, an increasing amount of evidence is steadily being acquired about the relationship of aneuploidy, deletions, and mutations, the influence of oncogenes, and the absence of tumor-suppressor genes in specific tumors. Chromosomes reported to be involved have included 7, 9p, 10, 17, and 22. Undoubtedly continued genetic inquiry will elucidate specific molecular events leading to the neoplastic changes in individual tumors.

A careful history and physical and neurologic examination supplemented by audiograms, visual fields utilizing tangent screen and perimetry, and neuroencephalograms when seizures are present or suspected must be the first steps in diagnosing and treating intracranial neoplasms. Also an interview with the patient's family is essential. Examination of the blood and cerebrospinal fluid may be useful in diagnosing and following the course of these tumors, but caution must be used at all times when performing a spinal tap which should follow all other diagnostic procedures. The symptoms associated with the presence of intracranial tumors are related in part to the rigid confines of the skull in which the brain is contained. An increase in intracranial pressure as a result of increasing size of a neoplasm can lead to headache even though the neoplasm is devoid of nerve endings responsive to pain. Supratentorial tumors tend to cause frontal and temporal headache, and infratentorial tumors can cause occipital headache and, at times, retroorbital pain. Other common symptoms are nausea and vomiting and other gastrointestinal problems and changes in personality. Also papilledema may be noted on physical examination. Other symptoms and signs depend in large part on the location of the neoplasm. Those in the sella are associated with abnormalities of orbital muscles and visual fields such as homonomous hemianopsia. Also alteration in the amounts of pituitary hormones secreted may give characteristic symptoms later. Focal seizures can be helpful in localizing the site of intracranial tumors. Herniation can occur through the tentorium cerebelli separating the cerebral hemispheres above from the cerebellum and brain stem below. When detected, emergency operative intervention is often required to prevent a fatal outcome. The symptoms mentioned and signs of motor and/or sensory abnormalities are very useful in elucidating the location and type of neoplasm involved.

Radiographic studies have come to occupy a major role in diagnosis of these tumors. Air contrast studies of cerebral ventricles have become obsolete with the advent of computerized tomography and nuclear magnetic resonance imaging alone and enhanced with contrast material. Although equally specific, the latter is superior for detecting neoplasms of the brain and assessing the presence of hemorrhage, air, and fluid. At times arteriograms may be useful to detect vascular tumors and the vascularization of others. Also MRI scanning is quite useful in the design of ports to be utilized in radiotherapy for these tumors.

The surgical approach to treatment and tissue diagnosis continues to be the initial management and constitutes the best chance for curing intracranial malignancies. The advances in imaging and instrumentation have made it even more effective, with almost all lesions approachable and the tentative diagnosis more accurate. MRI in several planes permits stereotactic localization of these lesions, and angiography indicates relationships to blood supply. Also embolization may aid the surgeon in resecting the neoplasm. It is imperative to obtain sufficient tissue for diagnosis even when a neoplasm cannot be either totally or partially resected. When the location is known, tissue is often obtained by endoscopic stereotactic biopsy. As soon as diagnostic studies are complete and the exact site, shape, and size of the flap with retained blood supply has been decided, attention must be directed to preliminary administration of corticosteroids and anticonvulsants with determination of levels of the latter. It is often advisable to restrain motion of the head with pin fixation especially when the operator is visualizing a magnified operative field. In addition to dexamethasone or other similar agent, mannitol and hyperventilation are used to reduce intracranial pressure and prevent edema. Shunting may be indicated in the presence of hydrocephalus. Only local anesthesia is usually necessary in adults, but general anesthesia in children is used. The choice of anesthetic agent includes only those without effect on intracranial pressure. Occipital scalp and bone flaps for infratentorial tumors may require C-1 and C-2 laminectomy for greater exposure. The surgical approach to most tumors arising in the sella is transsphenoidal. When the brain is exposed, intraoperative ultrasound study can confirm the location of a tumor below the surface if the surgeon requires this assistance. The usual technique of resection can be supplemented by ultrasonic aspiration when necessary. The laser is not used very often. Even when the entire neoplasm cannot be removed, reduction in its mass is often a valuable addition to other palliative measures. Occasionally a drain is left in place temporarily. Medication for combating potential seizures as well as edema and increased intracranial pressure must be continued postoperatively with discontinuation involving careful judgment. The possibility of combining operative and radiotherapeutic and/or chemotherapeutic treatment is reviewed before the surgeon initiates any surgical therapy.

The techniques available for irradiation are extensive, ranging from external beam irradiation to brachytherapy with implantation of radioactive material stereotactically and also include focal stereotactic irradiation with proton beam, linear accelerator, or gamma source. Photodynamic therapy consisting of injection of sensitizer and destruction of tumor cells taking up the sensitizer selectively by means of light activation is occasionally appropriate. Most primary intracranial tumors are unifocal, requiring reduced fields to be irradiated, eliminating the need to irradiate the whole brain. When prior partial excision has been accomplished, then only the margin is included. Experience has dictated the width indicated, and this depends on the type of tumor being irradiated. The brain is sensitive to irradiation, with the greatest problem in infancy through the first year or two of life. This limits the amount and number of fractionated doses and the total tumor dose. The ports and direction of the beam of irradiation are carefully arranged to maximize the tumor dosage and minimize the dosage delivered to the remainder of the brain. The most recent method for delivery is designated three-dimensional conformal irradiation. The target is always the tumor volume plus the additional margin thought to be at risk for microscopic spread.

The reactions to varying degrees of injury from irradiation are early and early and late delayed responses. The early increase in intracranial pressure and edema as a result of irradiation damage can be countered by corticosteroids and usually is limited and treatable. The early delayed response is thought to be the result of alteration in capillary permeability and temporary demyelinization of oligodendroglial cells. The late delayed response is the result of focal and/or diffuse injury to the white matter and can be fatal. The spinal cord is especially vulnerable to radiation myelopathy, and maintenance of position of the patient and accurate placement of the field of irradiation with each fractional dose is imperative. Some types of chemotherapy can increase injury from irradiation when used in combination. This has been amply documented for methotrexate, for example.

The use of chemotherapy for parenchymatous tumors of the brain is limited because of cerebral toxicity and the blood-brain barrier. Those agents most effective are able to cross it with relative ease. Access via the cerebrospinal fluid, usually through a transventricular reservoir, offers the advantage of concentrated dosage but can result in catastrophic complications. Intratumoral therapy is sometimes indicated for cystic tumors. Also, the intraarterial route for delivery has been used, but indications for this route have not been clarified.

GLIOMAS

The gliomas are the type of primary neoplasm found in the central nervous system most frequently. They are composed of one of the types of glial cells: astrocytes, ependymal cells, neuroglial types, and oligodendrocytes. The cells from which glial tumors arise supply the supporting structures for neurons (astrocytes), are associated with myelinization (oligodendrogliocytes), and line ventricular cavities and the central canal of the spinal cord (ependymal cells). Medulloblastomas are derived from neuroglial antecedents. Glioblastomas arise from malignant transformation of astrocytes, and they and astrocytomas together constitute the majority of gliomas. Various combinations of these precursors may be encountered in many of the tumors. Grades of these tumors range from grade ½, often exhibiting years of slow growth, to grade 4, with a history of weeks or months for tumors in this classification such as glioblastoma muliforme, which has an exceedingly poor prognosis. Grades I and II are low-grade tumors, and those of higher grade are high-grade tumors with greater chance for a lethal outcome. Typing is based on the degree and amount of nuclear atypia, endothelial proliferation, mitosis, and necrosis. The nomenclature for gliomas is somewhat confusing in that the terms, malignant glioma, glioblastoma multiforme, and astrocytoma grade IV, are often used interchangeably.

Except for juvenile pilocytic lesions and possibly subependymomas, astrocytomas are highly malignant tumors, and the first treatment is usually as extensive a surgical excision as possible even in cases of suitable recurrent tumors after careful diagnostic studies, planning, and preoperative preparation. The use of intraoperative ultrasound studies for localization, microscopic visualization of the operative field, and all the surgical instrumentation for resection should be utilized to remove the tumor from the center outward as far as possible, using the borders of white matter and cortical mapping as a guide for delineation of the margin and the extent to be resected. Preoperative embolization may be invaluable in solving problems of bleeding. Even when the extent of resection is limited, the operative resection is valuable in reducing intracranial pressure and edema, the population of remaining cells to be treated with radiotherapy and/or chemotherapy and biotherapy, and portions of the tumor that are most radioresistant and difficult to penetrate with chemotherapeutic agents.

Gliomas are radioresistant, but even anaplastic astrocytomas and glioblastomas do respond to radiotherapy in terms of increased survival, although much of the past evidence for this has been derived from retrospective studies. The usual management is to have irradiation therapy follow surgical resection, even when only partial removal is feasible. Because of the radioresistance of these tumors, the methods of irradiation have often been altered, using heavy particle beams, hyperfractionation and other methods of dividing and focusing the treatment, local hyperthermia, interstitial brachytherapy, various radiosensitizers, and the addition of chemotherapy. Tumor doses ranging from 6000 to 8000 cGy have been used, the dose depending on many factors related to the tumor and the method of irradiation. Reduction in dosage and delay in treatment of tumors in childhood may be wise in view of increased sensitivity and the dangers of neurologic damage to normal cerebral tissue in these young patients. Sensitization with halogenated pyrimidines introduced into the DNA of malignant gliomas has apparently improved the effectiveness of irradiation in initial studies. These neoplasms are also responsive to certain types of chemotherapy. PCV [procarbazine, lomustine (CCNU), and vincristine], procarbazine, streptozotocin, carmustine (BCNU), and lomustine alone and in some combinations are among those yielding the best results. Preferred current treatments of glioblastoma or anaplastic astrocytoma are lomustine, procarbazine, and vincristine; carmustine containing polymer water or without; and cisplatin.

Approximately one quarter of infratentorial tumors are cerebellar astrocytomas. They tend to be less malignant than supratentorial tumors and have symptoms related to their invasion of the vermis. In children enlargement of the head and symptoms of headache, nausea, and vomiting announce their presence. The most effective therapy is resection of both solid tumors and the mural lesion on the wall of cystic tumors. When it is not possible to remove the neoplasm completely, radiation is often added, especially in anaplastic lesions. Nitrosoureas have been used as palliative adjuvant therapy with some response.

Oligodendrogliomas appear in the cerebral hemispheres, lateral ventricles, and thalamus. They occur most often in midlife and can be anaplastic or differentiated or mixtures, including astrocytes and ependymal cells. A small portion are cystic. When resection of the tumor is possible, it should be done, but infiltration often extends beyond the point of possible excision. Irradiation may extend survival, but cure is not often accomplished. Chemotherapy with nitrosourea-based combinations has resulted in some responses. At the present time chemotherapy obtaining the best responses for anaplastic oligodendrogliomas consists of lomustine, procarbazine, and vincristine; carmustine; and cisplatin.

Almost two-thirds of ependymomas occur infratentorially, including the fourth ventricle, subarachnoid space, medulla, and cord. The supratentorial neoplasms are either parenchymal or intraventricular and have an unfortunate capacity for spreading by cellular dissemination. As much of the neoplasms as possible should be removed, either by means of a transcortical approach or suboccipital route with laminectomy of the first cervical vertebra. It is essential to leave the ventricular circulation intact at the termination of any surgical procedure. Radiation therapy is capable of extending survival, but anaplastic tumors such as ependymoblastomas are more resistant and have shorter survival times. The use of prophylactic irradiation of the spinal axis in addition to the primary site is somewhat controversial but is advocated by many radiologists. Chemotherapy has been used with responses even of recurrent and anaplastic neoplasms. Agents that have been used alone and in combinations include carmustine, carboplatin, diazoquinone, dibromodulcitol, etoposide, lomustine, procarbazine, and vincristine.

Astrocytomas, glioblatomas, and ependymomas are all gliomas that may occur in the brain stem. They can involve the midbrain, medulla, cranial nerves, and cord; and symptoms can include hydrocephalus, nausea and vomiting, somnolence, cranial nerve deficiencies, palsies, ataxia, and hemiplegia. Diagnosis has been aided greatly by magnetic resonance imaging (MRI) and stereotactic guided biopsies. Complete resection is not possible, but radiation improves rates of survival and symptomatology. Also, chemotherapy has been used with some responses that have not been of long duration but suggest that continuation of trials is amply justified.

Gliomas of the optic nerves, tracts, chiasm, and hypothalamus include a wide range of benign to anaplastic neoplasms ranging from piloid astrocytoma to glioblastoma and may be a feature of neurofibromatosis. Visual and oculo-motor symptoms, macrocephaly, and hemiparesis are among the conse-quences. When only one optic nerve is infiltrated, the entire structure is removed from the chiasm to the globe of the eye. When the chiasm is included, it is not resected. These patients are candidates for irradiation, but whether it is better to wait for the development or progression of symptoms is difficult to decide. Radiotherapy, using ports designed to protect the lens, can cause regression of symptoms and extension of the time before relapse. In children chemotherapy has been advocated to delay the necessity for radiotherapy, but the results of trials so far have been rather disappointing.

MEDULLOBLASTOMAS

Medulloblastomas are small cell cerebellar tumors possibly arising from neu-roepithelium arising in the roof of the ventricle. They are located chiefly in the midline or posterior vermis and lateral cerebellum. They may fill the fourth ventricle and are frequently associated with rapid increase in intracran-ial pressure and hydrocephalus, which must be assessed carefully before begin-ning therapy. More than half of the tumors appear in the first 10 years with a second increase a decade later. After staging the disease with magnetic resonance imaging or myelograms, the greatest hope for cure is complete resection of the neoplasm. The outlook is altered if no more than three quarters of the mass of tumor can be resected. The prognosis is poorer when the patient is in the first 4 years of life and, as would be expected, when metastases are present. Spinal metastases occur in approximately one-third of patients, but distant foci elsewhere are not frequent, appearing most fre-quently in long bones and ribs.

Corticosteroids are usually used to control increased intracranial pressure, and shunting is delayed until the time of operation. Most commonly a midline incision is made and extended through the foramen magnum. Diagnostic studies are completed preoperatively, and a decision made about which choice and sequence of operation, radiotherapy, and chemotherapy is indicated. It is possible frequently to relieve obstruction at the time of operation, obviating the need for external shunting. The primary objective of operation is complete resection of the tumor, including any portion of the tumor herniating over the spinal cord, using the dissecting microscope and modern instrumentation. Closure includes sufficient care to prevent subsequent leakage of cerebrospinal fluid. Radiotherapy is usually directed to the entire cerebrospinal axis because of the tendency of medulloblastomas to be distributed widely via the cerebro-spinal fluid. These tumors are very sensitive to irradiation, but nevertheless have a distressing tendency to recur. Both embryonal tumors and medulloblas-tomas respond to cisplatin, lomustine, and vincristine; lomustine, prednisone, and vincristine; and cisplatin, cyclophosphamide, etoposide, and vincristine.

Also, responses may be obtained with etoposide alone or with mechloreth-amine, vincristine, procarbazine, and prednisone (MOPP). Evaluation of techniques, sequences, and combinations of resection, radiotherapy, and chemotherapy is a continuing process.

PITUITARY TUMORS

Pituitary tumors originate in the sella turcica. Their symptoms result either from reduction or increase in secretions and invasion of adjacent structures or enlargement. They may be secretory adenomas or may be symptomatic because of their increasing size. Chromophobe tumors rarely become malignant and are symptomatic because of compression and secretory inhibition. These tumors expand the sella and may invade the cavernous and sphenoid sinuses and suprasellar cisterns and compress the optic chiasm. The enlarging tumor can compress the pituitary sufficiently to lead to clinical adrenal, gonadal, and thyroid deficiencies. Secretory tumors may be identified by the serum level of the hormone produced. Prolactinomas or compression of the pituitary stalk obstructing the flow of thalamic inhibitor result in high serum levels of prolactin and induce a clinical picture with features including galactorrhea, loss of libido and fertility, amenorrhea, and osteoporosis usually in young women. Acromegaly is induced by tumors producing increased serum levels of growth hormone, which is not suppressed by administration of glucose. Cushing's disease occurs when corticotropin is produced by an adenoma and serum cortisol levels are increased without suppression by administration of dexamethasone. Characteristic symptoms are moonface, buffalo hump, diabetes insipidus, hypertension, and abdominal striae. Adrenocorticotropic hormone (ACTH) can be measured in samples from the venous drainage of the cavernous sinus. Follicle-stimulating hormone, luteotropin, and thyrotropin are known products of pituitary adenomas, but they rarely are found.

In addition to symptoms and abnormal secretory levels, diagnosis of pituitary tumors may be determined by nuclear magnetic resonance scanning with the addition of gadolinium enhancement for detecting small lesions. Arachnoid and Rathke's cleft cysts, meningiomas, craniopharyngiomas, and metastatic tumors must be differentiated from pituitary adenomas since they can produce similar visual loss and hypopituitarism.

Bromocriptine is capable of reducing the serum level of prolactin and size of the tumor and can be used to defer or omit a surgical approach to therapy for prolactinomas. This treatment must be continued because symptoms, growth of the adenoma, and levels of prolactin increase with cessation of therapy. Operation is usually necessary only in those who cannot tolerate the drug. Bromocriptine may control acromegaly partially. Also somatostatin analogues can be effective but have the disadvantages of undesirable side effects and parenteral administration. Ketoconazole can be used to suppress the elaboration of cortisol in patients for whom operation is contraindicated. Resection through the nose and sphenoid sinus is successful in small tumors and almost totally successful in very large lesions of the pituitary with recurrence in a minority of cases. Radiotherapy can be done for those patients who refuse or are not suitable for operation and in cases with incomplete resection of the tumor. It is more successful in controlling the growth of these tumors and invasive sites than in alleviating the abnormal endocrine levels. One late sequella of radiation is the development of hypopituitarism which must be kept in mind during the lifetime follow-up.

NEUROFIBROMATOSIS

Neurofibromatosis occurs in two distinctive forms. Clinical features of type 1 are multiple fibromas, cafe-au-lait spots, and characteristic freckles of the skin, skeletal abnormalities and microcephaly, Lisch nodules in the iris, low-grade optic and cerebral astrocytomas, and learning disability. The fibromas are plexiform neurofibromas, and the neurofibromas associated with the syndrome probably originate from these plexiform precursors. Type 1 disease is encountered more frequently than type 2. The latter has few skin manifestations, but multiple cerebral and spinal tumors make the disease a formidable clinical problem. Bilateral Schwann cell tumors of the eighth cranial nerve, meningiomas (at times multiple), ependymomas, and early lens opacities are frequent features of type 2 disease. The gliomas are most frequently astrocytomas, but a mixture of gliomas may be present. They can involve one or both optic nerves, the optic chiasm, and hypothalamus. Some of the multiple neurofibromas throughout the body in patients with von Recklinghausen's disease, which is due to an autosomal dominant gene, may develop into schwannomas.

Both type 1 and type 2 neurofibromatosis are inherited diseases with variable penetrance. The first is due to an autosomal dominant gene (neurofibromin protein) on chromosome 17, and the second type is the result of an autosomal dominant gene (Merlin protein) on chromosome 22. In addition, tumor suppressor gene or genes present on chromosome 22 may be deleted, and this is thought to be responsible for the sporadic appearance of type 2 neurofibromatosis.

In addition to medical history and physical and auditory examination, magnetic resonance imaging of the brain and spinal axis is an invaluable diagnostic asset, especially when used with gadolinium enhancement. The management of the various neoplasms appearing with neurofibromatosis is discussed under the respective heading for each type.

ACOUSTIC NEUROMAS

Acoustic neuromas originate in the internal auditory canal and arise from vestibular nerve Schwann cells. Symptoms progress from early partial loss of hearing and may progress to complete deafness, vertigo, aural pain, facial weakness, dysphagia, and hydrocephalus. Many patients have type 2 familial neurofibromatosis and are susceptible to other tumors of the nervous system as well. Although they are benign and may grow slowly, acoustic neuromas compress the facial nerve with the usual distressing clinical picture. Cerebello-pontine neurilemmomas also may compress cranial nerves VII, IX, and X, but this rarely occurs.

Diagnosis usually rests on the results of magnetic resonance scanning with gadolinium enhancement. In those with only loss of hearing and a tumor that is apparently growing slowly, the choice of following the patient with magnetic resonance imaging and clinical examination is sometimes made. Most patients, however accept an operative approach to management. The facial nerve can be decompressed when the tumor is removed, and the paresis and related symptomatology will often regress. Operative approaches are translabrynthine (and occasionally through the middle cranial fossa) for small tumors with expectation of complete loss of hearing and very low morbidity and through a suboccipital craniotomy when there is a larger tumor with invasion of the posterior fossa and an attempt to preserve hearing is feasible. Radiotherapy can be used to treat recurrent tumors and as primary therapy in the elderly. Also, postoperative irradiation is advocated by many radiation oncologists after partial resection to inhibit progression of the tumor.

GLOMUS JUGULARE TUMORS

Glomus jugulare tumors arise from one or more sites in the glomus tissue of the jugular bulb. They grow very slowly but have an extensive blood supply. This makes resection of the tumors, which may pulsate, very difficult and at times mandates embolization following angiography immediately before operation. Angiography and magnetic resonance imaging confirm the diagnosis. These tumors can be secretory with syndromes similar to those of carcinoids and pheochromocytomas. Symptoms related to compression of the cranial nerves can lead to paresis of facial muscles and vocal cords as well as dysphagia and tinnitus. The fifth nerve is the one most often affected.

Operation requires great skill. The entire tumor is removed with vascular attachments after ligation of the jugular vein and sigmoid sinus via a suboccipital approach. Radiotherapy can be effective in treating recurrences and tumors not amenable to resection. Tumor dosages indicated are 5000 cGy or less.

CRANIOPHARYNGIOMAS

Craniopharyngiomas arise at the coalescence of the pituitary gland and infundibulum from Rathke's pouch cells. They may contain calcium and are detectable with computerized tomography and magnetic resonance imaging. Characteristic cysts appear, and the pituitary gland, optic chiasm, and hypothalamus are compressed with an increase in intracranial pressure. Visual defects, obesity, and retarded development occur in children.

These tumors may be treated either with resection or radiotherapy or both. Total resection can lead to complications of hypopituitarism, including diabetes insipidus, necessitating permanent replacement therapy if symptoms do not regress. Visual difficulties usually respond to the surgical procedure, however. Radiotherapy as primary treatment, subsequent to partial resection, and after recurrence elicits responses but is deferred until the age of 3 when possible. Also the cysts can be treated by stereotactic puncture and instillation of phosphorus 32 or yttrium 90.

PINEAL TUMORS

Up to half of pineal tumors are germinomas, and astrocytomas constitute approximately half of the remainder. The remaining tumors are those of the pineal parenchyma and embryonal carcinomas. Localization in the posterior third ventricle with ocular dysfunction and hydrocephalus may require shunting if cortisone administration fails. Although stereotactic biopsy for definitive diagnosis is desirable, the procedure is somewhat controversial at the present time. Radiotherapy with tumor dose of 25 Gy may result in regression and thus identification of a germinoma. Additional radiotherapy to the entire brain of up to 25 Gy then is administered. Refinement of surgical techniques and use of microsurgical approaches in recent years has reduced the discouraging rate of complications and mortality, and removal of pineal tumors is now feasible. It is mandatory in radioresistant tumors and useful for benign tumors and in conjunction with radiotherapy and chemotherapy of those that are radioresponsive. Germinomas are responsive to chemotherapy even after recurrence. Agents used alone or in various combinations are bleomycin, cisplatin, cyclophosphamide, dactinomycin, etoposide, methotrexate, and vinblastine. Recommended chemotherapy for germ cell tumors is cisplatin or carboplatin and etoposide. Although surgical intervention with modern methods is not thought to increase seeding, computerized tomograms or magnetic resonance imaging and examination of the cerebrospinal fluid must follow when there is suspicion that the spinal axis as well as the localized cerebral site is involved. When a diagnosis of disseminated germinomas or nongerminomas is made, systemic chemotherapy and cerebrospinal radiation must be considered.

MENINGIOMAS

Meningiomas are localized or appear as sheets of cells on the covering of the brain and spinal cord. Most are benign and grow slowly. Symptoms include headache and seizures and depend on the localization of the lesions which compress or surround adjacent structures. Computerized tomograms and magnetic resonance imaging along with arteriograms and analysis of cerebrospinal fluid are useful in establishing a presumptive diagnosis. The enlargement and advancement of these tumors slowly can compress the cranial nerves, cerebral hemispheres, and ventricles with a wide range of steadily advancing symptoms including proptosis, visual problems, loss of hearing, ataxia, and digital paresis. Close observation with repetition of diagnostic studies is used at times for asymptomatic meningiomas and other special cases, but microsurgical procedures are appropriate for the treatment of most cases. Complete resection is possible, complications are not prohibitive, and symptoms may regress postoperatively. However, the removal of the entire tumor may not be wise if the risk of increasing the symptoms and rate of complications is sufficiently great. Radiotherapy can be used following operation or, if the risk for operation is too great, alone.

CHORDOMAS

Chordomas arise from embryonic notochordal tissue at sites from the base of the skull to the sacrum and coccyx, including the vertebrae. Except for rare ecchordoses, these tumors originate within the bone and form an expanding tumor with an overlying mass of soft tissue at times. Cranial chordomas seldom appear; when they do, the location bears some relation to the clivus. Symptoms include a mass in the nasopharynx, visual loss, diplopia, lateral rectus palsy, facial hypesthesia, hydrocephalus, hypopituitarism, cervical pain, and other cranial nerve abnormalities. Symptoms of chordomas of the spine depend on the level of compression of the cord by the tumor(s). Usually symptoms begin with pain in the back. Those of the sacrum may compress the rectum with resultant tenesmus, bleeding, and changes in bowel habits. The treatment of chordomas at any site is resection usually followed by irradiation. Great care must be taken when operating on cranial chordomas to close the dura without leakage to prevent meningitis and to maintain the integrity of the rectum when resecting or taking biopsies of sacral lesions to prevent seeding into the lumen and the necessity for rectal resection. Radiotherapy has been extended to brachytherapy, charged particle beam irradiation, and gamma irradiation. Radiotherapy combats the tendency of these tumors to recur. Trials with chemotherapy have not been promising up to this time.

CHOROID PLEXUS TUMORS

Papillomas of the choroid plexus appear as irregular masses within the lateral, third, and fourth ventricles. They grow slowly, secrete cerebrospinal fluid, and become symptomatic when they obstruct the flow of cerebrospinal fluid and/ or produce excessive fluid and impede absorption. Seeding does occur but is usually not extensive. On the other hand, widespread seeding does occur as a common characteristic of choroid plexus carcinomas. Diagnosis and preoperative staging requires magnetic resonance imaging, study of the cerebrospinal fluid, and myelography. Symptomatology in patients, who most frequently are children, is chiefly that of increased intracranial pressure and, at times, nystagmus and locomotor ataxia.

Treatment with resection is the usual primary approach to therapy. The operative approach depends on the ventricular location of the tumor. Microsurgical technique and meticulous hemostasis are indispensible. If resection does not restore circulation of the cerebrospinal fluid, shunting may be necessary. Irradiation is used when the tumor is inoperable or the patient's condition does not permit or there is recurrence or incomplete resection. Because dissemination may be widespread, it may be wise to consider irradiating the entire cerebrospinal axis. Both systemic and intraventricular chemotherapy have been used with sporadic success. Among systemic agents used are cyclophosphamide, doxorubicin, and vincristine; and methotrexate and cytosine arabinoside are among those used as intraventricular adjuvant therapy.

HEMANGIOBLASTOMAS

Hemangioblastomas appear most frequently in midlife and occur in males more often than in females. They are vascular, usually grow slowly, may be either cystic or solid, and probably arise from primitive endothelial cells in the region of the fourth ventricle. Their distribution is in the cerebellum, spinal cord, cerebral hemispheres, and nerves and nerve roots in descending order of frequency. The cystic tumors are composed of a reactive wall and a mural tumor. In addition to occurring sporadically, these tumors appear as part of the Hippel-Lindau syndrome, which is inherited as an autosomal dominant gene with variable penetrance expressed as multiple hemangioblastomas, pheochromocytomas, retinal angiomatosis, cysts of the pancreas and kidney, and hypernephroma. When the diagnosis of hemangioblastoma is made in a case of the inherited disorder and treatment is completed, continued surveillance is indicated because of the likelihood of additional tumors. Clinical symptoms of hemangioblastomas include headache, torticollis, nausea, vomiting, diplopia, ataxis, and myelopathy. Also up to one-fifth of the patients have polycythemia.

Diagnostic workup includes nuclear magnetic resonance scanning, and gadolinium enhances visualization of the mural nodule in cystic tumors. Also, preoperative angiography may be indicated. Primary treatment of these tumors is resection. In the case of cystic tumors the neural nodular component is the object of treatment. Solid tumors, especially solid tumors of the brain stem, are exceedingly difficult to treat because of their vascularity. As a result of the high mortality reported for resection of lesions in that location, these tumors are irradiated without a positive tissue diagnosis at times. Adjuvant irradiation with tumor dose of 5500 cGy or less is indicated in cases not amenable to operation, those with incomplete removal of the hemangioblastoma, and those with recurrence.

DERMOID AND EPIDERMOID TUMORS

Dermoid and epidermoid tumors of the nervous system arise from embryonic skin cells. They are called epidermoid tumors when composed only of epithelial cells and dermoid tumors when epithelial cells, sebaceous glands, and hair follicles are included. The former are cystic, and both grow slowly. However, they are capable of displacing the orbit or brain when located in the orbital roof or skull. Intracranial tumors occur most often in the midline, and their increasing size compresses the cerebellum, cerebral hemispheres, and midbrain. They also occur in both the spinal canal and parenchyma of the cord. The intracranial and spinal dermoid tumors may exhibit a tract extending to the surface.

Diagnosis depends on clinical symptoms of compression of orbit, brain, spinal cord, and cauda equina and the appearance of computerized tomograms or magnetic resonance scans. The presence of a sinus tract extending from the surface is helpful in establishing the diagnosis as well. Treatment consists of ablative procedures. Tumors of the orbit and cranium are excised and often require plastic repair. Intracranial and spinal tumors are approached conservatively, especially when there are few or no symptoms. Reducing the size of the tumors may be sufficient to improve the symptoms without the appearance of undesirable sequellae as a result of resection. These complications of operation are more prone to occur after spinal than intracranial procedures.

PRIMITIVE NEUROECTODERMAL TUMORS

Primitive neuroectodermal tumors are rare malignancies requiring enhanced computerized tomography, myelograms, and examination of the cerebrospinal fluid for diagnosis. They include ependymoblastomas, medulloepitheliomas, neuroblastomas, pineoblastomas, and spongioblastomas. Treatment consists of surgical debulking and irradiation of the entire cerebrospinal axis in most cases. (Neuroblastomas may not require irradiation of the spine.) These tumors respond to chemotherapy with cyclophosphamide, lomustine, procarbazine, and teniposide alone and in various combinations with other drugs such as dexamethasone and methotrexate.

TUMORS OF THE SPINAL CORD

Tumors of the spinal cord may be secondary to intracranial tumors or primary in the cord. Extradural and both intra- and extramedullary intradural tumors of the spine are discussed under the headings of the various types of tumors of the nervous system and are mentioned in this section in summary fashion. Intradural tumors include meningiomas, extramedullary neurilemmomas, chordomas, and epidermoid tumors. Intramedullary tumors include ependymomas, astrocytomas, oligodendrogliomas, medulloblastomas, hemangiomas, and hemangioblastomas. Extradural tumors include metastatic tumors, chordomas, and occasionally neurilemmomas and meningiomas. Tumors of the spine appear in locations from the foramen magnum to the cauda equina and sacral level, but some are found more often in some portions than others. For example, meningiomas appear most frequently in the thoracic spine, chordomas appear most frequently in the sacral region, whereas astrocytomas are distributed throughout the spinal axis.

Infiltration and compression of the segmental nerve roots lead to pain in the region of sensory nerve distribution and weakness. As these tumors increase in size and compress the cord, a syndrome ensues consisting of pain contralateral to the area of the cord affected and weakness. When there is destruction of the parenchyma of the cord, weakness, progressive sensory loss, and absence of reflexes occurs. After tentative diagnosis and localization by means of computerized tomography, magnetic resonance imaging, and possibly ultrasound and angiography, most of these tumors are explored and resected utilizing microsurgical techniques after laminectomy. Those with extradural extension may necessitate a two-stage procedure. Adjunctive radiotherapy is used for cases with incomplete removal of the neoplasm, those not amenable to resection, recurrence of the tumor, and those with prohibitive risk for operative therapy. The tumor dosage usually used is no higher than 5500 cGy. It is possible to increase the dosage for treating tumors that have led to complete destruction of neural function and those involving the cauda equina. Presumably the same chemotherapeutic agents and their combinations will produce responses in tumors of the spinal cord when they are useful as palliation for their intracranial counterpart. The expectation of a response from intrathecal chemotherapy is limited to treating micrometastases.

PRIMARY LYMPHOMA

Primary non-Hodgkin's lymphoma is found sporadically with low incidence, but the prevalence is increasing rapidly in association with the presence of Epstein-Barr and AIDS viruses, hereditary conditions such as Wiscott-Aldrich and ataxia-telangiectasis syndromes, and acquired immunosuppression such as that resulting from lupus erythematosus and immunosuppressive drugs

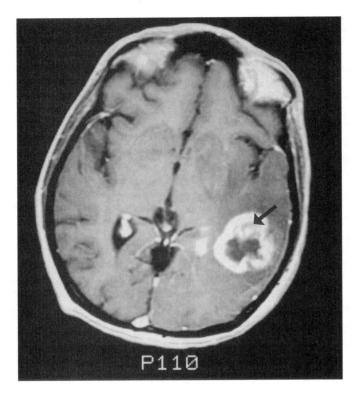

Figure 37 Nucleomagnetic resonance image of lymphoma of left parietal cerebral lobe.

utilized in organ transplantation. Symptoms include confusion, dementia, seizures, various neurologic abnormalities depending on localization of the lesion(s), headache, nausea, and vomiting. Diagnosis is reached by clinical examination, history, magnetic resonance imaging, examination of cerebrospinal fluid, and stereotactic needle biopsy. When the single lesion is very large with high intracranial pressure, it may be necessary to reduce the size of the tumor surgically. The largest of multiple tumors may also require this treatment. In addition, shunting may be indicated in some cases with high pressure and hydrocephalus that cannot be relieved otherwise. Irradiation of the whole brain with tumor dosage in the range of 4000 cGy without inclusion of the spinal axis is used in all but exceptional cases. Responses are obtained when intrathecal and systemic single and multiple chemotherapeutic agents are used adjuvant to radiation therapy. Primary lymphoma of the central nervous system responds to chemotherapy with cyclophosphamide, doxorubicin, vincristine, and prednisone (CHOP); also methotrexate in high dosage intravenously with or without intrathecal methotrexate or cytarabine. In acquired disease, other effects of the causal condition must be treated as well.

THIRTEEN

SECONDARY NEOPLASMS AND AIDS, GRAFTING, RADIATION, AND CHEMOTHERAPY

The incidence of AIDS, first diagnosed in 1981, has steadily increased in the global population at an alarming rate since that time. The groups originally found to be infected most often were intravenous drug users, homosexuals, and recipients of transfusions of infected blood. Heterosexuals, children of infected mothers, and medical personnel exposed to contaminated blood and body fluids now have become infected in increasing numbers. When the immunosuppression is not severe early in the course of the disease, it is labeled AIDS-related complex, which then progresses to the clinical syndrome of AIDS. When the immunodeficiency virus invades a cell, the viral DNA is converted to RNA by reverse transcriptase and is integrated into the cell where it multiplies. A receptor on the helper/inducer CD4 lymphocytes makes them attractive to the AIDS virus, which destroys these cells after invasion and replication. This impairs the immune response of the host sufficiently for the patients to become susceptible to ordinarily rare infections and tumors as a result of the immunoincompetence. Infection with these viruses has resulted in a worldwide plague consisting of a fatal disease for which all therapeutic measures have proved only to be palliative. Unless effective new drugs or improved manipulation of cellular components, such as the CD4 receptor and chemokine receptor 5 (CKR5), are found, the current distressing mortality is likely to continue.

Infecting organisms that are ordinarily combated effectively by helper CD4 T cells are those causing the greatest havoc in patients with AIDS. Among those encountered are *Aspergillus, Candida, Cryptococcus,* cytomegalovirus, hepatitis and herpes viruses, *Histoplasma, Legionella, Listeria, Mucor, Mycobacterium, Nocardia, Pneumocystis carinii, Salmonella typhimurium, Strongyloides, Toxoplasma,* and *Zygomycetes.* These infections lead to a multiplicity of medical and surgical problems in these debilitated patients. Leukoencephalopathy is an additional problem often encountered.

NEOPLASMS IN PATIENTS WITH AIDS

In addition to many other clinical problems, the characteristic immunosuppression in AIDS leads to an increase in the appearance of secondary tumors including melanomas, basal and squamous carcinomas, and astrocytomas. Those appearing most frequently are Kaposi's sarcoma and non-Hodgkin's lymphoma. The former was known as an unusual cutaneous tumor appearing in Mediterranean men. In AIDS patients it may become quite widespread and extend into the alimentary tract, lungs, and liver. With gastrointestinal involvement, management is especially difficult and leads to obstruction, ileocolitis, perforation, hemorrhage, and malabsorption. The prognosis can be very poor, and surgical intervention may be necessary. Recommended chemotherapy for Kaposi's sarcoma is daunomycin; liposomal doxorubicin; and bleomycin, doxorubicin, and vincristine or vinblastine (ABV). Single agents eliciting responses alone are doxorubicin; etoposide; interferon alfa; paclitaxel; vinblastine; and vincristine. When used as chemotherapy for Kaposi's sarcoma in patients with AIDS, management requires great skill. The lymphomas may cause obstruction and hemorrhage and also may require operative removal of tumors or bypass. Chemotherapy and radiation treatment have the major disadvantage of increasing immunosuppression, which can lead directly to a fatal outcome.

SECONDARY NEOPLASMS FOLLOWING ALLOGRAFTING

An increase in the numbers, unusual behavior, and distribution of secondary neoplasms is also a complication of organ and bone marrow allografting. The types of neoplasms encountered in increased numbers most often include squamous carcinoma of the skin, non-Hodgkin's lymphoma, Kaposi's sarcoma, carcinoma of vulva and perineum, carcinoma in situ of the cervix, carcinoma of the kidney, and hepatoma. Those appearing with the least time of induction are Kaposi's sarcomas, which may appear within the first year. On the other hand, carcinomas of the vulva and perineum may not be found until a decade after transplantation. The neoplasms treated most easily and successfully are carcinomas in situ of the uterine cervix, low-grade malignancies of the skin, and carcinomas in situ of the vulva and perineum. Recipients of nonrenal allografts are more prone to develop potentially life-threatening neoplasms, chiefly lymphomas, difficult to treat successfully. Lymphoproliferative disorders and solid tumors are seen with increased frequency following bone marrow transplantation. Xenografting and effective manipulation of the immune system to meet the problem of secondary tumors now encountered after allografting are goals not yet achieved.

SECONDARY NEOPLASMS FOLLOWING IRRADIATION

Data for secondary neoplasms resulting from nuclear bomb explosions which may be as much as 5 Gy whole body irradiation and the incidence of cancer in uranium miners have substantiated the carcinogenic effects of irradiation in human populations. This information and that obtained following radiotherapy alone and with chemotherapy confirm the increased incidence of neoplasms such as leukemia and carcinomas of the lung, breast, thyroid, bone, connective tissue, and stomach in survivors following radiotherapy for a primary cancer. There is a clear relationship between the incidence of secondary tumors and dosage to the site and with the passage of time. Leukemias begin to appear within a few years, but solid tumors may occur as long as 2 decades later. Irradiation during childhood is especially risky for subsequent sequellae including additional tumors. Radiodiagnostic studies including the use of radioisotopes are known to cause some increase in secondary cancers, but the numbers are very small in comparison to those following radiotherapy.

SECONDARY NEOPLASMS FOLLOWING CHEMOTHERAPY

The large numbers of patients given chemotherapy with or without radiotherapy for carcinoma of the breast, Hodgkin's disease, and tumors in childhood with prolonged survival have provided the opportunity for cohort, case-control, and other studies leading to much objective evidence for the causal relationship between chemotherapy and the appearance of secondary neoplasms. The predominant type of neoplasm is acute nonlymphocytic leukemia. Secondary leukemias after treatment of Hodgkin's disease are related most often to cumulative dosage of alkylating agents. The number of leukemias occurring after treatment of neoplasms of the breast with alkylating agents such as melphalan is 10 times greater than the number following treatment with cyclophosphamide. The primary neoplasm in childhood whose treatment results in the greatest incidence of secondary cancer is retinoblastoma followed by Hodgkin's disease, rhabdomyosarcoma, Ewing's tumor, Wilms' tumor, and Hodgkin's disease. The secondary malignancy occurring with greatest frequency following treatment of these tumors is bone sarcoma followed by rhabdomyosarcoma, leukemia, and tumors of the brain, thyroid, and breast. The secondary tumors often differ in behavior, response to treatment, and other characteristics compared with primary neoplasms. There is a relationship between total dosage of chemotherapeutic agent and the number of secondary neoplasms appearing. The response in terms of the etiology of secondary cancer following transplantation, radiotherapy, and chemotherapy undoubtedly is modified by host factors such as smoking, age at the time of exposure, acquired immunodeficiencies, and genetic abnormalities of chromosomes, oncogenes, and suppressor genes. Since the risk of secondary neoplasms is greater after treatment with some chemotherapeutic compounds than after treatment with others, this basis for selection of the regimen to use is an additional consideration in the choice of agent(s) when justified by expected extended length of survival.

REFERENCES

INTERNET ACCESS

Compendiums

Ferguson, T.: *Health Online.* Reading, Mass.: Addison-Wesley, 1996, p. 308.
Hogarth, M., and Hutchinson, D.: *An Internet Guide for the Health Professional.* Pub.
    by authors, 1996, p. 191.
Rosenfeld, L., Janes, J., and Vander Kolk, M.: *The Internet Compendium.* Neal-Schu-
    man, 1995, p. 529.

WebSites and Other Resources*

American Society of Clinical Oncology OnLine World Wide Web Site
    http://www.asco.org
Brain tumors
    http://132-183.1.64/abta/primer.htm
Breast cancer information center
    http://nysernet.org/bcic/
Breast cancer information clearing house
    http://www.rad.uhipi.it:7080/works/hcc/prentation-
Cancer net
    gopher.nik.gov/11/clin/cancernet

*Some sites require a fee.

Grateful med
  http://www.rlm.nih.gov/factsheets.dir/grateful.html
Gynecology oncology handbook
  http.//gynoncology.obgyn.washington.edu/documentation/
  GYN%20onc%20Handbook.html
Harvard med. library
  hollis.harvard.edu
Hepatocellular CA
  http://www.rad.uhipi.it:7080/works/hcc/prentation-hcc.html
Jefferson Cancer Center clinical trials
  http://www.jci.tju.edu/jcc/JCCProt.html
Libraries nationwide
  http://lcweb.loc.gov/23950/
Medline guide
  http://;www.sils.umich.edu/~nscherer/Medline/MedlineGuide.html
Michigan cancer center
  http://www.cancer.med.umich.edu
National cancer center Tokyo
  gopher.ncc.go.jp
News Groups
  sci.med.diseases.cancer
  alt.support.cancer
  1-800-4CANCER
  sci.med
  alt.support.cancer.prostate
  alt.support.ostomy
Oncolink. U. Pennsylvania cancer resource
  http://www.oncolink/upenn/edu/
  http://cancer.med.upenn.edu
Pain, practice guidelines for cancer
  http://www.stat.washington.edu/TALARIA/TALARIA.html
Pediatric cancer
  http://oncolink.upenn.edu/disease/pediatric.html
Pediatric oncology group
  http://pog.ufl.edu/
Sloan-Kettering Institute
  http://www.ski.mskcc.org/
Telescan (European)
  http://telescan.nki.nl:80/
TransWeb (transplantation)
  http://www.med.umich.edu:80/trans/transweb/
TX cancer data
  txcancer.mda.uth.tum.edu
UCSF Galen Library
  http://www.library.ucsf.edu
University of Texas M.D. Anderson Cancer Center
  http://utmdacc.uth.tmc.edu/MDA/mdainfo.html
U.S. National Library of Medicine
  gopher.nlm.nih.gov

U.S. National Library of Medicine HyperDoc
  http://www.nlm.nih.gov/
Virtual hospital
  http://www.vh.radiology.uiowa.edu/

BIBLIOGRAPHY

Cancer of the Skin and Melanoma

Barth, A., and Morton, D.L.: The role of adjuvant therapy in melanoma management. *Cancer* (Suppl) **75:**726–734, 1995.

Bridgewater, J.A., and Gore, J.E.: Biological response modifiers in melanoma. *Brit Med Bull* **51:**631–646, 1995.

Evans, R.A.: Elective lympyh node dissection for malignant melanoma: The tumor burden of nodal disease (Rev). *Anticanc Res* **15:**575–579, 1995.

Goldberg, I.H.: Basal cell carcinoma (Rev). *Lancet* **347:**663–667, 1996.

Grevey, S.C., Zax, R.H., and McCall, M.W.: Melanoma and Mohs' micrographic surgery (Rev). *Adv Dermatol* **10:**175–198, 1995.

Harris, M.N., Shapiro, R.L., and Roses, D.F.: Malignant melanoma. Primary surgical management (excision and node dissection) based on pathology and staging. *Cancer* **75:**715–725, 1995.

Ho, R.C.: Medical management of stage IV malignant melanoma. (Rev). *Cancer* **75:**735–741, 1995.

Johnson, T.M., Smith, J.W., Nelson, B.R., and Chang, A.: Current therapy for cutaneous melanoma. *J Am Acad Dermatol* **32:**689–707, 1995.

Marks, R.: Squamous cell carcinoma (Rev). *Lancet* **347:**735–738, 1996.

Rudenstam, C.M.: Open trials in cutaneous malignant melanoma (Rev). *Eur J Surg Oncol* **22:**128–130, 1996.

Stone, C.A., and Goodacre, T.E.: Surgical management of regional lymph nodes in primary cutaneous malignant melanoma (Rev). *Brit J Surg* **82:**1015–1022, 1995.

Urist, M.M.: Management of patients with intermediate-thickness melanoma (Rev). *Annu Rev Med* **47:**211–217, 1996.

Whooley, B.P., and Wallack, M.K.: Surgical management of melanoma. *Surg Oncol* **4:**1878–1895, 1995.

Carcinoma of the Breast

Bearman, S.I.: High-dose chemotherapy with autologous hematopoietic progenitor cell support for metastatic and high-risk primary breast cancer (Rev). *Sem Oncol* (Suppl 2) **23:**60–67, 1996.

Daniel, Y., Inbar, M., Bar-Am., A., and Peyser, M.R.: The effect of tamoxifen treatment on the endometrium (Rev). *Fertil Steril* **65:**1083–1089, 1996.

Fisher, B., Redmond, C., Poisson, R., et al.: Eight year results of a randomized clinical trial comparing total mastectomy and lumpectomy with or without irradiation in the treatment of breast cancer. *N Engl J Med* **320:**822–828, 1989.

DiFronzo, L.A., and O'Connell, T.X.: Breast cancer in pregnancy and lactation (Rev). *Surg Clin North Am* **76:**267–278, 1996.

Harris, L., and Swain, S.M.: The role of primary chemotherapy in early breast cancer (Rev). *Sem Oncol* **23:**31–42, 1996.

Hayes, D.F.: Serum (circulating) tumor markers for breast cancer. (Rev). *Rec Results Cancer Res* **140:**101–113, 1996.

Hughes, K.S., Lee, K.A., and Rolfs, A.: Controversies in the treatment of ductal carcinoma in situ (Rev). *Surg Clin North Am* **76:**243–265, 1996.

Kaufmann, M.: Review of known prognostic variables (Rev). *Rec Results Cancer Res* **140:**77–87, 1996.

Law, T.M., Hesketh, P.J., Porter, K.A., Lawn-Tsao, L., and Lopez, M.J.: Breast cancer in elderly women: Presentation, survival, and treatment options (Rev). *Surg Clin North Am* **76:**289–308, 1996.

Leonard, R.C.: High-dose chemotherapy for breast cancer: The case for trials in adjuvant therapy (Rev). *J Roy Soc Med* **89:**337–339, 1996.

Lopez, M.J., and Porter, K.A.: Inflammatory breast cancer (Rev). *Surg Clin North Am* **76:** 411–429, 1996.

Macmillan, R.D., Purushotham, A.D., and George, W.D.: Local recurrence after breast-conserving surgery for breast cancer (Rev). *Brit J Surg* **83:**149–155, 1996.

Noguchi, M., Kinne, D.W., and Miyazaki, I.: Breast-conserving controversies and consensus (Rev). *J Surg Oncol* **62:** 228–234, 1996.

Radford, D.M., and Zehnbauer, B.A.: Inherited breast cancer (Rev). *Surg Clin North Am* **76:**205–220, 1996.

Recht, A.: Selection of patients with early stage invasive breast cancer for treatment with conservative surgery and radiation therapy (Rev). *Sem Oncol* **23:**19–30, 1996.

Sabel, M., and Aichinger, H.: Recent developments in breast imaging (Rev). *Phys Med Biol* **41:**315–368, 1996.

Seidman, A.D.: Chemotherapy for advanced breast cancer: a current perspective (Rev). *Sem Oncol* (Suppl 2) **23:**55–59, 1996.

Styblo, T.M., and Wood, W.C.: Adjuvant chemotherapy in the node-negative breast cancer patient (Rev). *Surg Clin North Am* **76:**327–341, 1996.

Veronesi, U. and Zurrida, S.: Breast cancer surgery: A century after Halsted (Rev). *J Cancer Res Clin Oncol* **122:**74–77, 1996.

Williams, W.L. Jr., Powers, M., and Wagman, L.D.: Cancer of the male breast (Rev). *J Natl Med Assoc* **88:**439–443, 1996.

Winchester, D.P.: Breast cancer in young women (Rev). *Surg Clin North Am* **76:**279–287, 1996.

Neoplasms of the Head and Neck

Alvi, A., and Stegnjajic, A.: Sternocleidomastoid myofascial flap for head and neck reconstruction. *Head Neck* **16:**326–330, 1994.

Armstrong, J., Harrison, I., Sprio, R., et al.: The role of postoperative radiation therapy in maligant salivary gland tumors: A matched pair analysis using historic controls. *Int J Rad Oncol Biol Phys* **15:**176–180, 1988.

Awde, J.D., Kogon, S.L., and Morin, R.J.: Lip cancer: A review. *J Can Dent Assoc* **62:**634–636, 1996.

Benninger, M.S., Enrique, R.R., and Nichols, R.D.: Symptom-directed selective endoscopy and cost containment for evaluation of head and neck cancer. *Head Neck* **15:**532–536, 1993.

Chang, L., Stevens, K.R., Moss, W.T., et al.: Squamous cell carcinoma of the pharyngeal walls treated with radiotherapy (Rev). *Int J Rad Oncol Biol Phys* **35:**477–483, 1996.

Dreyfuss, A.L., et al.: Continuous infusion high-dose leucovorin with 5-fluorouracil and cisplatin for untreated stage IV carcinoma of the head and neck. *Ann Intern Med* **112:**167–172, 1990.

Ervin, Tk.J., et al.: An analysis of induction chemotherapy in the multidisciplinary treatment of squamous cell carcinoma of the head and neck. *J Clin Oncol* **5:**10–20, 1987.

Fee, W.E. Jr., Gilmer, P.A., and Goffinet, D.R.: Surgical management of recurrent nasopharyngeal carcinoma after radiation failure at the primary site. *Laryngoscope* **98:**1220–1226, 1988.

Givens, C.D., Johns, M.E., and Cantrell, R.W.: Carcinoma of the tonsil. *Arch Otolaryngol* **107:**730–734, 1981.

Ishiyami, A., Eversole, L.R., Ross, D.A., et al.: Papillary squamous neoplasms of the head and neck. *Laryngoscope* **104:**1446–1452, 1994.

Ioannides, D., Fossion, E., Boeck, W., et al.: Surgical management of the osteoradionecrotic mandible with free vascularised composite flaps. *J Cranio-Maxillo-Facial Surg* **22:**330–334, 1994.

Kempf, H.G., Becker, G., Weber, B.P., et al.: Diagnostic and clinical outcome of neurogenic tumours in the head and neck area. *J Oto-Rhino-Laryngol Related Spec* **57:**273–278, 1995.

Milroy, C.M., and Ferlito, A.: Immunohistochemical markers in the diagnosis of neuroendocrine neoplasms of the head and neck (Rev). *Ann Otol Rhinol Laryngol* **104:**413–418, 1995.

Myers, E.N., and Alvi, A.: Management of carcinoma of the supraglottic larynx: evolution, current concepts, and future trends (Rev). *Laryngoscope* **106:**559–567, 1996.

Qin, D.X., Hu, Y.H., Yan, J.H., et al.: Analysis of 1379 patients with nasopharyngeal carcinoma treated by radiation. *Cancer* **61:**1117–1124, 1988.

Rafla, S.: Malignant parotid tumors: Natural history and treatment. *Cancer* **40:**136–144, 1977.

Shohet, J.A., and Duncavage, J.A.: Management of the frontal sinus with inverted papilloma (Rev). *Otolaryngol-Head Neck Surg* **114:** 649–652, 1996.

Sugarman, P.R., Joseph, B.K., and Savage, N.W.: The role of oncogenes, tumour suppressor genes and growth factors in oral squamous cell carcinomas: A case of apoptosis versus proliferation (Rev). *Oral Dis* **1:**2–88, 1995.

Toohill, R.F., et al.: Cisplatin and 5-fluorouracil as neoadjuvant therapy in head and neck cancer. *Arch Otolaryngol* **113:**758–761, 1987.

Zimmer, W., and DeLuca, S.A.: Primary tracheal neoplasms: recognition, diagnosis and evaluation (Rev). *Am Fam Physician* **45:**2651–2657, 1992.

Thyroid Neoplasms

Azadian, A., Rosen, I.B., Walfish, P.G., and Asa, S.L.: Management considerations in Hürthle cell carcinoma (Rev). *Surgery* **118:**711–714, 1995.

Clark, O.H.: Recurrent thyroid cancer (Rev). *J Endocrin Invest* **18:**167–169, 1995.

Farid, N.R., Zou, M., and Shi, Y.: Genetics of follicular thyroid cancer (Rev). *Endocrin Metabol Clin North Am* **24:**865–883, 1995.

Grebe, S.K., and Hay, I.D.: Follicular thyroid cancer (Rev). *Endocrin Metabol Clin North Am* **24:**761–801, 1995.

Houston, R.S., and Stratton, M.R.: Genetics of non-medullary thyroid cancer (Rev). *Quart J Med* **88:**685–693, 1995.

Ladenson, P.W.: Optimal laboratory testing for diagnosis and monitoring of thyroid nodules, goiter, and thyroid cancer (Rev). *Clin Chem* **42:**183–187, 1996.

Moley, J.F.: Medullary thyroid cancer (Rev). *Surg Clin North Am* **75:**405–420, 1995.

Patwardhan, N., Cataldo, T., and Braverman, L.E.: Surgical management of the patient with papillary cancer (Rev). *Surg Clin North Am* **75:**449–464, 1995.

Sweeney, D.C., and Johnston, G.S.: Radioiodine therapy for thyroid cancer (Rev). *Endocrin Metab Clin North Am* **24:**803–839, 1995.

Takahashi, M.: Oncogenic activation of the ret protooncogene in thyroid cancer (Rev). *Crit Rev Oncogen* **6:**35–46, 1995.

Tezelman, S., and Clark, O.H.: Current management of thyroid cancer. (Rev). *Advan Surg* **28:**191–221, 1995.

Vasen, H.F., and Vermey, A.: Hereditary medullary thyroid carcinoma (Rev). *Cancer Detect Prevent* **19:**143–150, 1995.

Parathyroid Cancer

Cohn, K., Silverman, M., Corrado, J., and Sedgewick, C.: Parathyroid carcinoma: The Lahey Clinic experience. *Surgery* **98:**1095, 1985.

Kitapci, M.T., Tastekin, G., Turgut, M., et al.: Preoperative localization of parathyroid carcinoma using Tc-99m MIBI. *Clin Nucl Med* **18:**217–219, 1993.

Rosen, I.B., Young, J.E., Archibald, S.D., et al.: Parathyroid cancer: Clinical variations and relationship to autotransplantation. *Can J Surg* **37:**465–469, 1994.

Sandelin, K., Tullgren, O., and Farnebo, L.O.: Clinical course of metastatic parathyroid cancer. *World J Surg* **18:**594–688, 1994.

Shen, W., Duren, M., Morita, E., et al.: Reoperation for persistent or recurrent primary hyperparathyroidism (Rev). *Arch Surg* **131:**861–867, 1996.

Sloan, D.A., Schwartz, R.W., Mcgrath, P.C., and Kenady, D.A.: Diagnosis and management of thyroid and parathyroid hyperplasia and neoplasia (Rev). *Curr Opin Oncol* **7:**47–55, 1995.

Wassif, W.S., Moniz, C.F., Friedman, E., et al.: Familial isolated hyperparathyroidism: A distinct genetic entity with an increased risk of parathyroid cancer. *J Clin Endocrinol Metabol* **77:**1485–1489, 1993.

Neoplasms of the Adrenal

Brown, J.P., Albala, D.M., and Jahoda, A.: Laparoscopic surgery for adrenal lesions (Rev). *Sem Surg Oncol* **12:**96–99, 1996.

Brunt, L.M., Doherty, G.M., Norton, J.A., et al.: Laparoscopic adrenalectomy compared to open adrenalectomy for benign adrenal neoplasms. *J Am Coll Surg* **183:**1–10, 1996 (Comment in *J Am Coll Surg* **183:**71–73, 1996).

Gross, M.D., Shapiro, B., Francis, I.R., et al.: Scintigraphic evaluation of clinically silent adrenal masses. *J Nucl Med* **35:**1145–1152, 1954 (Comment in *J Nucl Med* **35:**1152–1154, 1994, and **36:**1727–1728, 1995).

Guazzoni, G., Montorsi, F., Bergamaschi, F., et al.: Effectiveness and safety of laparoscopic adrenalectomy. *J Urol* **152:**1375–1378, 1994.

Gutierrez, M.L., and Crooke, S.T.: Mitotane (*o,p*-DDD). *Cancer Treat Rev* **7:**49, 1980.

Huch Boni, R.A., Debatin, J.F., and Krestin, G.P.: Contrast-enhanced MR imaging of the kidneys and adrenal glands (Rev). *Mag Res Imag Clin North Am* **4:**101–131, 1996.

Lamberts, S.W.: Endocrine tumors (Rev). *Canc Chemother Biol Response Mod* **16:**511–523, 1996.

Lin, S.R., Lee, Y.J., and Tsai, J.H.: Mutations of the *p53* gene in human functional adrenal neoplasms. *J Clin Endocrin Metabol* **78:**483–491, 1994.

Percarpio, B., and Knowlton, A.H.: Radiation therapy of adrenal cortical carcinoma. *Acta Radiol Ther Phys Biol* **15:**288, 1976.

Sullivan, M., Boileau, M., and Hodges, C.V.: Adrenal cortical carcinoma. *J Urol* **120:**660, 1978.

Carcinoids

Davis, K.P., Hartman, L.K., Keeney, G.L., and Shapiro, H.: Primary ovarian carcinoid tumors (Rev). *Gynecol Oncol* **61:**259–265, 1996.

Lamberts, S.W., Van Der Lely, A.J., De Herder, W.W., and Hofland, L.J.: Octreotide (Rev). *N Engl J Med* **334:**246–254, 1966.

Perry, R.R., and Vinik, A.I.: Endocrine tumors of the gastrointestinal tract, (Rev). *Annu Rev Med* **47:**57–68, 1996.

Thompson, G.B., vanHeerden, J.A., Martin, J.K., et al.: Carcinoid tumors of the gastrointestinal tract: Presentation, management, and prognosis. *Surgery* **98:**1054, 1985.

Pheochromocytoma

Beierwaltes, W.H., Sisson, J.C., Shapiro, B., et al.: Malignant potential of pheochromocytoma. *Proc Am Assoc Cancer Res* **27:**647, 1986.

Cooper, M.J., Helman, L.J., and Israel, M.A.: Molecular biology and the pathogenesis of neuroblastoma and pheochromocytoma. *Cancer Cells* **7:**95, 1989.

Fink, I.J., Reinig, J.W., Dwyer, A.J., et al.: MR imaging of pheochromocytomas. *J Comput Assist Tomogr* **9:**454, 1985.

Glowniak, J.V., Shapiro, B., Sisson, J.C., et al.: Familial extra-adrenal pheochromocytoma. *Arch Intern Med* **145:**145–257, 1985.

Greenberg, M., Moawad, A.H., Wietles, B.M., et al.: Extraadrenal pheochromocytoma. Detection during pregnancy using MR imaging. *Radiology* **161:**475, 1986.

Irvin, G.I., Fishman, I.M., Sher, J.A., et al.: Pheochromocytoma lateral vs. anterior operative approach. *Ann Surg* **209:**774–776, 1989.

Shapiro, B., Copp, J.E., Sisson, J.C., et al.: Iodine-131 metaiodobenzylguanidine for locating suspected pheochromocytoma: Experience in 400 cases. *J Nucl Med* **26:**576, 1985.

Sheps, S.G., Jiang, N.S., Klee, G.G., and Heerden, J.A.: Recent developments in the diagnosis and management of pheochromocytoma. *Proc Mayo Clin* **65:**88, 1990.

Multiple Endocrine Neoplasms

Bordi, C.: Endocrine tumours of the stomach (Rev). *Path Res Pract* **191:**373–380, 1995.

Gagel, R.F.: Putting the bits and pieces of the RET proto-oncogene puzzle together (Rev). *Bone* **17** (Suppl):13S–16S, 1995.

Goodfellow, P.J., and Wells, S.A. Jr.: RET gene and its implications for cancer (Rev). *J Natl Cancer Inst* **87:**1515–1523, 1995.

Holloway, K.B., and Flowers, F.P.: Multiple endocrine neoplasia 2B (MEN 2B/MEN 3) (Rev). *Dermatol Clin* **13:**99–103, 1995.

Kousseff, B.G.: Multiple endocrine neoplasia 2 (MEN 2/MEN 2a) (Sipple syndrome) (Rev). *Dermatol Clin* **13:**91–97, 1995.

Metz, D.C.: Multiple endocrine neoplasia type I. (Rev). *Sem Gastrointest Dis* **6:**56–66, 1995.

Mulligan, L.M., and Ponder, B.A.: Genetic basis of endocrine disease: Multiple endocrine neoplasia type 2 (Rev). *J Clin Endocrinol Metabol* **80:**1989–1995, 1995.

Padberg, B., Schroder, S., Capella, C., et al.: Multiple endocrine neoplasia type 1 (MEN 1) revisited. (Rev). *Virchow's Archiv* **426:**541–548, 1995.

Perry, R.R., and Vinik, A.I.: Endocrine tumors of the gastrointestinal tract (Rev). *Annu Rev Med* **47:**57–68, 1996.

Rindi, G.: Clinicopathologic aspects of gastric neuroendocrine tumors (Rev). *Am J Surg Pathol* **1** (Suppl):S20–S29, 1995.

Takahashi, M.: Oncogenic activation of the RET proto-oncogene in thyroid cancer. (Rev). *Crit Rev Oncogen* **6:**35–46, 1995.

Teh, B.T., Grimmond, S., Shepherd, J., et al.: Multiple endocrine neoplasia type I: Clinical syndrome to molecular genetics. (Rev). *Aust N Z J Surg* **65:**708–713, 1995.

Paragangliomas

Bak, J., Olsson, Y., Grimelius, L., and Spannare, B.: Paraganglioma of the cauda equina. A case report and review of literature. *APMIS* **104:**234–240, 1996.

Nguyen, Q.A., Gibbs, P.M., and Rice, D.H.: Malignant nasal paraganglioma: A case report and review of the literature. *Otolaryngol-Head Neck Surg* **113:**157–161, 1995.

Skodt, V., Jacobsen, G.K., and Helsted M.: Primary paraganglioma of the lung. Report of two cases and review of the literature. *APMIS* **103:**597–603, 1995.

Tomic, S., and Warner, T.: Pancreatic somatostatin-secreting gangliocytic paraganglioma with lymph node metastases. (Rev). *Am J Gastroenterol* **91:**607–608, 1996.

Neoplasms of the Lung

Burt, M., Wronski, A., Arbit, E., and Salicich, J.H.: Resection of brain metastases from non-small cell lung carcinoma. *J Thorac Cardiovasc Surg* **103:**399–441, 1992.

Crawford, J.: Update: Vinorelbine (Navelbine) in non-small cell lung cancer (Rev). *Sem Oncol* **23** (Suppl 5):2–7, 1996.

Cohen, M.C., and Kaschula, R.O.: Primary pulmonary tumors in childhood: a review of 31 years' experience and the literature. *Pediat Pulmonol* **14:**222–232, 1992.

Davila, D.G., Dunn, W.F., Tazelaar, H.D., and Pairolero, P.C.: Bronchial carcinoid tumors (Rev). *Mayo Clin Proc* **68**:795–803, 1993.

Edelman, M.J., and Gandara, D.R.: Promising new agents in the treatment of non-small cell lung cancer (Rev). *Canc Chemother Pharmacol* **37**:385–393, 1996.

Ettinger, D.S.: Ifosfamide in the treatment of small-cell lung cancer (Rev). *Sem Oncol* **23** (Suppl 6):2–6, 1996.

Flint, A.: Detection of pulmonary neoplasms by bronchial washings. Are cell blocks a diagnostic aid? *Acta Cytol* **37**:21–23, 1993.

Goldberg, B.B., Steiner, R.M., Lie, J.B., et al.: US-assisted bronchoscopy with use of miniature transducer-containing catheters. *Radiology* **190**:233–237, 1994 (Comment in *Radiology* **192**:579–580, 1994).

Grillo, H.C., and Mathiesen, D.J.: Primary tracheal tumors: Treatment and results. *Annu Thorac Surg* **49**:69–77, 1990.

Hancock, B.J., Di Lorenzo, M., Youssef, S., et al.: Childhood primary pulmonary neoplasms (Rev). *J Pediatr Surg* **28**:1133–1136, 1993.

Hays, M.M., Zhang, D.Y., and Brown, W.: Transthoracic fine-needle aspiration biopsy cytology of pulmonary neoplasms. *Diag Cytopathol* **10**:315–319, 1994.

Johnson, D.H.: Ifosfamide in non-small cell lung cancer (Rev). *Sem Oncol* **23** (Suppl 6):7–10, 1996.

Loehrer, P.J. Sr.: The role of ifosfamide in small-cell lung cancer (Rev). *Sem Oncol* **23** (Suppl 7):140–144, 1996.

Marchevsky, A.M.: Lung tumors derived from ectopic tissues (Rev). **12**:172–184, 1995.

Muller, D.L., and Allen, M.S.: Rare pulmonary neoplasms. *Mayo Clin Proc* **68**:492–498, 1993.

Nestle, U., Nieder, C., Abel, U., et al.: A palliative accelerated irradiation regimen (PAIR) for advanced non-small-cell lung cancer (Rev). *Radiother Oncol* **38**:195–203, 1996.

Radermecker, M.A., Ghaye, B., Dekoster, G., and Limet, R.: "A priori" resectability of non-small cell pulmonary neoplasms in relation to the new international classification (Rev). *Rev Med Liege* **50**:264–267, 1995.

Shahidi, H., and Kvale, P.A.: Long-term survival following surgical treatment of solitary brain metastasis in non-small cell lung cancer (Rev). *Chest* **109**:1271–1276, 1996.

Shepherd, F.A., et al.: Is there ever a role for salvage operation in small-cell lung cancer. *J Thorac Cardiovasc Surg* **101**:196–200, 1991.

Thatcher, N., Niven, R.M., and Anderson, H.: Aggressive vs. nonaggressive therapy for metastatic non-small cell lung cancer (Rev). *Chest* **109** (Suppl):S87–S92, 1996.

Mesothelioma

Aisner, J., et al.: Current approach to malignant mesothelioma of the pleura. *Chest* **107** (Suppl 6):3325–3445, 1995.

Ball, D.L., and Cruickshank, D.G.: The treatment of malignant mesothelioma of the pleura: Review of a 5-year experience with special reference to radiotherapy. *Am J Clin Oncol* **13**:4–9, 1990.

DeValle, M.J., Faber, L.P., and Kittle, C.F.: Extrapleural pneumonectomy for diffuse malignant mesothelioma. *Ann Thorac Surg* **42**:612, 1986.

Colleoni, M., et al.: Surgery followed by intracavitary plus systemic chemotherapy in malignant pleural mesothelioma. *Tumori* **82**:53–56, 1996.

Harvey, J.C., et al.: Diffuse malignant mesothelioma: Options in surgical treatment. *Compr Ther* **21:**13–19, 1995.

Hunt, K.J., et al.: Treatment of malignant mesothelioma with methotrexate and vinblastine with or without platinum chemotherapy. *Chest* **109:**1239–1242, 1996.

Lippman, M.: Deposition and retention of inhaled fibres: Effects on incidence of lung cancer and mesothelioma. *Occup Environ Med* **51:**793–798, 1994.

Martini, N., McCormach, P.M., Baines, M.S., et al.: Pleural mesothelioma. *Ann Thorac Surg* **43:**113, 1987.

Moreno de la Sante, P., et al.: Therapy options in malignant mesothelioma. *Curr Opin Oncol* **17:**134–137, 1995.

Robinson, L.A., et al: Localized pleural mesothelioma. The clinical spectrum. *Chest* **106:**1611–1615, 1994.

Sugarbaker, D.J., Lee, T.H., Coupe, G., et al.: Extrapleural pneumonectomy, chemotherapy, and radiotherapy in the treatment of diffuse malignant pleural mesothelioma. *J Thorac Cardiovasc Surg* **102:**10–15, 1991.

Mediastinal Neoplasms

Boston, B.: Chemotherapy of invasive thymoma. *Cancer* **38:**49, 1976.

Ginsberg, R.J.: Mediastinal germ cell tumors: The role of surgery (Rev). *Sem Thorac Cardiovasc Surg* **4:**51–54, 1992.

Golbey, R.B.: Mediastinal germ cell tumors. A continuing odyssey (Rev). *Chest Surg Clin North Am* **4:** 195–200, 1994.

Kantoff, P.: Surgical and medical management of germ cell tumors of the chest (Rev). *Chest* **103** (Suppl):331–333, 1993.

Monden, Y., Nakahara, K., Kagotani, K., et al.: Myasthenia gravis with thymoma: Analysis of and postoperative prognosis for 65 patients with thymomatous myasthenia gravis. *Ann Thorac Surg* **38:**46, 1984.

Nakahara, K., Ohno, K., Hashimoto, K., et al.: Thymoma: Results with complete resection and adjuvant postoperative radiation in 141 consecutive patients. *J Thorac Cardiovasc Surg* **95:**1041, 1988.

Rodriguez, J., Pugh, W. C., Romaguera, J.E., and Cabanillas, F.: Primary mediastinal large cell lymphoma (Rev). *Hematol Oncol* **12:**175–184, 1994.

Neoplasms of the Esophagus

Bates, B.A., Detterbeck, F.C., Bernard, S.A., et al.: Concurrent radiation therapy and chemotherapy followed by esophagectomy for localized esophageal carcinoma. (Rev). *J Clin Oncol* **14:**156–163, 1996.

Burdette, W.J.: Palliative operation for carcinoma of cervical and thoracic esophagus. *Ann Surg* **173:**714–732, 1971.

Burdette, W.J., and Jess, R.: Carcinoma of the cervical esophagus. *J Thorac Cardiovasc Surg* **63:**41–53, 1972.

Clark, G.W., and DeMeester, T.R.: Surgical management of Barrett's esophagus (Rev). *Ann Chir Gynecol* **84:**139–144, 1995.

Coleman, J.J. 3d: Reconstruction of the pharynx and cervical esophagus (Rev). *Sem Surg Oncol* **11:**208–220, 1995.

Fink, U., Stein, H.J., Wilke, H., et al.: Multimodal treatment for squamous cell esophageal cancer (Rev). *World J Surg* **19**:198–204, 1995.

Gossot, D., Cattan, P., Fritsch, S., et al.: Can the morbidity of esophagectomy be reduced by the thoracoscopic approach? (Rev). *Surg Endosc* **9**:1113–1115, 1995.

Horstmann, O., Verreet, P.R., Becker, H., et al.: Transhiatal oesophagectomy compared with transthoracic resection and systematic lymphadenectomy for the treatment of oesophageal cancer (Rev). *Eur J Surg* **161**:557–567, 1995.

Iizuka, T.: Multimodal treatment of oesophageal carcinoma (Rev). *Ann Surg Gynecol* **84**:1216–1221, 1995.

Kelsun, D.P., and Ilson, D.H.: Chemotherapy and combined-modality therapy for esophageal cancer (Rev). *Chest* **107** (Suppl): 2245–2325, 1995.

Lightdale, C.J.: Detection of anastomotic recurrence by endoscopic ultrasonography (Rev). *Gastrointest Endosc Clin North Am* **5**:595–600, 1995.

Milhaire, J.P., Labat, J.P., Lozac, H.P., et al.: Preoperative concomitant radiochemotherapy in squamous cell carcinoma of the esophagus: Results of a study of 56 patients (Rev). *Int J Rad Oncol Biol Phys* **34**:429–437, 1996.

O'Rourke, I., Tait, N., Bull, C., et al.: Oesophageal cancer: Outcome of modern surgical management (Rev). *Aust N Z J Surg* **65**:11–16, 1995.

Recht, A.: The role of radiation therapy in treating patients with potentially resectable carcinoma of the esophagus (Rev). *Chest* **107** (Suppl):2335–2405, 1995.

Reed, C.E.: Comparison of different treatments for unresectable esophageal cancer (Rev). *World J Surg* **19**:828–835, 1995.

Tilamus, H.W.: Changing patterns in the treatment of carcinoma of the esophagus (Rev). *Scand J Gastroenterol* **212** (Suppl):38–42, 1995.

Neoplasms of the Infradiaphragmatic Gastrointestinal Tract

Adam, Y.G., and Efron, G.: Trends and controversies in the management of carcinoma of the stomach. *Surg Gynecol Obstet* **169**:371–385, 1990.

Allum, H., Powell, J., McConkey, C., and Fielding, J.W.L.: Gastric cancer: A 25 year review. *Br J Surg* **76**:535–540, 1989.

Anonymous: World progress in surgery: Management of adenocarcinoma of the low rectum. *World J Surg* **16**:428–515, 1992.

Avradopoulos, K.A., Vezeridis, M.P., and Wanebo, H.J.: Pelvic exenteration for recurrent rectal cancer (Rev). *Adv Surg* **29**:215–233, 1996.

Basha, G., and Penninck, F.: Exfoliated tumour cells and locally recurrent colorectal cancer (Rev). *Acta Chir Belg* **96**:66–70, 1996.

Bertagnolli, M.M., and DeCosse, J.J.: Laparoscopic colon resection for cancer—an unfavorable view. (Rev). *Adv Surg* **29**:155–164, 1996.

Bleiberg, H.: Role of chemotherapy for advanced colorectal cancer: New opportunities (Rev). *Sem Oncol* **23** (Suppl 3):42–50, 1996.

Brennan, M.F., and Karpeh, M.S. Jr.: Surgery for gastric cancer: The American view (Rev). *Sem Oncol* **23**:352–359, 1996.

Cavenna, E.: Outcome of restorative perineal graciloplasty with simultaneous excision of the anus and rectum for cancer. A ten-year experience with 81 patients. *Dis Colon Rectum* **39**:182–190, 1996.

Chen, F., and Stewart, M.: The morbidity of defunctioning stomata (Rev). *Aust N Z J Surg* **66**:218–221, 1996.

Chiarugi, M., Buccianti, P., Sidoti, F., et al.: Single and double stapled anastomoses in rectal cancer surgery; a retrospective study on the safety of the technique and its indication (Rev). *Acta Chir Bel* **96:**31–36, 1996.

Cortina, R.: Management and prognosis of carcinoma of the appendix (Rev). *Dis Colon Rectum* **38:**848–852, 1995.

Deans, G.T., and Spence, R.A.: Neoplastic lesions of the appendix (Rev). *Br J Surg* **82:**299–306, 1995.

Doci, R., Gennari, L., Bignami, P., et al.: One hundred patients with hepatic metastases from colorectal cancer treated by resection: Analysis of prognostic determinants. *Br J Surg* **78:**797–801, 1991.

Fountzilas, G., Gossios, K., Zisiadis, A., et al.: Prognostic variable in patients with advanced colorectal cancer treated with fluorouracil and leucovorin-based chemotherapy (Rev). *Med Pediat Oncol* **26:**305–317, 1996.

Fukushima, M.: Adjuvant therapy of gastric cancer: The Japanese experience (Rev). *Sem Oncol* **233:**69–78, 1996.

Gonderson, L.L.: Past, present, and future of intraoperative irradiation for colorectal cancer (Rev). *Int J Radiat Oncol Biol Phys* **34:**741–744, 1996.

Hirata, K., Kitahara, K., Momosaka, Y., et al.: Diffuse ganglioneuromatosis with plexiform neurofibromas limited to the gastrointestinal tract involving a large segment of small intestine (Rev). *J Gastroenterol* **31:**263–267, 1996.

Kelsen, D.P.: Adjuvant and neoadjuvant therapy for gastric cancer (Rev). *Sem Oncol* **23:**379–389, 1996.

Kerr, D.J., Gray, R.: Adjuvant chemotherapy for colorectal cancer (Rev). *Br J Hosp Med* **55:**259–262, 1996.

Lang, H., Jahne, J., Flemming, P., et al.: *Pseudomyxoma peritonei* of appendiceal origin. *Eur J Surg* **161:**355–360, 1995.

Martenson, J.A., Lipsitz, S.R., Wagner, H. Jr., et al.: Initial results of a phase II trial of high dose radiation therapy, 5-fluorouracil, and cisplatin for patients with anal cancer: An Eastern Cooperative Oncology Group study. *Int J Rad Oncol Biol Phys* **35:**745–749, 1996.

Maruyama, K., Sasako, M., Kinoshita, T., et al.: Surgical treatment for gastric cancer: The Japanese approach (Rev). *Sem Oncol* **23:**360–368, 1996.

Minsky, B.D.: The role of radiation therapy in gastric cancer (Rev). *Sem Oncol* **23:**390–396, 1996.

Noguchi, M., and Miyazaki, I.: Prognostic significance and surgical management of lymph node metastasis in gastric cancer (Rev). *Br J Surg* **83:**156–161, 1996.

Passman, M.A., Pommier, R.F., and Vetto, J.T.: Synchronous colon primaries have the same prognosis as solitary colon cancers (Rev). *Dis Colon Rectum* **39:**329–334, 1996.

Paterson, I.M., Easton, D.F., Corbishly, C.M., et al.: Changing distribution of adenocarcinoma of the stomach. *Br J Surg* **74:**481–482, 1987.

Ross, P.J., and Cunningham, D.: Chemotherapy of metastatic bowel cancer (Rev). *Br J Hosp Med* **55:**263–266, 1996.

Sager, P.M., and Pemberton, J.H.: Surgical management of locally recurrent rectal cancer (Rev). *Br J Surg* **83:**293–304, 1996.

Touboul, E., Schlienger, M., Buffat, L., et al.: Conservative versus nonconservative treatment of epidermoid carcinoma of the anal canal for tumors longer than or equal to 5 cm. *Cancer* **75:**786–793, 1995.

Vaughn, D.J., and Treat, J.: Cancers of the large bowel and hepatobiliary tract (Rev). *Cancer Chemother Biol Response Mod* **16:**495–510, 1996.

Wanebo, H.J., Chu, D.D., Avradopoulos, K.A., and Vezeridis, M.P.: Current perspectives on repeat hepatic resection of colorectal carcinomas; a review. *Surgery* **119:**361–371, 1996.

Wils, J.: The treatment of advanced gastric cancer (Rev). *Sem Oncol* **23:**397–406, 1996.

Zoetmulder, F.A., and Baris, G.: Wide resection and reconstruction preserving fecal continence in recurrent anal cancer. Report of three cases. *Dis Colon Rectum* **38:**80–84, 1995.

Hepatic Cancer

Bluemke, D.A., Soyer, P.A., Chan, B.W., et al.: Spiral CT during arterial portography: Technique and applications. *Radiographics* **15:**623–637, 1995.

Gazelle, G.S., and Haage, J.R.: Hepatic neoplasms: Surgically relevant segmental anatomy and imaging techniques. *Am J Roentgenol* **158:**1015–1018, 1992.

John, T.G., and Garden, O.J.: Needle track seeding of primary and secondary liver carcinoma after percutaneous liver biopsy. *Surgery* **6:**199–203, 1993.

Kane, R.A., Hughes, L.A., Cua, E.J., et al.: The impact of intraoperative ultrasonography on surgery for liver neoplasms. *J. Ultrasound Med* **13:**1–6, 1994.

Lee, C.S., et al.: Surgical treatment of 109 patients with symptomatic and asymptomatic hepatocellular carcinoma. *Surgery* **99:**481–490, 1986.

Powers, C., Ros, P.R., Stoupis, C., et al.: Primary liver neoplasms: NMR imaging with pathologic correlation. *Radiographics* **14:**459–482, 1994.

Slomka, M., and Radwan, P.: The evaluation of clinical results of hepatic artery embolization. *Materia Med Polona* **24:**193–195, 1992.

Tang, Z.Y., Yu, Y.Q., Zhou, X.D., et al.: Surgery of small hepatocellular carcinoma: Analysis of 144 cases. *Cancer* **64:**536–541, 1989.

Tumors of the Pancreas

DiBartolomeo, M., Bajetta, E., Bochicchio, A.M., et al.: A phase II trial of dacarbazine, fluorouracil, and epirubicin in patients with neuroendocrine tumours. A study by the Italian Trials in Medical Oncology Group. *Ann Oncol* **6:**77–79, 1995.

Blandamura, S., Costantin, G., Nitti, D., and Boccato, P.: Intraoperative cytology of pancreatic masses. A 10-year experience. *Acta Cytolog* **39:**23–27, 1995.

Cameron, J.L., Crist, D.W., Sitzmann, J.V., et al.: Factors influencing survival following pancreaticoduodenectomy for pancreatic cancer. *Am J Surg* **161:**120–125, 1991.

Fuhrman, G.M., Charnsangavej, C., Abbruzzese, J.L., et al.: Thin-section contrast-enhanced computed tomography accurately predicts the resectability of malignant pancreatic neoplasms. *Am J Surg* **167:**104–111, 1994.

Hahn, S.A., and Kern, S.E.: Molecular genetics of exocrine pancreatic neoplasms (Rev). *Surg Clin North Am* **75:**857–869, 1995.

Howard, T.J., Zinner, M.J., Stabile, B.E., and Passaro, E.: Gastrinoma excision for cure: A prospective analysis. *Ann Surg* **211:**9–14, 1990.

Jaksic, T., Yaman, M., Thorner, P., et al.: A 20-year review of pediatric pancreatic tumors (Rev). *J Pediat Surg* **27:**1315–1317, 1992.

Karlson, B.M., Forsman, C.A., Wilander, E., et al.: Efficiency of percutaneous core biopsy in pancreatic tumor diagnosis. *Surgery* **120:**75–79, 1996.

Khoursheed, M., Crotch-Harvey, M., and Gould, D.A.: Embolization in the palliation of complications of inoperable primary pancreatic neoplasms. *Clin Radiol* **49:**784–786, 1994.

Lee, W.J., Park, Y.T., Choi, J.S., et al.: Solid and papillary neoplasms of the pancreas. *Yonsei Med J* **37:**131–141, 1996.

Legaspi, A., and Brennan, M.F.: Management of islet-cell carcinoma. *Surgery* **104:**1018–1022, 1988.

Lichtenstein, D.R., and Carr-Locke, D.L.: Mucin-secreting tumors of the pancreas (Rev). *GI Endosc Clin North Am* **5:**237–258, 1995.

Long, P.P., Hruban, R.H., Lo, R., et al.: Chromosome analysis of nine endocrine neoplasms of the pancreas. *Cancer Genet Cytogen* **77:**55–59, 1994.

Moosa, A.R., and Gamagami, R.A.: Diagnosis and staging of pancreatic neoplasms (Rev). *Surg Clin North Am* **75:**871–890, 1995.

Pitt, H.A.: Curative treatment for pancreatic neoplasms. Standard resection (Rev). *Surg Clin North Am* **75:**891–904, 1995.

Reber, H.A., Ashley, S.W., and McFadden, D.: Curative treatment for pancreatic neoplasms. Radical resection. *Surg Clin North Am* **75:**905–912, 1995.

Sciannameo, F., Ronca, P., Alberti, D., and Uccellini, R.: Therapeutic strategies in the surgical management of pancreatic neoplasms in the elderly. *Panminerva Medica* **35:**93–95, 1993.

Shepherd, J.J., Challis, D.R., Davies, P.F., et al.: Multiple endocrine neoplasm, type 1. Gastrinomas, pancreatic neoplasms, microcarcinoids, the Zollinger-Ellison syndrome, lymph nodes, and hepatic metastases. *Arch Surg* **128:**1133–1142, 1993.

Skogseid, B., Grama, D., Rastad, J., et al.: Operative tumour yield obviates preoperative pancreatic tumour localization in multiple endocrine neoplasia type 1. *J Intern Med* **238:**281–288, 1995.

Thoeni, R.F., and Blankenberg, F.: Pancreatic imaging. Computed tomography and magnetic resonance imaging (Rev). *Radiat Clin North Am* **31:**1085–1113, 1993.

Warshaw, A.L., Zhuo-yun, G., Wittenberg, J., and Waltman, A.C.: Preoperative staging and assessment of resectability of pancreatic cancer. *Arch Surg* **125:**230–233, 1990.

Neoplasms of the Biliary Tract

Alden, M.E., and Mohiuddin, V.: The impact of radiation dose in combined external beam and intraluminal Ir-192 brachytherapy for bile duct cancer. *Int J Rad Oncol Biol Phys* **28:**945–951, 1994.

Cameron, J.L., Pitt, H.A., Zinner, M.J., et al.: Management of proximal cholangiocarcinomas by surgical resection and radiotherapy. *Am J Surg* **159:**91–98, 1990.

Donohue, J.H., Nagorney, D.M., Grant, C.S., et al.: Carcinoma of the gallbladder: Does radical resection improve outcome? *Arch Surg* **125:**237–241, 1990.

Fritz, P., Brambs, H.J., Schraube, P., et al.: Combined external beam radiotherapy and intraluminal high dose rate brachytherapy on bile duct carcinomas. *Int J Rad Oncol Biol Phys* **29:**855–861, 1994.

Houry, S., Schlienger, M., Huguier, M., et al.: Gallbladder carcinoma: Role of radiation therapy. *Br J Surg* **76:**448–450, 1989.

Hsue, V., Wong, C.S., Moore, M., et al.: A phase I study of combined radiation therapy with 5-fluorouracil and low dose folinic acid in patients with locally advanced pancreatic or biliary carcinoma. *Int J Rad Oncol Biol Phys* **34:**445–450, 1996.

Kamada, T., Saitou, H., Takamura, A., et al.: The role of radiotherapy in the management of extrahepatic bile duct cancer: An analysis of 145 consecutive patients treated with intraluminal and/or external beam radiotherapy. *Int J Rad Oncol Biol Phys* **34:**767–774, 1996.

Kuvshinoff, B.W., Armstrong, J.G., Fong, Y., et al.: Palliation of irresectable hilar cholangiocarcinoma with biliary drainage and radiotherapy. *Br J Surg* **221:**788–797, 1995.

Leung, J., Guiney, M., and Das, R.: Intraluminal brachytherapy in bile duct carcinomas. *Aust N Z J Surg* **66:**74–77, 1996.

Mahe, M., Stampfli, C., Romestaing, P., et al.: Primary carcinoma of the gall-bladder: Potential for external radiation therapy. *Radiother Oncol* **33:**204–208, 1994.

Montemaggi, P., Morganti, A.G., and Dobelbower, R.R. Jr.: Role of intraluminal brachytherapy in extrahepatic bile duct and pancreatic cancers: Is it just for palliation? *Radiology* **1998:**61–66, 1996.

Moreno-Gonzales, E., Gomez, R., Loinaz, C., et al.: Surgical resection of biliary tract malignancies after interventional radiology treatment. *J Surg Oncol* **3:**200–202, 1993.

Nimura, Y., Hagakawa, N., Kamiya, J., et al.: Combined portal vein and liver resection for carcinoma of the biliary tract. *Br J Surg* **78:**727–731, 1991.

Ogura, Y., Mizumoto, R., Isaji, S., et al.: Radical operations for carcinoma of the gallbladder: Present status in Japan. *World J Surg* **15:**337–343, 1991.

Pitt, H.A., Nakeeb, A., Abrams, R.A., et al.: Perihilar cholangiocarcinoma. Postoperative radiotherapy does not improve survival. *Ann Surg* **221:**788–797, 1995.

Reding, R., Buard, J., Lebeau, G., and Launois, B.: Surgical management of 552 carcinomas of the extrahepatic bile ducts. *Ann Surg* **213:**236–241, 1991.

Saunder, K.D., Longmire, W.P. Jr., Tompkins, R.K., et al.: Diffuse bile duct tumors: Guidelines for management. *Ann Surg* **57:**816–820, 1991.

Schoenthaler, R., Castro, J.R., Halberg, F.E., and Phillips, T.L.: Definitive postoperative irradiation of bile duct carcinoma with charged particles and/or photons. *Int J Rad Oncol Biol Phys* **27:**75–82, 1993.

Yeo, C.J., Pitt, H.A., and Cameron, J.L.: Cholangiocarcinoma. *Surg Clin North Am* **70:**1429–1447, 1990.

Neoplasms of the Kidney and Ureters

Abeshouse, B.S.: Primary benign and malignant tumors of the ureter. *Am J Surg* **91:**237–271, 1956.

Ala-Opas, M. Y., and Martikainen, P.M.: Multilocular renal cyst. Report of two cases and review of the literature. *Ann Chir Gynaecol* **84:**318–322, 1995.

Arranz Arija, J.A., Carrion, J.R., Garcia, F.R., et al.: Primary renal lymphoma: Report of 3 cases and review of the literature. *Am J Nephrol* **14:**148–153, 1994.

Bosniack, M.A.: Observation of small incidentally detected renal masses (Rev). *Sem Urol Oncol* **13:**267–272, 1995.

Clericuzio, C.L., and Johnson, C.: Screening for Wilms' tumor in high-risk individuals (Rev). *Hematol Oncol Clin North Am* **9:**1253–1265, 1995.

Cummings, K.B.: Nephroureterectomy: Rationale in the measurement of transitional cell carcinoma of the upper urinary tract. *Urol Clin North Am* **18:**569–578, 1991.

Curry, N.S.: Small renal masses (lesions smaller than 3 cm): Imaging evaluation and management. *Am J Roentgenol* **164:**355–362, 1995.

Fichtner, J., and Hohenfellner, R.: Damage to the urinary tract secondary to irradiation (Rev). *World J Urol* **13:**240–242, 1995.

Grabstald, H., Whitmore, W.F., and Melamed, M.R.: Renal pelvic tumors. *JAMA* **218:**845–853, 1971.

Herts, B.R., and Baker, M.E.: The current role of percutaneous biopsy in the evaluation of renal masses (Rev). *Sem Urol Oncol* **13:**254–261, 1995.

Huch Boni, R.A., Debatin, J.F., and Krestin, G.P.: Contrast-enhancing MR imaging of the kidneys and adrenal glands (Rev). *Mag Reson Imag Clin North Am* **4:**101–131, 1996.

Jereb, B., Burgers, J.M., Tournade, M.F., et al: Radiotherapy in the International Society of Pediatric Oncology nephroblastoma studies: A review. *Med Pediat Oncol* **22:**221–227, 1994.

Jitkusawa, S., Nakamura, K., Nakayama, M., et al.: Transitional cell carcinoma of kidney extending into renal vein and inferior vena cava. *Urology* **25:**310–312, 1985.

Johnson, D.E., DeBerardinis, M., and Ayala, A.G.: Transitional cell carcinoma of the renal pelvis. Radical or conservative surgical treatment? *South Med J* **67:**1183–1186, 1974.

Kawashima, A., Goldman, S.M., and Sandler, C.M.: The indeterminate renal mass (Rev). *Rad Clin North Am* **34:**997–1015, 1996.

Licht, M.R.: Renal adenoma and oncocytoma (Rev). *Sem Urol Oncol* **13:**262–266, 1995.

Long, J.P., Anglard, P., Gnarra, J.R., et al.: The use of molecular genetic analysis in the diagnosis of renal cell carcinoma (Rev). *World J Urol* **12:**69–73, 1994.

Marshall, M.E., Mohler, J.L., Edmonds, K., et al.: An updated review of the clinical development of coumarin (1,2-benzopyrone) and 7-hydroxycoumarin (Rev). *J Cancer Res Clin Oncol* **120** (Suppl):S39–S42, 1994.

Meadows, L.M., Lindley, C., and Ozer, H.: Treatment of gastrointestinal and renal adenocarcinomas with interferon-alpha (Rev). *Biotherapy* **4:**179–187, 1992.

Mickisch, G.H.: Chemoresistance of renal cell carcinoma: 1986–94 (Rev). *World J Urol* **12:**214–223, 1994.

Motzer, R.J., Bander, N.H., Nanus, D.M.: Renal-cell carcinoma. *N Engl J Med* **335:**865, 1996.

Ritchie, M.L., Kelalis, P.P., Haase, G.M., et al.: Preoperative therapy for intracaval and atrial extension of Wilms' tumor (Rev). *Cancer* **71:**4104–4110, 1993.

Savage, P.D.: Renal cell carcinoma (Rev). *Curr Opin Oncol* **7:**275–280, 1995.

Wagle, D.G., Moore, R.H., and Murphy, G.P.: Primary carcinoma of the renal pelvis. *Cancer* **33:**1642–1648, 1974.

Wilhelm, M., Krause, U., Kovacs, G.: Diagnosis and prognosis of renal-cell tumors: A molecular approach (Rev). *World J Urol* **13:**143–148, 1995.

Wood, D.J., and Herr, H.W.: The evolving role of surgery in the management of renal cell carcinoma. *Sem Urol* **7:**172–180, 1989.

Yagoda, A., Petrylak, D., and Thompson, S.: Cytotoxic chemotherapy for advanced renal cell carcinoma (Rev). *Urol Clin North Am* **20:**303–321, 1993.

Neoplasms of the Urinary Bladder

Barentz, J.O., Ruizs, S.H., and van Erning, L.J.: Magnetic resonance imaging of urinary bladder cancer: An overview and new developments (Rev). *Mag Reson Q* **9:**235–258, 1993.

Bowles, W.T., and Cordonnier, J.J.: Total cystectomy for carcinoma of the bladder. *J. Urol* **90:**731, 1963.

Cloudhary, G.: Human health perspectives on environmental exposure to benzidine: A review. *Chemosphere* **32:**267–291, 1996.

Cohen, S.M., and Johansson, S.L.: Epidemiology and etiology of bladder cancer (Rev). *Urol Clin North Am* **19:**421–428, 1992.

Kroft, S.H., and Oyasu, R.: Urinary bladder cancer: mechanisms of development and progression (Rev). *Lab Invest* **71:**258–274, 1994.

Moon, R.C., Detrisac, C.J., Thomas, C.F., and Kelloff, G.J.: Chemoprevention of experimental bladder cancer (Rev). *J Cell Biochem* (Suppl) **16I:**134–138, 1992.

Novick, A.C., and Stewart, B.H.: Partial cystectomy in the treatment of primary and secondary carcinoma of the bladder. *J. Urol* **116:**570, 1976.

Rosin, M.P., Saad el Din Zaki, S., Ward, A.J., and Anwar, W.A.: Involvement of inflammatory reactions and elevated cell proliferation in the development of bladder cancer in schistosomiasis patients (Rev). *Mutation Res* **305:**283–292, 1994.

Sternberg, C.N.: Bladder preservation—A prospect for patients with urinary bladder cancer (Rev). *Acta Oncol* **34:**588–597, 1995.

Neoplasms of the Prostate

Catalona, W.J., and Bigg, S.W.: Nerve-sparing radical prostatectomy. Evaluation of results after 250 patients. *J Urol* **143:**538, 1990.

Catalona, W.K., et al.: Measurement of prostate specific antigen as a screening test for prostate cancer. *N Engl J Med* **324:**1156–1161, 1991.

D'Amico, A.V., and Coleman, C.N.: Role of interstitial radiotherapy in the management of clinically organ-confined prostate cancer: The jury is still out (Rev). *J Clin Oncol* **14:**304–315, 1996.

Das, S.: Laparoscopic staging pelvic lymphadenectomy: Extraperitoneal approach (Rev). *Sem Surg Oncol* **12:**134–138, 1996.

Donahue, R.E., Man, J.H., Whitesel, J.A., et al.: Pelvic lymph node dissection: Guide to patient management in clinically locally confined adenocarcinoma of the prostate. *Urol* **20:**559–565, 1982.

Dreicer, R., Cooper, C.S., and Williams, R.D.: Management of prostate and bladder cancer in the elderly (Rev). *Urol Clin North Am* **23:**87–97, 1996.

Epstein, J.I.: The diagnosis and reporting of adenocarcinoma of the prostate in core needle biopsy specimens (Rev). *Cancer* **78:**350–356, 1996.

Hanks, G.E.: Optimizing the radiation treatment and outcome of prostate cancer. *Int J Radiat Oncol Biol Phys* **11:**1235–1245, 1985.

Lee, F., Littrup, P.J., Torp-Pedersen, S.T., et al.: Prostate cancer: Comparison of transrectal ultrasound and digital rectal examination for screening. *Radiology* **168:**389–394, 1988.

Moore, R.G., Partin, A.W., and Kavoussi, L.R.: Role of laparoscopy in the diagnosis and treatment of prostate cancer (Rev). *Sem Surg Oncol* **12:**139–144, 1996.

Stamey, T.A., Villers, A.A., McNeal, J.E., et al.: Positive surgical margins at radical prostatectomy: Importance of the apical dissection. *J Urol* **143:**1166–1173, 1990.

Zippe, C.D.: Cryosurgery of the prostate: Techniques and pitfalls (Rev). *Urol Clin North Am* **23:**147–163, 1996.

Urethral Neoplasms

Drew, P.A., Murphy, W.M., Civantos, F., and Speights, V.O.: The histogenesis of clear cell adenocarcinoma of the lower urinary tract. Case series and review of the literature. *Hum Pathol* **27:**248–252, 1996.

Hofmockel, G., Dammrich, J., Manzanilla Garcia, H., et al.: Primary non-Hodgkin's lymphoma of the male urethra. A case report and review of the literature. *Urol Int* **55:**177–180, 1995.

Mordkin, R.M., Skinner, D.G., and Levine, A.M.: Long-term disease-free survival after plasmacytoma of the urethra: A case report and review of the literature. *Urology* **48:**149–150, 1996.

Oliva, E., and Young, R.H.: Nephrogenic adenoma of the urinary tract: A review of the microscopic appearance of 80 cases with emphasis on unusual features. *Mod Pathol* **8:**722–730, 1995.

Neoplasms of the Penis

Ben-Yosef, R., and Kapp, D.S.: Cancer metastatic to the penis: Treatment with hyperthermia and radiation therapy and review of the literature. *J Urol* **148:**67–71, 1992.

Bissada, N.K.: Conservative extirpative treatment of cancer of the penis (Rev). *Urol Clin North Am* **19:**283–290, 1992.

Cabanas, R.M.: Anatomy and biopsy of sentinel lymph nodes (Rev). *Urol Clin North Am* **19:**267–276, 1992.

Gerbaulet, A., and Lambin, P.: Radiation therapy of cancer of the penis. Indication, advantages, and pitfalls (Rev). *Urol Clin North Am* **19:**325–332, 1992.

Jackson, S.M.: The treatment of carcinoma of the penis. *Br J Surg* **53:**33, 1966.

Rozan, R., Albuisson, E., Giraud, B., et al.: Interstitial brachytherapy for penile carcinoma: A multicentric survey (259 patients). *Radiother Oncol* **36:**83–93, 1995.

Shammas, F.V., Ous, S., and Fossa, S.D.: Cisplatin and 5-fluorouracil in advanced cancer of the penis. *J Urol* **147:**630–632, 1992.

Neoplasms of the Testis

Bokemeyer, C., Duczyk, M.A., Kohne, H., et al.: Hematopoietic growth factors and treatment of testicular cancer: Biological interactions, routine use and dose-intensive chemotherapy (Rev). *Ann Hematol* **72:**1–9, 1996.

Crown, J.: High-dose chemotherapy of solid tumors (Rev). *Ann Oncol* **6** (Suppl 1):11–14, 1995.

Epstein, B.E., Order, S.E., and Zinreich, C.S.: Staging, treatment, and results in testicular seminoma: A 12-year report. *Cancer* **65:**405–411, 1990.

Motzer, R.J.: Adjuvant chemotherapy for patients with stage II nonseminomatous testis cancer (Rev). *Sem Oncol* **22:**641–646, 1995.

Nichols, C.R.: Ifosfamide in the treatment of germ cell tumors (Rev). *Sem Oncol* **23** (Suppl 6):65–73, 1996.

Roth, B.J.: The role of ifosfamide in the treatment of testicular and urothelial malignancies (Rev). *Sem Oncol* **23** (Suppl 7):19–27, 1996.

Staubitz, W.J., Early, K.S., Magoss, I.V., and Murphy, G.P.: Surgical management of testis tumors. *J Urol* **111:**205, 1974.

Thomas, G.M., Rider, W.D., Dembo, A.J., et al.: Seminoma of the testis: Results of treatment and patterns of failure after radiation therapy. *Int J Radiat Oncol Biol Phys* **8:**165–174, 1982.

Zeitman, A.L., Coen, J.J., Ferry, J.A., et al.: The management and outcome of stage IAE non-Hodgkin's lymphoma of the testis (Rev). *J Urol* **155:**943–946, 1996.

Neoplasms of Uterus and Uterine Cervix

Averette, H.E., Lichtenger, M., Sevin, B.U., and Girtanner, R.E.: Pelvic exenteration: A 15-year experience in a general hospital. *Am J Obstet Gynecol* **150:**179, 1984.

Burke, T.W., Fowler, W.C. Jr., and Morrow, C.P.: Clinical aspects of risk in women with endometrial carcinoma (Rev). *J Cell Biochem* (Suppl) **23:**131–136, 1995.

Clark, K.: Endometrial cancer: risk factors and diagnosis (Rev). *W Va Med J* **92:** 28–30, 1996.

Denehy, T.R., Eastman, R., SanFilippo, L., et al.: Bolus mitomycin C and 5-FU with sequential radiation for poor-prognosis locally advanced cervical cancer (Rev). *Gynecol Oncol* **60:**64–71, 1996.

Gurney, H., Murphy, D., and Crowther, D.: The management of primary fallopian tube carcinoma. *Br J Obstet Gynecol* **97:**822, 1990.

Kuo, D.Y., and Runowicz, C.D.: Gynaecologic effects of tamoxifen (Rev). *Med Oncol* **12:** 87–94, 1995.

Kupelian, P.A., Eifel, P.J. Tornos, C., et al.: Treatment of endometrial carcinoma with radiation therapy alone (Rev). *Int J Rad Oncol Biol Phys* **27:**817–824, 1993.

Meigs, J.V.: Carcinoma of the cervix—The Wertheim operation. *Surg Gynecol Obstet* **78:**192, 1944.

Morton, G.C., and Thomas, G.M.: Does adjuvant chemotherapy change the prognosis of cervical cancer? (Rev). *Curr Opin Obstet Gynecol* **8:**17–20, 1996.

Rotman, M., Aziz, H.J., Halpern, J., et al.: Endometrial carcinoma. Influence of prognostic factors on radiation management (Rev). *Cancer* **71** (Suppl):1471–1479, 1993.

Rutledge, F.N.: The role of radical hysterectomy in adenocarcinoma of the endometrium. *Gynecol Oncol* **2:**331, 1974.

Shimm, D.S., Wang, C.C., Fuller, A.F. Jr., et al.: Management of high-grade stage-I adenocarcinoma of the endometrium: Hysterectomy following low dose external beam pelvic irradiation. *Gynecol Oncol* **25:**183, 1986.

Thigpen, T., Vance, R., Khansur, T., and Malamud, F.: The role of ifosfamide and systemic therapy in the management of carcinoma of the cervix (Rev). *Sem Oncol* **23** (Suppl 6):56–64, 1996.

Wren, B.: Hormonal therapy and genital tract cancer (Rev). *Curr Opin Obstet Gynecol* **8:**38–41, 1996.

Neoplasms of the Ovary

Davis, K.P., Hartmann, L.K., Keeney, G.L., and Shapiro, H.: Primary ovarian carcinoid tumors (Rev). *Gynecol Oncol* **61:**259–265, 1996.

Lorigan, P.C., Crosby, T., and Coleman, R.E.: Current drug treatment guidelines for epithelial ovarian cancer. *Drugs* **51:**571–584, 1996.

Markman, M.: Ifosfamide in the treatment of ovarian cancer. *Sem Oncol* **23** (Suppl 6):47–49, 1996.

Miralles, R.M.: Pelvic masses and endoscopic surgery: Diagnosis (Rev). *Eur J Obstet Gynecol Reprod Biol* **65:**75–79, 1996.

Muderspach, L., Muggia, F.M., and Conti, P.S.: Second-look laparotomy for stage III epithelial ovarian cancer: Rationale and current issues (Rev). *Cancer Treat Rev* **21:**499–511, 1996.

Smith, J.P., and Day, T.G.: Review of ovarian cancer at the University of Texas Systems Cancer Center. *Am J Obstet Gynecol* **135:**984, 1979.

Wijnen, A.J., and Rosenshein, M.D.: Surgery in ovarian cancer. *Arch Surg* **115:**863–868, 1980.

Cancer of the Vagina

Brown, G.R., Fletcher, G.H., and Rutledge, F.N.: Irradiation of in situ and invasive squamous cell carcinoma of the vagina. *Cancer* **28:**1278–1283, 1971.

Herbst, A.L., Green, T.J., and Ulfelder, H.: Primary carcinoma of the vagina. An analysis of 68 cases. *Am J Obstet Gynecol* **106:**210–218, 1970.

Perez, C.A., Camel, H.M., Galakatos, A.E., et al.: Definitive irradiation in carcinoma of the vagina. Long-term evaluation of results. *Int J Radiat Oncol Biol Phys* **15:**1283, 1988.

Underwood, P.J., and Smith, R.T.: Carcinoma of the vagina. *JAMA* **217:**46–52, 1971.

Wharton, J.T., Rutledge, F.N., Gallagher, H.S., and Fletcher, G.H.: Treatment of clear cell adenocarcinoma in young women. *Obstet Gynecol* **45:**365–368, 1975.

Neoplasms of the Vulva

Acosta, A.A., Given, F.T., Frazier, A.B., et al.: Preoperative radiation therapy in the management of squamous cell carcinoma of the vulva. *Am J Obstet Gynecol* **132:**198–206, 1978.

Boronow, R.C., Hickman, B.T., Reagan, M.T., et al.: Combined therapy as an alternative to exenteration for locally advanced vulvovaginal cancer. II. Results, complications, and dosimetric and surgical considerations. *Am J Clin Oncol* **10:**171–181, 1987.

Di Saia, P.J., Creasman, W.T., and Rich, W.M.: An alternate approach to early cancer of the vulva. *Am J Obstet Gynecol* **133:**825–832, 1979.

Durrant, K.R., Mangione, C., Lacave, A.J., et al.: Bleomycin, methotrexate, and CCNU in advanced inoperable squamous cell carcinoma of the vulva: A phase II study of the EORTC Gynaecological Cancer Cooperative Group (GCCG). *Gynecol Oncol* **37:**359–362, 1990.

Frankendal, B., Larsson, L.G., and Westling, P.: Carcinoma of the vulva. Results of an individualized treatment schedule. *Acta Radiol Ther Phys Biol* **12:**165–174, 1973.

Stillman, F.H., Sedlis, A., and Boyce, J.G.: A review of lower genital intraepithelial neoplasia and the use of topical 5-fluorouracil. *Obstetr Gynecol Surv* **40:**190–220, 1985.

Thomas, G., Dembo, A., DePetrillo, A., et al.: Concurrent radiation and chemotherapy in vulvar carcinoma. *Gynecol Oncol* **34:**263, 1989.

Acute Lymphocytic Leukemia

Bassan, R., Lerede, T., Rambaldi, A., and Barbui, T.: Role of anthracyclines in the treatment of adult acute lymphoblastic leukemia (Rev). *Acta Haematol* **95:**188–192, 1996.

Copelan, E.A., and McGuire, E.A.: The biology and treatment of acute lymphoblastic leukemia in adults. *Blood* **85:**1151, 1995.

Gokbuget, N., and Hoelzer, D.: High-dose methotrexate in the treatment of adult acute lymphoblastic leukemia (Rev). *Ann Hematol* **72:**194–201, 1996.

Acute Myelocytic Leukemia

Cline M.J.: Molecular basis of leukemia. *N Engl J Med* **330:**228, 1994.

Estey, E.: Treatment of refractory AML (Rev). *Leukemia* **10:**932–936, 1996.

Foon, K.A., and Gale, R.P.: Therapy of acute myelogenous leukemia. *Blood Rev* **6:**15, 1992.

Warrell, R.P. Jr.: Pathogenesis and management of acute promyelocytic leukemia (Rev). *Ann Rev Med* **47:**555–565, 1996.

Chronic Lymphocytic Leukemia

Caligaris-Cappio, F.: B-chronic lymphocytic leukemia: A malignancy of anti-self B cells. *Blood* **87:**2615–2620, 1996.

Cheson, B.D., Bennett, J.M., Grever, M., et al.: National Cancer Institute-sponsored Working Group guidelines for chronic lymphocytic leukemia: Revised guidelines for diagnosis and treatment. *Blood* **87:**4990–4997, 1996.

Hoyer, J.D., Ross, C.W., Li, Cy, et al.: True T-cell chronic lymphocytic leukemia: A morphologic and immunophenotypic study of 25 cases (Rev). *Blood* **87:**3520–3521, 1996.

Kay, N.E., Ranheim, E.A., and Peterson, L.C.: Tumor suppressor genes and clonal evolution in B-CLL (Rev). *Leukemia Lymphoma* **18:**41–49, 1995.

Robertson, L.E., Denny, A.W., Huh, Y.O., et al.: Natural killer cell activity in chronic lymphocytic leukemia patients treated with fludarabine. *Cancer Chemother Pharmacol* **37:**445–450, 1996.

Savin, A., and Piro, O.: Newer purine analogs for the treatment of hairy-cell leukemia. *N Engl J Med* **330:** 691, 1994.

Solal-Celingy, P., Brice, P., Brousse, N., et al.: Phase II trial of fludarabine monophosphate as first-line treatment in patients with advanced follicular lymphoma: A multicenter study by the Groupe d'Etude des Lymphomes de l'Adulte. *J Clin Oncol* **14:**514–519, 1996.

Chronic Myelocytic Leukemia

Applebaum, F.R., Clift, R., Buckner, C.D., et al.: Allogeneic marrow transplantation for chronic myeloid leukemia (Rev). *Med Oncol* **11:**69–74, 1994.

Cervantes, F., and Rozman, C.: Benign hematopoietic progenitors in chronic myeloid leukemia: Current status and future prospects (Rev). *Ann Hematol* **69:**99–105, 1994.

Clift, R.A., Buckner, C.D., Thomas, E.D., et al.: Marrow transplantation for patients in accelerated phase of chronic myeloid leukemia (Rev). *Blood* **84:**4368–4373, 1994.

Kantarjian, H.M., O'Brien, S., and Anderline, P.: Treatment of CML; Current status and investigational options (Rev). *Blood* **87:**3069–3081, 1996.

Kumar, L.: Leukemia: Management of relapse after allogeneic bone marrow transplantation (Rev). *J Clin Oncol* **12:**1710–1717, 1994.

Lanza, F., and Bi, S.: Role of *p53* in leukemogenesis of chronic myeloid leukemia (Rev). *Stem Cell* **13:**445–452, 1995.

Nakai, H., and Misawa, S.: Chromosome 17 abnormalities and inactivation of the *p53* gene in chronic myeloid leukemia and their prognostic significance (Rev). *Leukemia Lymphoma* **19:**213–221, 1995.

Pui, C.H., and Crist, W.M.: Treatment of childhood leukemias (Rev). *Curr Opin Oncol* **7:**36–44, 1995.

Silla, L.M., Whiteside, T.L., and Ball, E.D.: The role of natural killer cells in the treatment of chronic myeloid leukemia (Rev). *J Hematotherapy* **4:**269–279, 1995.

Malignant Non-Hodgkin's Lymphoma

Aisenberg, A.C.: Coherent view of non-Hodgkin's lymphoma. *J Clin Oncol* **13:**2656, 1995.

Armitage, J.O.: Treatment of non-Hodgkin's lymphoma. *N Engl J Med* **328:**1023, 1993.

Boiardi, A., Silvani, A., Valentini, S., et al.: Chemotherapy as first treatment for primary malignant non-Hodgkin's lymphoma of the central nervous system preliminary data. *J Neurol* **241:**96–100, 1993.

Lehne, G., Hannisdal, E., Langholm, R., and Nome, O.: A 10-year experience with splenectomy in patients with malignant non-Hodgkin's lymphoma at the Norwegian Radium Hospital. *Cancer* **74:**933–939, 1994.

Uyl-de Groot, C.A., Hagenbeek, A., Verdonck, L.F., et al.: Cost-effectiveness of ABMT in comparison with CHOP chemotherapy in patients with intermediate- and high-grade malignant non-Hodgkin's. *Bone Marrow Transpl* **16:**463–470, 1995.

Seifert, E., Schulte, F., and Stolte, M.: Long-term results of treatment of malignant non-Hodgkin's lymphoma of the stomach. *Z Gastroenterol* **30:**505–508, 1992.

Seifert, E., Schulte, F., Weismuller, J., et al.: Endoscopic and bioptic diagnosis of malignant non-Hodgkin's lymphoma of the stomach. *Endoscopy* **25:**497–501, 1993.

Hodgkin's Disease

Carbone, A., and Cloghini, A.: The immunodiagnosis of Hodgkin's disease (Rev). *Int J Biol Markers* **11:**1–5, 1996.

DeVita, V.T., and Hubbard, S.M.: Hodgkin's disease (Rev). *N Engl J Med* **328:**560, 1993.

Frezza, G., Barbieri, E., Ainzani, P.L., et al.: Supradiaphragmatic early stage Hodgkin's disease: Does mantle radiation therapy still have a role? (Rev). *Haematologica,* **81:**138–142, 1996.

Longo, D.L.: The case against the routine use of radiation therapy in advanced-stage Hodgkin's disease (Rev). *Cancer Invest* **14:**353–360, 1996.

Prosnitz, L.R., Wu, J.J., and Yahalom, J.: The case for adjuvant radiation therapy in advanced Hodgkin's disease (Rev). *Cancer Invest* **14:**361–370, 1996.

Teasch, H., and Diehl, V.: Hodgkin's disease: From basic science to clinical application (Rev). *Leukemia* **10:**74–77, 1996.

Neoplasms of Plasma Cells

Alexanian, R., and Dimopoulos, M.: The treatment of multiple myeloma. *N Engl J Med* **330:**484, 1994.

Blade, J., Kyle, R.A., and Greipp, P.R.: Multiple myeloma in patients younger than 30 years. Report of 10 cases and review of the literature. *Arch Intern Med* **156:**1463–1468, 1996.

Handelsman, H.: Haematopoietic stem-cell transplantation in multiple myeloma. *Cancer Treat Rev* **22:**119–125, 1996.

Jacobs, P., Wood, L., LeRoux, I., et al.: Waldenström's macroglobulinemia treated by sequential hemibody irradiation. *J Clin Apheresis* **3:**181–184, 1987.

Kantarjian, H.M. Alexanian, R., Kotter, C.A., et al.: Fludarabine therapy in macroglobulinemic lymphoma. *Blood* **75:**1928–1931, 1990.

Seligman, M., Mihaesco, E., Preud'homme, J.L., et al.: Heavy chain disease: Current findings and concepts. *Immunol Rev* **48:**145–167, 1979.

Neoplasms of Bone

Bloem, J.L., and Kroon, H.M.: Osseous lesions (Rev). *Radiol Clin North Am* **31:**261–278, 1993.

Delamarter, R.B., Sachs, B.L., Thompson, G.H., et al.: Primary neoplasms of the thoracic and lumbar spine. *Clin Orthop Rel Res* **256:**87–100, 1990.

Kanis, J.A.: Bone and cancer: Pathophysiology and treatment of metastases (Rev). *Bone* **17** (Suppl):101S–105S, 1995.

Kostuik, J.P., Errico, T.J., Gleason, T.F., and Errico, C.E.: Spinal stabilization of vertebral column tumors. *Spine* **13:**250–256, 1988.

Nicholson, H.S., Mulvihill, J.J., and Byrne, J.: Late effects of therapy in adult survivors of osteosarcoma and Ewing's sarcoma. *Med Pediat Oncol* **20:**6–12, 1992 (Comment in *Med Pediat Oncol* **22:**296–297, 1994).

Manabe, S., Tateishi, A., Abe, M., and Ohno, T.: Surgical treatment of metastatic tumours of the spine. *Spine* **14:**41–47, 1989.

Postma, A., Kingma, A., De Ruiter, J.H., et al.: Quality of life in bone tumor patients comparing limb salvage and amputation of the lower extremity. *J Surg Oncol* **51:**47–51, 1992.

Schmidt, R.G.: Management of extremity metastatic bone cancer. *Curr Prob Cancer* **19:**166–182, 1995.

Weinstein, J.N., and McLain, R.F.: Primary tumours of the spine. *Spine* **12:**843–851, 1987.

Sarcoma

Bernstein, S.C., and Roenigk, R.K.: Leiomyosarcoma of the skin. Treatment of 34 cases (Rev). *Dermatol Surg* **22:** 631–635, 199.

Cariero, F., Gipponi, M., Peressini, A., et al: Radiation-associated angiosarcoma: Diagnostic and therapeutic implications—two case reports and a review of the literature. *Cancer* **77:**2496–2502, 1996.

Fish, F.S.: Soft tissue sarcoma in dermatology (Rev). *Dermatol Surg* **22:**268–273, 1996.

Hollowood, K., and Fletcher, C.D.: Malignant fibrous histiocytoma: Morphologic pattern or pathologic entity? (Rev). *Sem Diag Pathol* **12:**210–220, 1995.

Hollowood, K., and Fletcher, C.D.: Soft tissue sarcomas that mimic benign lesions (Rev). *Sem Diag Pathol* **12:**87–97, 1995.

Moore, M.P., and Kinne, D.W.: Breast sarcoma (Rev). *Surg Clin North Am* **76:**383–392, 1996.

Suit, H.: Tumors of the connective and supporting tissues (Rev). *Radiother Oncol* **34:**93–104, 1995.

Suster, S.: Primary sarcomas of the lung (Rev). *Sem Diagn Pathol* **12:**140–157, 1995.

Washecka, R.M., Mariani, A.J., Zuna, R.E., et al.: Primary intratesticular sarcoma. Immunohistochemical ultrastructural and DNA flow cytometric study of three cases with a review of the literature. *Cancer* **77:**1524–1528, 1996.

Solid Tumors of Childhood

Altman, R.P., Randolph, J.G., and Lilly, J.R.: Sacrococcygeal teratoma. *J Pediat Surg* **9:**389–398, 1974.

Dale, P.S., Webb, H.W., and Wilkinson, A.H., Jr.: Resection of the inferior vena cava for recurrent Wilms' tumor. *J Pediat Surg* **30:**121–122, 1995.

de Kraker, J., Weitzman, S., and Voute, P.A.: Preoperative strategies in the management of Wilms' tumor (Rev). *Hematol Oncol Clin* **9:**1275–1285, 1995.

Farhi, D.C., Odell, C.A., and Shurin, S.B.: Myelodysplastic syndrome and acute myeloid leukemia after treatment for solid tumors of childhood. *Am J Clin Path* **100:**270–275, 1993.

Grosfield, J.L: Neuroblastoma: A 1990 overview. *Pediat Surg Int* **6:**9–13, 1991.

Grundmann, E., Ueda, Y., Schneider-Stock, R., and Roessner, A.: New aspects of cell biology in osteosarcoma. *Pathol Res Pract* **191:**563–570, 1995.

Imamura, J., Bartram, C.R., Berthold, F., et al.: Mutation of the *p53* gene in neuroblastoma and its relationship with *N-myc* amplification. *Cancer Res* **53:**4053–4058, 1993.

Kung, F.H., Desai, S.J., Dickerman, J.D., et al.: Ifosfamide/carboplatin/etoposide (ICE) for recurrent malignant solid tumors of childhood: A Pediatric Oncology Group Phase I/II study. *J Pediat Hematol Oncol* **17:**265–269, 1995.

Lukens, J.N.: Progress resulting from clinical trials. Solid tumors in childhood cancer (Rev). *Cancer* **74:**2710–2718, 1994.

Marina, N.M., Krance, R., Ribeiro, R.C., and Crist, W.M.: Diagnosis and treatment of the most common solid tumors in childhood (Rev). *Primary Care Clin Off Pract* **19:**871–889, 1992.

Pui, C.H., Hudson, M., Luo, X., et al.: Serum interleukin-2 receptor levels in Hodgkin's disease and other solid tumors of childhood. *Leukemia* **7:**1242–1244, 1993.

Raney, R.B., Gehan, E.A., Haya, D.M., et al.: Primary chemotherapy with or without radiation therapy, surgery, or both for children with localized residual sarcoma of the bladder, prostate, or vagina. *Cancer* **66**:2072–2078, 1990.

Siimes, M.A., Rautonen, J., Makipernaa, A., and Sipila, I.: Testicular function in adult males surviving childhood malignancy. *Pediatr Hematol Oncol* **12**:231–241, 1995.

Takeuchi, S., Bartram, C.R., Ludwig, R., et al.: Mutations of *p53* in Wilms' tumors. *Mod Pathol* **81**:483–487, 1995.

Neoplasms of the Brain and Spinal Cord

Allen, E.D., Byrd, S.E., Darling, C.F., et al.: The clinical and radiological evaluation of primary brain tumors in children, Part I: Clinical evaluation. *J Natl Med Assoc* **85**:445–451, 1993.

Allen, E.D., Byrd, S.E., Darling, C.F., et al.: The clinical and radiological evaluation of primary brain neoplasms in children, Part II: Radiological evaluation. *J Natl Med Assoc* **85**:546–553, 1993.

Black, P.M.: Brain tumors, II, *N Engl J Med* **324**:1471–1476, 1991.

Di Rocco, C., and Iannelli, A.: Intracranical supratentorial tumors: Classification, clinical findings, surgical management (Rev). *Rays* **21**:9–25, 1996.

Drugs of choice for cancer chemotherapy. *Med Lett Drugs Therap* **39**:21–28, 1997.

Filley, C.M., and Kleinschmidt-DeMasters, B.K.: Neurobehavioral presentations of brain neoplasms. *West J Med* **163**:19–25, 1995.

Finlay, J., August, C., Packer, R., et al.: High dose chemotherapy with marrow rescue in children with malignant brain tumors. *J. Neuro-Oncol* **7**:511, 1989.

Hoack, H.C., Bang, F., and Laurberg, P.: Impaired growth hormone secretion in patients operated for pituitary adenomas. *Growth Reg* **4**:63–67, 1994.

Kaye, A.H., Murstyn, G., and Apuzzo, M.S.: Photoradiation therapy and it's potential in the management of neurological tumors. *J Neurosurg* **69**:1–14, 1988.

Klibanski, A., and Zerva, N.T.: Diagnosis and management of hormone secreting pituitary adenomas. *N Engl J Med* **324**:822–831, 1991.

Kuric, J.: Spinal cord tumors (Rev). *Crit Care Nurs Clin Am* **7**:151–157, 1995.

Leeds, N.E., and Jackson, E.F.: Current imaging techniques for the evaluation of brain neoplasms (Rev). *Curr Opin Oncol* **6**:254–261, 1994.

Luk, I.S., Chan, J.K., Chow, S.M., and Laung, S.: Pituitary adenoma presenting as sinonasal tumor: Pitfalls in diagnosis. *Human Pathol* **27**:605–609, 1996.

Madsen, J.R., and Scott, R.M.: Chiari malformations, syringomyelia, and intramedullary spinal cord tumors (Rev). *Curr Opin Neurol Neurosurg* **6**:559–563, 1993.

McCollough, W.M., Narcus, R.B. Jr., Rhoton, A.L. Jr., et al.: Long-term followup of radiotherapy for pituitary adenoma: The absence of late recurrence after ≥4500 cGy. *Int J Rad Oncol Biol Phys* **21**:607, 1991.

Miller, D.C., Hochberg, F.H., Harris, N.L., et al.: Pathology with clinical correlations of primary central nervous system non-Hodgkin's lymphoma. The Massachusetts General Hospital experience 1958–1989. *Cancer* **74**:1383–1397, 1994.

Morantz, B.A.: Radiation therapy in the treatment of cerebral astrocytomas. *Neurosurg* **20**:275–282, 1987.

Murovick, J., and Sundaresan, N.: Pediatric spinal axis tumors (Rev). *Neurosurg Clin* **3**:947–958, 1992.

Newton, H.B., Newton, C.L., Gatens, C., et al.: Spinal cord tumors: Review of etiology, diagnosis, and multidisciplinary approach to treatment (Rev). *Cancer Pract* **3:**207–218, 1996.

Panagopoulos, K.P., El-Azouzi, M., Chisolm, H.L., et al.: Intracranial epidermoid tumors. *Arch Neurol* **47:**813–816, 1990.

Ravesz, T., Scaravilli, T., Coutinho, L., et al.: Reliability of histological diagnosis including grading in gliomas biopsied by image-guided stereotactic technique. *Brain* **116:**781–793, 1993.

Roos, K.L., and Muckway, M.: Neurofibromatosis (Rev). *Dermatol Clin* **13:** 105–111, 1995.

Sankhla, S.K., and Nadkarni, J.S., and Bhagwati, S.N.: Adoptive immunotherapy using lymphokine-activated killer (LAK) cells and interleukin-2 for recurrent malignant primary brain tumors. *J Neuro-Oncol* **27:**133–140, 1996.

Steinbok, P., Cochrane, D.D., and Poskitt, K.: Intramedullary spinal cord tumors in children (Rev). *Neurosurg Clin North Am* **3:**931–945, 1992.

Thornton, A.F. Jr., Sandler, H.M., Ten Haken, R.K., et al.: The clinical utility of magnetic resonance imaging in 3-dimensional treatment planning of brain neoplasms. *Int J Rad Oncol Biol Phys* **24:**767–775, 1992.

Tien, R.D., Felsberg, G.J., Friedman, H., et al.: NMR imaging of high-grade cerebral gliomas: value of diffusion-weighted echoplanar pulse sequences. *Am J Roentgenol* **162:**671–677, 1994.

Tomita, T., and McLone, D.G.: Medulloblastoma in childhood: Results of radical resection and low dose neuraxis radiation therapy. *J Neurosurg* **64:**238–242, 1986.

Wu, J.K., Ye, Z., and Darras, B.T.: Frequency of *p53* tumor suppressor gene mutations in human primary brain tumors. *Neurosurg* **33:**824–830, 1993.

Secondary Neoplasms

Deeg, H.J., and Witherspoon, R.P.: Risk factors for the development of secondary malignancies after marrow transplantation (Rev). *Hematol Oncol Clin North Am* **7:**417–429, 1993.

Draper, G.J., Sanders, B.M., and Kingston, J.E.: Second primary neoplasms in patients with retinoblastoma. *Br J Cancer* **53:**661–671, 1986.

Fisher, B., Rockette, H., Fisher, E.R., et al.: Leukemia in breast cancer patients following adjuvant chemotherapy or postoperative radiation: The NSABP experience. *J Clin Oncol* **3:**1640–1658, 1985.

Gertz, M.A., Noel, P., and Kyle, R.A.: Second malignancies after chemotherapy and transplantation (Rev). *Crit Rev Oncol Hematol* **14:**107–125, 1993.

Green, M.H., Harris, E.L., Gershenson, D.M., et al.: Melphalan may be a more potent leukemogen than cyclophosphamide. *Ann Intern Med* **105:**36–67, 1986.

Krown, S.E.: AIDS associated malignancies (Rev). *Cancer Chemother Biol Resp Mod* **16:**491–561, 1996.

Penn, I.: Depressed immunity and the development of cancer (Rev), *Cancer Detect Prevent* **18:**241–252, 1994.

Penn, I.: Sarcomas in organ allograft recipients (Rev). *Transplantation* **60:**1485–1491, 1995.

Swinnen, L.J.: Transplant immunosuppression-related malignant lymphomas (Rev). *Cancer Treat Res* **66:**95–110, 1993.

Tan-Shalaby, J., and Tempero, M.: Malignancies after liver transplantation: A comparative review (Rev). *Semin Liver Dis* **15:**156–164, 1995.

Tucker, M.A., D'Angio, D. J., Boice, J.D., et al.: Bone sarcomas linked to radiotherapy and chemotherapy in children. *N Engl J Med* **317:**588–593, 1987.

Zalla, M.J.: Kaposi's sarcoma. An update. *Dermatologic Surg* **22:**274–287, 1996.

INDEX

ISBN 0-07-008992-2

9 780070 089921

90000>